How to improve your ART success rates

An evidence-based review of adjuncts to IVF

How to improve your ART success rates

An evidence-based review of adjuncts to IVF

Edited by

Gab Kovacs

International Medical Director, Monash IVF, and Professor of Obstetrics and Gynaecology,
Monash University, Toorak, Victoria, Australia

CAMBRIDGE
UNIVERSITY PRESS

CAMBRIDGE UNIVERSITY PRESS
Cambridge, New York, Melbourne, Madrid, Cape Town,
Singapore, São Paulo, Delhi, Tokyo, Mexico City

Cambridge University Press
The Edinburgh Building, Cambridge CB2 8RU, UK

Published in the United States of America by Cambridge University Press, New York

www.cambridge.org
Information on this title: www.cambridge.org/9781107648326

First published 2011

Printed in the United Kingdom at the University Press, Cambridge

A catalogue record for this publication is available from the British Library

ISBN 978-1-107-64832-6 Paperback

Contents

Section 7. Ancillary treatments

Section 8. Assessment of results

Contributors

Mohamed Aboulghar, MD
Professor of Obstetrics and Gynecology, Faculty of Medicine, Cairo University, Egypt; Clinical Director, The Egyptian IVF Center, Maadi, Cairo, Egypt

Ahmed Abou-Setta, MD, PhD
Alberta Research Centre for Health Evidence, University of Alberta, Edmonton, Alberta, Canada

Mary E. Abusief, MD
Reproductive Endocrinology and Infertility Specialist, Fertility Physicians of Northern California, Palo Alto and San Jose, California, USA

G. David Adamson, MD
Director, Fertility Physicians of Northern California, Palo Alto and San Jose, California, USA

R. J. Aitken, PhD, ScD, FRSE
Discipline of Biological Sciences, ARC Centre of Excellence in Biotechnology and Development and Hunter Medical Research Institute, University of Newcastle, Callaghan, Australia

Hesham Al-Inany, MD, PhD
Department of Obstetrics & Gynecology, Cairo University, Cairo, Egypt

Baris Ata, MD, MCT
Clinical and Research Fellow, Division of Reproductive Endocrinology and Infertility, Department of Obstetrics and Gynecology, McGill University, Montreal, Canada

Hamdy Azab, MD
Department of Obstetrics & Gynecology, Cairo University, Cairo, Egypt

Adam Balen, MD, DSc, FRCOG
Professor of Reproductive Medicine and Surgery, Leeds Centre for Reproductive Medicine, Leeds, UK

David H. Barad, MD, MS
Clinical Director, ART Program and CHR Research, Center for Human Reproduction (CHR) New York, USA; Assoc. Clin. Professor, Departments of Epidemiology and Social Medicine and Obstetrics, Gynecology and Women's Health, Albert Einstein College of Medicine, Bronx, New York, USA

Pedro N. Barri, MD, PhD
Service of Reproductive Medicine, Department of Obstetrics and Gynecology, Catedra de Investigacion en Obstetricia y Ginecología, Institut Universitari Dexeus, Barcelona, Spain

C. Blockeel, MD
UZ Brussels, Belgium

Giuseppe Botta, PhD, MD
Clinica Ruesch, Napoli, Italy

Mark Bowman, MBBS, PhD, FRANZCOG, CREI
Medical Director, Sydney IVF and Clinical Associate Professor, University of Sydney, Australia

Chris Brewer, BMedSc, MB ChB
Research Registrar, Leeds Centre for Reproductive Medicine, Leeds, UK

Dominique M. Butawan, MD
Department of Obstetrics and Gynecology, Division of Reproductive Endocrinology, University of Tennessee Health Science Center, Memphis, Tennessee, USA

Sandra A. Carson, MD
Professor of Obstetrics and Gynecology and Director, Division of Reproductive Endocrinology and Infertility, The Warren Alpert Medical School at Brown University, Women & Infants Hospital of Rhode Island, Providence, Rhode Island, USA

Hai Ying Chen, MD, MSc
McGill Reproductive Centre, McGill University Health Centre, Montreal, Canada

Anne Clark, MPS, MBChB, FRCOG, FRANZCOG, APP, CREI
Fertility First, 50–52 Gloucester Road, Hurstville, NSW 2220, Australia

Buenaventura Coroleu, B, MD, PhD
Head of the Service of Reproductive Medicine Department of Obstetrics, Gynecology and Reproduction Institut Universitari Dexeus, Barcelona, Spain

S. Das, MD, MRCOG, DFSRH
Consultant Gynaecologist, Bolton Hospital NHS Foundation Trust, Bolton, Greater Manchester, UK

C. Dechanet, MD
Médecine de la Reproduction, Département de Gynécologie-Obstétrique, Pôle Naissances et Pathologies de la Femme, Academic hospital A. de Villeneuve (CHU Montpellier), Faculté de Médecine, Université Montpellier, France

H. Déchaud, MD, PhD
Médecine de la Reproduction, Département de Gynécologie-Obstétrique, Pôle Naissances et Pathologies de la Femme, Academic hospital A. de Villeneuve (CHU Montpellier), Faculté de Médecine, Université Montpellier, France

Cora de Klerk, MSc
Senior Researcher, Erasmus MC, The Netherlands

Sheryl de Lacey, RN, BAppSci(Nurs), MA, PhD
Associate Professor, School of Nursing & Midwifery, Flinders University, Adelaide, Australia

S. Deutsch-Bringer, MD
Médecine de la Reproduction, Département de Gynécologie-Obstétrique, Pôle Naissances et Pathologies de la Femme, Academic hospital A. de Villeneuve (CHU Montpellier), Faculté de Médecine, Université Montpellier, France

P. Devroey, MD, PhD
Global Fertility Academy, Germany

Didier Dewailly, MD
Department of Endocrine Gynaecology and Reproductive Medicine, Hôpital Jeanne de Flandre, and Faculty of Medicine of Lille, Université de Lille II, France

Hakan E. Duran, MD
University of Iowa Carver College of Medicine, Iowa City, Iowa, USA

Walid El Sherbiny, MD
Department of Obstetrics & Gynecology, Cairo University, Cairo, Egypt

Tarek El-Toukhy, MRCOG
Assisted Conception Unit, Guy's and St Thomas' Hospital NHS Foundation Trust, London, UK

Johannes L. H. Evers, MD, PhD, FRCOG
Centre for Reproductive Medicine and Biology, Research School for Oncology and Developmental Biology GROW, Maastricht University Medical Centre, Maastricht, The Netherlands

Cynthia Farquhar, MB ChB, MSCOG, FRANZCOG, MD
Postgraduate Professor of Obstetrics and Gynaecology and Co-ordinating Editor of the Cochrane Menstrual Disorders and Subfertility Group, Department of

Obstetrics and Gynaecology, University of Auckland, New Zealand

Rodney D. Franklin, PharmD
Department of Pharmacy Practice, School of Pharmacy, University of Mississippi, Jackson, Mississippi, USA

Juan A. Garcia-Velasco, MD, PhD
Director and Associate Professor of Obstetrics and Gynecology, IVI-Madrid, Rey Juan Carlos University, Madrid, Spain

David K. Gardner, DPhil
Department of Zoology, University of Melbourne, Parkville, Victoria, Australia

Norbert Gleicher, MD
President and Medical Director, Center for Human Reproduction (CHR), New York, USA; President, Foundation for Reproductive Medicine, New York, USA; and Visiting Professor, Department of Obstetrics, Gynecology and Reproductive Sciences, Yale University School of Medicine, New Haven, Connecticut, USA

Gedis Grudzinskas, BSc, MD, FRACOG, FRCOG
Harley Street, London, UK

Roger Hart, MD FRANZCOG, MRCOG, CREI
Professor of Reproductive Medicine, School of Women's and Infant's Health, The University of Western Australia, King Edward Memorial Hospital, Perth, Australia

B. Hédon, MD
Professor, Médecine de la Reproduction, Département de Gynécologie-Obstétrique, Pôle Naissances et Pathologies de la Femme, Academic hospital A. de Villeneuve (CHU Montpellier), Faculté de Médecine, Université Montpellier, France

Colin M. Howles, PhD, CBIol, MSB, FRSM
Vice President of Regional Medical Affairs, Fertility and Endocrinology Global Business Unit, Merck Serono S.A., Geneva, Switzerland

Jack Yu Jen Huang, MD, PhD
The Ronald O. Perelman and Claudia Cohen Center for Reproductive Medicine, Weill Cornell Medical College of Cornell University, New York, USA

N. P. Johnson, MD, CREI, FRCOG, FRANZCOG
Department of Obstetrics and Gynaecology, University of Auckland, New Zealand

Hey-Joo Kang, MD
The Ronald O. Perelman and Claudia Cohen Center for Reproductive Medicine, Weill Cornell Medical College of Cornell University, New York, USA

Gab Kovacs, MD, FRCOG, FRANZCOG, CREI
International Medical Director, Monash IVF, and Professor of Obstetrics and Gynaecology, Monash University, Toorak, Victoria, Australia

Ben Kroon, BHB, MBChB, FRANZCOG
Queensland Fertility Group, Brisbane, Australia

Anver Kuliev, MD, PhD
Director of Research, Reproductive Genetics Institute, Chicago, Illinois, USA

William H. Kutteh, MD, PhD
Department of Obstetrics and Gynecology, Division of Reproductive Endocrinology, University of Tennessee Health Science Center, Memphis, Tennessee, USA

Nick Macklon, MD, PhD, FRCOG
Chair in Obstetrics and Gynaecology at the University of Southampton, and Consultant Gynaecologist and Director of Complete Fertility Centre Southampton, UK

Ragaa Mansour, MD, PhD
Director, The Egyptian IVF-ET Center, Cairo, Egypt

Lamiya Mohiyiddeen, MBBS, MRCOG, MD
Department of Reproductive Medicine, St Mary's Hospital, CMFT University Hospitals NHS Trust, Manchester, UK

Lisa J. Moran, BSc (Hons), BND, PhD
Research Fellow, The Robinson Institute, Discipline of Obstetrics and Gynaecology, The University of Adelaide, Australia

David Mortimer, PhD
Oozoa Biomedical Inc, Caulfeild Village, West Vancouver, BC, Canada

Sharon T. Mortimer, PhD
Oozoa Biomedical Inc, Caulfeild Village, West Vancouver, BC, Canada

Luciano G. Nardo, MD, MRCOG
Consultant, Department of Reproductive Medicine, St Mary's Hospital, CMFT University Hospitals NHS Trust, Manchester; North West Fertility, GyneHealth, Manchester, UK

Robert J. Norman, BSc, MB ChB, MD, FRANZCOG, FRCOG, FRCPA, CREI
Professor in Obstetrics and Gynaecology The University of Adelaide, Australia

Willem Ombelet, MD, PhD
Genk Institute for Fertility Technology, Department of Obstetrics and Gynaecology, Genk, Belgium

Luk Rombauts, MD, PhD, FRANZCOG, CREI
Clinical Research Director, Monash IVF, and Senior Clinical Lecturer, Department of Obstetrics and Gynaecology, Monash University, Toorak, Victoria, Australia

Zev Rosenwaks, MD
The Ronald O. Perelman and Claudia Cohen Center for Reproductive Medicine, Weill Cornell Medical College of Cornell University, New York, USA

Francisco J. Ruiz Flores, MD
Clinical Fellow, IVI-Madrid, Rey Juan Carlos University, Madrid, Spain

Anthony J. Rutherford, MBBS, FRCOG
Leeds NHS Teaching Hospitals, Leeds, UK

Gavin Sacks, MA, BM, BCh, DPhil, MRCOG, FRANZCOG
Clinical Director, IVFAustralia, A Conjoint Senior Lecturer, University of New South Wales, Sydney, Australia

Denny Sakkas, Phd
Molecular Biometrics®, Inc., Research and Development, New Haven, Connecticut and Department of Obstetrics, Gynecology, and Reproductive Sciences, Yale University School of Medicine, New Haven, Connecticut, USA

M. W. Seif, PhD, FRCOG
Academic Unit of Obstetrics, Gynaecology & Reproductive Health, University of Manchester at St Mary's Hospital, Manchester, UK

Ayse Seyhan, MD
Clinical and Research Fellow, Department of Obstetrics and Gynecology, McGill University, Montreal, Canada

Caroline Smith, PhD, MSc, BSc (Hons), LicAc
Associate Professor of Complementary Medicine, Centre for Complementary Medicine Research, University of Western Sydney, Penrith South DC, NSW, Australia

Kate Stern, MBBS, FRANZCOG, FRCOG, CREI
Endocrine and Metabolic Service, Royal Women's Hospital, Melbourne and Melbourne IVF, Melbourne, Australia

Elizabeth A. Sullivan, MD, MBBS, MPH, MMed (Sexual Health), FAFPHM
Associate Professor, Perinatal and Reproductive Epidemiology and Research Unit, the University of New South Wales, Australia

Sesh Kamal Sunkara, MBBCh, MRCOG
Assisted Conception Unit, Guy's and St. Thomas' Hospital NHS Foundation Trust, London, UK

Seang Lin Tan, MD, MBBS, FRCOG, FRCSC, FACOG, MMed(O&G), MBA
MUHC Reproductive Centre, Department of Obstetrics and Gynecology, McGill University, Montreal, Quebec, Canada and Montreal Reproductive Centre, Montreal Canada

Mohamed Taranissi, FRCOG
Assisted Reproduction and Gynaecology Centre, London, UK

Kelton P. Tremellen, MBBS (Hons), PhD, FRANZCOG, CREI
Deputy Medical Director, Repromed, and Associate Professor, School of Pharmacy and Medical Sciences, University of South Australia, Australia

Wendy S. Vitek, MD
Fellow, Reproductive Endocrinology and Infertility, The Warren Alpert Medical School at Brown University, Women & Infants Hospital of Rhode Island, Providence, Rhode Island, USA

V. Vloeberghs, MD
Leuven University Fertility Center, Department Obstetrics and Gynecology, UZ Gasthuisberg, Leuven, Belgium

Bradley J. Van Voorhis, MD
The F. K. "Ted" Chapler Professor of Reproductive Medicine, University of Iowa Carver College of Medicine, Iowa City, Iowa, USA

S. F. van Voorst, MSc
Department of Obstetrics and Gynaecology, Erasmus Medical Centre Rotterdam, The Netherlands

Amr Wahba, MD
Department of Obstetrics & Gynecology, Cairo University, Cairo, Egypt

Yueping A. Wang, BMed, MPH
Biostatistician, Perinatal and Reproductive Epidemiology and Research Unit, The University of New South Wales, Australia

Klaus E. Wiemer, PhD
KEW Technology, Woodinville, WA, USA

Section 1 Patient selection and preparation

Chapter 1

Pre-treatment hormone assessment to optimize IVF outcomes

Kelton P. Tremellen

Introduction

There is considerable debate and substantial individual variation in clinical practice regarding what hormones should be assessed in all patients prior to commencing in vitro fertilization (IVF) treatment. While it would appear logical to measure multiple hormones such as gonadotropins (luteinizing hormone [LH]; follicle stimulating hormone [FSH]), steroids (testosterone, 17 hydroxy-progesterone), prolactin, and thyroid function (thyroid stimulating hormone [TSH]; thyroxine [FT4]) in all women with suspected anovulation (irregular menstrual cycle), the utility of such an extensive hormone analysis in the average ovular patient about to commence IVF for male or tubal factor infertility is less certain. In today's environment of escalating medical costs it is imperative that we only order tests that have potential clinical value. Furthermore, abnormal test results can produce anxiety in the patient, an undesirable outcome at a time when the patient is already under considerable psychological distress. The focus of this chapter is to explore the evidence behind which hormone tests should be a mandatory prerequisite for all women about to undergo their first cycle of IVF treatment.

Hormone assessments of ovarian reserve

It is well known that the response to controlled ovarian hyperstimulation (COH) during IVF treatment is highly variable, even among women of similar age. This undoubtedly reflects the wide variation in ovarian reserve between different women, which is primarily determined by the size of the primordial follicular pool. Unfortunately history and examination have a very poor sensitivity in predicting ovarian responsiveness to COH. Therefore performing hormone assessments of ovarian reserve before commencing a first cycle of IVF treatment may be useful. Firstly, these tests may allow for a more accurate prediction of a woman's anticipated response to COH, allowing for tailoring of the starting dose of gonadotropin stimulation. Secondly, since it is well recognized that low ovarian reserve has a significant negative influence on the chances of pregnancy during IVF treatment, hormone assessment of ovarian reserve can give couples better information on the likely benefits/success of treatment beyond maternal-age prognostic assessment.

The traditional hormones used for assessment of ovarian reserve include early follicular phase FSH/estradiol, serum inhibin B, and anti-mullerian hormone (AMH) [1]. A recent review of over 2000 cycles of IVF from 20 individual studies has concluded that AMH is a

How to Improve Your ART Success Rates, ed. Gab Kovacs. Published by Cambridge

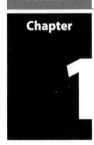

better marker for predicting ovarian response to COH than patient age, day 3 FSH, estradiol and inhibin B [2]. All of the available data show a strong positive correlation between basal serum AMH levels and the number of retrieved oocytes in women undergoing ovarian stimulation [2]. This observation is not surprising since AMH is produced by the granulosa cells of the small antral follicles, with several studies reporting an excellent correlation between serum AMH levels and ultrasound-assessed antral follicle counts. It is these small antral follicles (2–10 mm) that are recruited as mature oocytes in response to gonadotropin stimulation during IVF treatment. Not only is AMH a more accurate measure of ovarian response to COH, its concentration in serum does not fluctuate significantly during the menstrual cycle, unlike other hormonal assessments of ovarian reserve (FSH, inhibin B, and estradiol) [2]. This makes it a more practical measure of ovarian reserve since it can be sampled at any time that the patient attends clinic, unlike FSH, estradiol, and inhibin B that are only accurate if taken in the early follicular phase of the menstrual cycle [1].

While serum AMH appears to be an excellent marker of quantitative ovarian reserve, it appears to have very limited usefulness as a marker of oocyte quality. Serum AMH levels do not predict embryo morphology or the rate of embryo aneuploidy [2]. Furthermore, recent data from studies of natural conception show no correlation between serum AMH and rates of miscarriage or genetic abnormality in the foetus [3, 4]. Similar studies have also failed to find a correlation between FSH levels and embryo aneuploidy [5]. Therefore, hormone assessments of ovarian reserve should not be used to judge oocyte quality, but only to predict qualitative ovarian reserve.

It may be useful to correctly predict the occurrence of a poor response as this may avoid treatment in women destined not to respond to COH, thus reducing the financial and emotional costs associated with cancelled cycles. Traditionally a day 3 FSH exceeding 15 IU/l has been seen as a very poor prognostic sign and has been used by many clinics to exclude patients from IVF treatment [1]. Several authors have investigated the utility of AMH in the prediction of poor response to FSH. The reported sensitivity and specificity for predicting poor response are in the range 44–97% and 41–100% respectively, depending on the "cut off" serum AMH value used in the individual study [2]. In our own clinic we have reported that a serum AMH of less than 14 pmol/l (1.96 ng/ml) has a sensitivity and specificity of 73% for predicting a poor response (≤ four oocytes) to ovarian stimulation [6]. If serum AMH measurements suggest low ovarian reserve, it has been our practice to double the starting dose of gonadotropin stimulation from 150 to 300 IU/day in young women in their first cycle of IVF treatment. While this approach would be expected to increase the oocyte yield, no randomized control trial has yet been conducted to confirm this benefit. A small retrospective observational study has reported that increasing the starting dose of gonadotropin stimulation in young patients with predicted poor response did not result in a significant improvement in oocyte yield or pregnancy rates, but also reassuringly did not produce any dangerous levels of ovarian hyperstimulation [7]. Therefore, the clinical utility of predicting poor ovarian reserve using serum AMH may only be in helping prepare patients for a poor oocyte response in their first cycle of IVF treatment.

Serum AMH levels in women with polycystic ovarian syndrome (PCOS) are on average two to three times higher than their age matched ovulatory peers, with serum AMH having a relatively high sensitivity and specificity (92% and 67% respectively) for diagnosing the presence of polycystic ovaries on scan [2]. Since PCOS or polycystic ovaries are a very significant risk factor for the development of ovarian hyperstimulation syndrome (OHSS), serum AMH is highly likely to predict the occurrence of OHSS during IVF treatment. Our group was the first to report this association between high serum AMH and the development of OHSS [8]. Since then, four prospective studies have been published on the topic, each reporting a relevant value for AMH for the prediction of hyper-response and OHSS [2]. The results of these publications suggest that once serum AMH exceeds approximately 30 pmol/l (4.2 ng/ml), or is in the top quartile of serum AMH results for their age, the patient is at considerable risk of OHSS. Unfortunately no randomized controlled trial has analyzed if reducing the starting dose of gonadotropin stimulation does reduce the incidence of OHSS, while still maintaining good pregnancy rates. It was standard practice in our unit to reduce the starting dose of gonadotropin stimulation from 150 IU/day to 100–125 IU/day in young patients (< 36 years of age) if the serum AMH was greater than 30 pmol/l. However, it became evident that the optimal "therapeutic window" in these PCOS patients is quite narrow, with 150 IU FSH producing an excessive response, while 100–112 IU FSH often producing an inadequate response. Therefore it has now become our standard practice to place all young women with high AMH (> 30 pmol/l) on a starting dose of 125 IU of FSH in a gonadotropin-releasing hormone (GnRH) antagonist cycle of IVF. The use of a GnRH antagonist has been shown to half the risk of hospitalization with severe OHSS, while also giving the treating doctor the opportunity to use a GnRH agonist trigger to further minimize the severity of OHSS if an exaggerated response to stimulation is still observed despite the reduction in starting dose of gonadotropin stimulation [9].

The vast majority of studies suggest that serum AMH has a very poor performance for predicting pregnancy outcome during a stimulated cycle of IVF [2]. Only one prospective study has reported a fall in pregnancy rates derived from both fresh and subsequent frozen embryo transfers once the serum AMH concentration dropped below 7.8 pmol/l (1.1 ng/ml) [10]. A retrospective study has reported a similar significant reduction in cumulative pregnancies (fresh plus frozen embryo transfers) once the serum AMH fell below 14 pmol/l [6]. These observations are a consequence of the relationship between AMH and quantitative response to COH. Women with higher AMH produce a greater number of oocytes during IVF treatment, with a resulting greater number of good quality embryos available for cryopreservation. However, extreme caution should be shown when using AMH to exclude women from IVF treatment based on predicted poor reserve since there have been documented cases of live-birth pregnancy in women with undetectable levels of serum AMH.

Assessment of thyroid dysfunction

There are several logical reasons for testing thyroid function in all women presenting for IVF treatment. Firstly, undiagnosed hypothyroidism is relatively common in the infertile population, affecting 5–6% of women with idiopathic or anovulatory infertility and 2% of women with tubal or male factor infertility [11]. Hyperthyroidism is significantly less common, affecting between 0.1 and 1% of women in the reproductive age group [12]. The treatment of women with previously undiagnosed hypothyroidism with thyroxine replacement can itself result in natural conception, removing the need for IVF treatment. Furthermore, undiagnosed hypothyroidism may adversely affect the IVF cycle as it has been linked with failed oocyte fertilization despite the use of good quality sperm [13]. Finally, untreated hypothyroidism may lead to pregnancy complications such as miscarriage, growth restriction, and pre-term delivery, plus a possible reduction in the neuropsychomotor development of the child conceived by fertility treatment [12]. It has been suggested that thyroid function is best assessed in infertile women with both a TSH and FT4 test, since isolated hypo-FT4 (normal TSH) has been reported in up to 2% of pregnancies and may still interfere with the child's neurological development [12].

Compared to natural conception, IVF treatment itself may exacerbate hypothyroidism since the supra-physiological levels of estradiol seen during COH will result in an increase in production of thyroxine-binding globulin, thereby reducing the concentration of biologically active free thyroxine hormone. It would therefore appear prudent to order a screening TSH and FT4 test on all women before commencing IVF treatment [12].

Miscellaneous hormone assessment

Two previous studies have analyzed the utility of measuring hormones such as prolactin, LH, FSH, estradiol, progesterone, testosterone, DHEAS (dehydroepiandrosterone sulfate), 17 hydroxy-progesterone, and androstenedione in ovulatory women prior to IVF treatment [14,15].While a mild elevation in prolactin levels was more commonly observed in women about to commence IVF treatment than a fertile reference population, there was no significant difference in hormone levels between those women who became pregnant during the IVF cycle and those who did not. The minor increase in serum prolactin seen in these ovulatory women probably reflects an anxiety related "stress" response common in infertile patients. Furthermore, another study has shown that treatment of minor elevations in prolactin

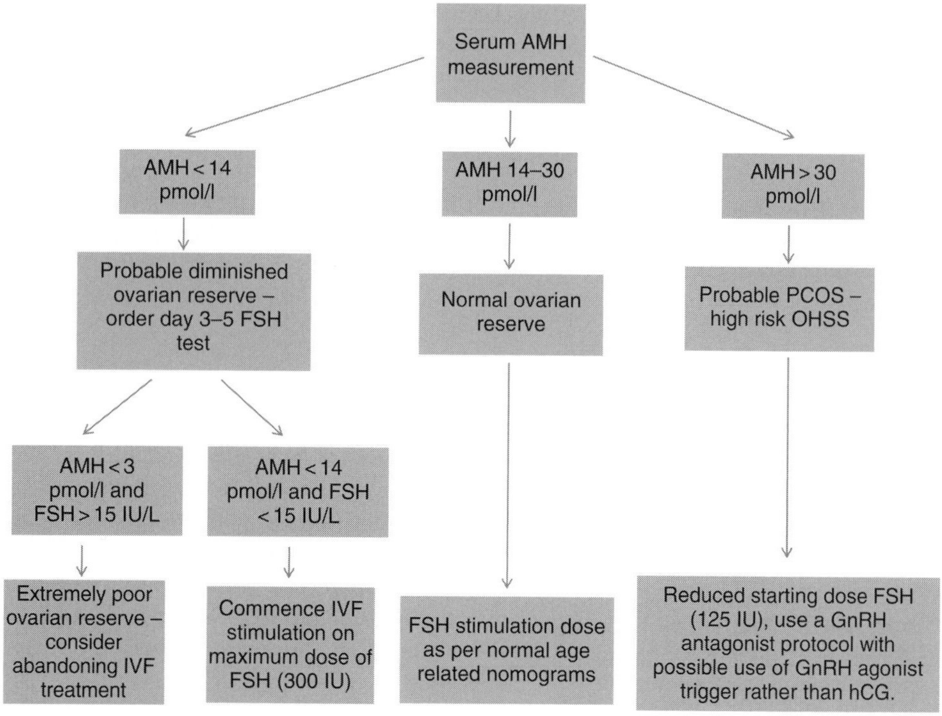

Figure 1.1 Use of serum anti-mullerian hormone (AMH) to tailor controlled ovarian hyperstimulation treatment in patients undergoing their first cycle of IVF.

The serum AMH measurement thresholds depicted are for the Immunotech AMH assay platform. Conversion units: 1 ng/ml AMH = 7.14 pmol/l.

using dopamine agonist therapy before IVF actually worsens embryology outcomes [16], thereby providing no justification for the routine assessment of prolactin or any of these other reproductive steroids/gonadotropins prior to IVF treatment in ovulatory women.

Conclusion

The literature would suggest that measurement of serum AMH and TSH/FT4 should be a mandatory part of the infertility "work-up" in any woman undergoing IVF treatment for the first time. Serum AMH allows for the best assessment of likely ovarian response to COH, with the added advantage of being able to be sampled at any time in the menstrual cycle. For those women with low AMH, an additional day 3–5 FSH assessment may be appropriate as it may identify those women with a very poor chance of successful pregnancy (FSH > 15 IU/L). Serum AMH measurements can be used to predict patients response to COH in their first cycle of IVF and individualize their treatment regime, as outlined in Figure 1.1. Patients identified as having abnormal thyroid function should have this corrected before commencing IVF treatment so as optimize IVF embryology and pregnancy outcomes.

References

1. Broekmans FJ, Kwee J, Hendriks DJ, Mol BW, Lambalk CB. A systematic review of tests predicting ovarian reserve and IVF outcome. *Hum Reprod Update* 2006;**12**:685–718.
2. La Marca A, Sighinolfi G, Radi D, Argento C, Baraldi E, Artenisio AC, *et al.* Anti-Mullerian hormone (AMH) as a predictive marker in assisted reproductive technology (ART). *Hum Reprod Update* 2010;**16**:113–30.
3. Plante BJ, Beamon C, Schmitt CL, Moldenhauer JS, Steiner AZ. Maternal antimullerian hormone levels do not predict fetal aneuploidy. *J Assist Reprod Genet* 2010;**27**:409–14.
4. Tremellen K, Kolo M. Serum anti-Mullerian hormone is a useful measure of quantitative ovarian reserve but does not predict the chances of live-birth pregnancy. *Aust N Z J Obstet Gynaecol* 2010;**50**:568–72.
5. Massie JA, Burney RO, Milki AA, Westphal LM, Lathi RB. Basal follicle-stimulating hormone as a predictor of fetal aneuploidy. *Fertil Steril* 2008;**90**:2351–5.
6. Lekamge DN, Barry M, Kolo M, Lane M, Gilchrist RB, Tremellen KP. Anti-Müllerian hormone as a predictor of IVF outcome. *Reprod Biomed Online* 2007;**14**:602–10.
7. Lekamge DN, Lane M, Gilchrist RB, Tremellen KP. Increased gonadotrophin stimulation does not improve IVF outcomes in patients with predicted poor ovarian reserve. *J Assist Reprod Genet* 2008;**25**(11–12):515–21.
8. Tremellen KP, Kolo M, Gilmore A, Lekamge DN. Anti-mullerian hormone as a marker of ovarian reserve. *Aust N Z J Obstet Gynaecol* 2005;**45**:20–24.
9. Devroey P, Aboulghar M, Garcia-Velasco J, Griesinger G, Humaidan P, Kolibianakis E, *et al.* Improving the patient's experience of IVF/ICSI: a proposal for an ovarian stimulation protocol with GnRH antagonist co-treatment. *Hum Reprod* 2009;**24**: 764–74.
10. Nelson SM, Yates RW, Fleming R. Serum anti-Müllerian hormone and FSH: prediction of live birth and extremes of response in stimulated cycles – implications for individualization of therapy. *Hum Reprod* 2007;**22**:2414–21.
11. Arojoki M, Jokimaa V, Juuti A, Koskinen P, Irjala K, Anttila L. Hypothyroidism among infertile women in Finland. *Gynecol Endocrinol* 2000;**14**:127–31.
12. Krassas GE, Poppe K, Glinoer D. Thyroid function and human reproductive health. *Endocr Rev* 2010;**31**:702–55.

13. Cramer DW, Sluss PM, Powers RD, McShane P, Ginsburgs ES, Hornstein MD, *et al.* Serum prolactin and TSH in an in vitro fertilization population: is there a link between fertilization and thyroid function? *J Assist Reprod Genet* 2003;**20**:210–5.

14. Laufer MR, Floor AE, Parsons KE, Kuntz KM, Barbieri RL, Friedman AJ. Evaluation of hormonal testing in the screening for in vitro fertilization (IVF) of women with tubal factor infertility. *J Assist Reprod Genet* 1995;**12**:93–6.

15. Zollner U, Lanig K, Steck T, Dietl J. Assessment of endocrine status in patients undergoing in-vitro fertilization treatment. Is it necessary? *Arch Gynecol Obstet* 2001;**265**:16–20.

16. Doldi N, Papaleo E, De Santis L, Ferrari A. Treatment versus no treatment of transient hyperprolactinemia in patients undergoing intracytoplasmic sperm injection programs. *Gynecol Endocrinol* 2000;**14**:437–41.

Chapter 2

Role of pelvic ultrasonography in the selection and preparation of patients for IVF

Didier Dewailly

The main value of ultrasound in the context of IVF is to provide information on the status of the ovarian reserve. Ultrasound can also assess the state of the uterus and investigate possible stigma of endometriosis. Its value in assessing the chances of embryo implantation is so far more limited. Besides selection and preparation of patients, it has obvious applications in monitoring patients and performing ultrasound-guided procedures. These aspects are covered in other chapters.

Evaluation of the ovarian reserve

The assessment of ovarian reserve (OR) is based on a series of clinical, biological, and ultrasound criteria. The ultrasound parameters used for this evaluation are antral follicle count (AFC), the ovarian volume, and the ovarian blood flow by Doppler measurement. This assessment predicts the risk of poor response (PR) or excessive response to controlled ovarian hyperstimulation (COH). It is of great importance for counseling the patients and for setting the COH protocol.

Prediction of poor response to COH

A poor response to COH is defined by cycle cancellation or by fewer than three mature follicles and/or insufficient rise in estradiol serum levels (<500 pg/mL) during COH and/or by fewer than four oocytes at follicle puncture.

The antral follicle count: recent evolutions and disputed issues

In recent years, the follicle count has emerged as a key marker of ovarian reserve, but its place is now endangered by the advent of the anti-Müllerian hormone (AMH) assay. (This is discussed in detail in Chapter 1.) Anti-Müllerian hormone has the advantage of being a marker of all the growing follicles up to 5 mm. With ultrasound, only follicles of diameter greater than 1 mm are counted. However, it is considered that the number of such follicles is a good reflection of the stock of primordial follicles. In good agreement, the AFC decreases with age. Among visible follicles on ultrasound between days 2 and 5, it seems that the follicles of 2–6 mm are more predictive of the ovarian response than those of 7–10 mm. Follicles between 2 and 6 mm are best correlated with AMH and the number of oocytes collected at the puncture.

How to Improve Your ART Success Rates, ed. Gab Kovacs. Published by Cambridge University Press.

A recent meta-analysis has re-evaluated the predictive value of the AFC [1]. With a threshold of greater than or equal to four follicles per ovary, the sensitivity and specificity for predicting the cancellation of the cycle are 66.7 and 94.7% respectively. The risk of cancellation is multiplied by 37 if AFC is <4.

Which threshold?

In the majority of studies, the threshold was set at three or four follicles per ovary [1]. The continuing improvement in image resolution now allows detection and enumeration of follicles less than 2 mm in diameter. This will lead to reconsideration of the former thresholds when using the newest equipment. In addition, there is interobserver variability which implies that each center should determine its own reference threshold. Finally, inter-cyclical variability of the AFC is important, especially in young and infertile women. One measure of low AFC in a young woman (age <25) must be interpreted with caution and should be checked.

What about 3D ultrasound?

The "multi-planar" method still requires manual counting after image acquisition. Counting time in 3D ultrasound (U/S) is significantly shorter but apparently only because the 3D needs a second manual tracking. Interestingly, the AFC can be done retrospectively by "navigating" within the ovary in three planes on the saved volume acquisitions. This is helpful in case of discordance between U/S and clinical/biological data. Some software allows automatic counting of the follicles on the volume acquisitions but at present, they are not reliable enough for follicles smaller than 10 mm. The superiority of 3D over 2D ultrasound to determine accurately the AFC is therefore not evident, but the literature on this matter is still scarce. Whether the 3D mode is more reproducible between observers still awaits confirmation. It seems that the AFC is slightly lower in 3D than in 2D.

AFC or AMH or both?

Antral follicle count and AMH are very well correlated to each other. Therefore, AMH and AFC are equally effective in predicting PR and the number of oocytes collected [1]. In a recent study [2], receiving operator characteristic (ROC) curves for predicting PR were superimposable (area under the curve of 0.905 and 0.935 for AMH and AFC, respectively). The combination of AMH and AFC did not increase the strength of prediction of PR. The main advantage of AMH is its very low variability between cycles, lower than that of AFC. Indeed, in one study [3], the concordance of the AFC between the different phases of the cycle was modest, with a variation of 34% over the cycle for follicles of 2–5 mm and 31% for those of 2–10 mm, while the AMH varied by only 13% in the same cycle with much smaller variations (72% of repeated samples remained in the same quintile against 41% for AFC). In this study, measurements of the AFC were made by the same observer. It is therefore possible that this variation is even greater among different observers.

As for all other markers of OR, including AMH, AFC is not a valid test for predicting pregnancy.

Ovarian volume

Even with 3D U/S, the ovarian volume does not appear an appropriate test for OR testing before IVF. The ROC curve of the AFC is significantly better than the ovarian volume for prediction of PR in IVF [1].

Doppler

Increased stromal blood flow has also been suggested as a more relevant predictor of ovarian response to hormonal stimulation than parameters such as ovarian or stromal volume, but the evidence is still scarce in the literature [1].

Prediction of the ovarian hyperstimulation syndrome

Ultrasound is also very useful to predict the risk of ovarian hyperstimulation syndrome (OHSS). Identifying women at risk allows the protocols to be adapted and surveillance to be increased in order to reduce the morbidity and even the mortality due to this event. Women carrying this risk are those endowed with a high number of growing ovarian follicles, whether or not they have the full blown polycystic ovary syndrome (PCOS). Once again, the AFC appears to be the most efficient U/S parameter for predicting this risk [4]. However, the threshold is not yet universally agreed, for the same reasons as stated above on the prediction of PR. The earlier proposal of a threshold of 14 [4] should certainly be revised upwards with new equipment. It is not known whether the AFC is proving to be a better marker than AMH, as an increased serum level of the latter is also predictive of the risk for OHSS [4].

Some data indicate that Doppler study of ovarian blood flow may have some value in predicting the risk for OHSS during gonadotropin therapy but this has not been confirmed.

Prediction of implantation

Ultrasound techniques were tested to study endometrial receptivity. The measurement of endometrial thickness and echogenicity has little predictive value. The measurement of endometrial volume by 3D U/S does not appear to be superior. The Doppler study of uterine arteries, whether carried out on the day of human chorionic gonadotropin administration or the day of transfer, does not appear to have sufficient predictive power. Finally, more recently, the study of endometrial and sub-endometrial blood flow, coupled with the 3D U/S, has been disappointing [5].

Ancillary uses of ultrasound

Sonosalpingography

In comparison to hysterosalpingography, this technique has the advantage of not being irradiating and gives information at the same time about the morphology of the myometrium and ovaries. However, in case of tubal occlusion, it does not describe the internal tubal morphology, nor does it indicate the level of the obstruction. So far, it has not replaced hysterosalpingography in the routine clinical work-up.

Diagnosis of ovarian diseases

Ultrasonography is now a must in the investigation of ovulation disorders, along with clinical findings and hormonal assays. The determination of the AFC contributes greatly to the diagnosis of the PCOS and the primary ovarian failure (POF), along with the clinical/biological data.

Detection of uterine and tubo-peritoneal lesions

Ultrasound is highly sensitive in detecting those lesions that are responsible for infertility through interference with egg migration and implantation and/or with sperm progression, such as fibroids, polyps, synechiae, or malformations. Conversely, it is less sensitive than laparoscopy in detecting mild pelvic adhesions or peritoneal endometriosis. These aspects are covered in greater detail in other chapters.

Conclusion

Pelvic ultrasonography is now a must in the selection and preparation of patients for IVF. However, AFC is at the crossroads. Whether it will still be used to complement (or instead of) the AMH assay depends on its technological evolution and, more particularly, on the possibility of automatic counting of the small follicles (<10 mm) with sufficient accuracy and reproducibility.

References

1. Gibreel A, Maheshwari A, Bhattacharya S, Johnson NP. Ultrasound tests of ovarian reserve; a systematic review of accuracy in predicting fertility outcomes. *Hum Fertil (Camb)* 2009;**12**:95–106.
2. Jayaprakasan K, Deb S, Batcha M, Hopkisson J, Johnson I, Campbell B, *et al.* The cohort of antral follicles measuring 2–6 mm reflects the quantitative status of ovarian reserve as assessed by serum levels of anti-Mullerian hormone and response to controlled ovarian stimulation. *Fertil Steril* 2010;**94**:1775–81.
3. van Disseldorp J, Lambalk CB, Kwee J, Looman CW, Eijkemans MJ, Fauser BC, *et al.* Comparison of inter- and intra-cycle variability of anti-Mullerian hormone and antral follicle counts. *Hum Reprod* 2010;**25**:221–7.
4. Humaidan P, Quartarolo J, Papanikolaou EG. Preventing ovarian hyperstimulation syndrome: guidance for the clinician. *Fertil Steril* 2010;**94**:389–400.
5. Ng EH, Chan CC, Tang OS, Yeung WS, Ho PC. Changes in endometrial and subendometrial blood flow in IVF. *Reprod Biomed Online* 2009;**18**:269–75.

Chapter 3

Is pre-IVF laparoscopy/ hysteroscopy worthwhile?

B. Hédon, C. Dechanet, S. Deutsch-Bringer and H. Déchaud

Introduction

When considering IVF or other assisted procreation techniques in order to try and alleviate a patient's subfertility, there are a number of clinical requirements to consider. The way the patient is prepared is part of the quality management of the whole procedure and can contribute significantly to the global efficacy of the programme. IVF is an invasive and costly procedure. Optimizing its results is obligatory.

Moreover, as IVF is not a first-line therapy, it usually comes after a number of other "classical" treatments have failed to help the patient become pregnant. Even when IVF is the only treatment that can be considered, it is necessary to explain why this is so to the couple. To do this, the physician has to to rely on accurate evaluations. It is against this background that laparoscopy and hysteroscopy may be considered. However, it should be noted that practices differ widely from one center to the other.

In some centers commencing IVF would not be accepted until after thorough investigations, including systematic evaluation of the uterine cavity (hysteroscopy) and of the pelvis (laparoscopy), had been performed.

However, the patient often considers these investigations as even more invasive than the IVF procedure itself and can be reluctant to accept them, particularly if they have already been performed during the initial phase of infertility management.

Clearly, the variety of clinical situations precludes any systematic attitude; therefore decisions for every patient shoud be made on an individual basis and considering the balance between benefits and risks.

This paper reviews the literature in order to bring some light to bear on these issues.

Hysteroscopy

Diagnosis

This is more and more frequently an office procedure [1, 2]. The diagnostic performance of hysteroscopy is undisputed for the uterine cavity itself. It gives a fair appreciation of the volume and the morphology of the cavity and also gives insight on the endometrium, both surface appearance and thickness. Alternative investigations would be hysterography and ultrasonography 2D or preferably 3D, without or preferably with contrast medium.

How to Improve Your ART Success Rates, ed. Gab Kovacs. Published by Cambridge University Press.

There are numerous reports comparing the diagnostic efficacy of hysteroscopy with hysterosalpingography, always in favor of hysteroscopy. The difference is less significant when compared with ultrasonography with contrast medium, but the discussion is mainly about matters of practicability and of personal experience.

But more than the type of investigation of the uterine cavity, the questions to be answered are:

- is it always necessary to investigate the uterine cavity before a patient enters an IVF programme, and, if yes, how?
- if not routinely, when is prior hysteroscopy useful?
- does hysteroscopic therapy of intra-uterine anomalies improve pregnancy results of ART?

Congenital or acquired pathologies of the uterine cavity undoubtedly significantly decrease the potential results of assisted procreation [3]. Prevalence of endometrial and uterine cavity anomalies can be as high as 38% of patients [4, 5], in particular when there have been previous ART failures [6, 7].

Treatment

On the therapeutic side, there are reports that show a significant improvement in fertility results after hysteroscopic surgery of intrauterine conditions [8], although this is not always the case [9].

These findings, together with the simplicity of the office procedure, make a strong case in favor of routine investigation of the uterine cavity by hysteroscopy before entering an ART program.

However, many centers would disagree with such a systematic attitude. They would argue that the prevalence of subclinical pathologic anomalies of the uterine cavity varies widely depending on individual risk factors of the patient and that many so-called anomalies do not significantly interfere with embryo implantation. Moreover, even though hysteroscopy would be indicated if a uterine cavity anomaly is suspected, hysterosalpingography or ultrasonography would suffice for an initial screening.

In the absence of proper randomized controlled trials (RCTs), no definitive attitude can be recommended. Existing recommendations do not consider hysteroscopy as a routine investigation, and require its use for confirmation of doubtful pathology and for the relevant therapy only (ESHRE 2000, RCOG 2004).

Indications for pre-IVF hysteroscopy

1. Uterine cavity assessment should be part of routine investigations when exploring the infertile couple. In the absence of clinical symptoms (normal menses, no breakthrough bleeding, normal uterus at clinical examination), the type of investigation (ultrasonography, hysterography, or hysteroscopy) should be left to the personal experience and organization of the physician. There should be very few exceptions to this approach, and only if the cause of infertility is clearly of male origin and if there is no history of familial uterine pathology and the patient is less than 35 years of age.
2. In all other cases:
   - more than 35 years of age
   - abnormal uterine bleeding

  - abnormal clinical findings or any other suspicious finding, hysteroscopy should be the gold standard in order to evaluate the potential of the uterine cavity and eventually treat any anomaly before entering an ART program.
3. Hysteroscopy should become compulsory in case of a history of two prior ART failures.
4. The therapeutic indications do not differ before IVF from what they are at the end of the fertility work-up. Intra-uterine polyps should be resected. Sub-mucous myomas should be resected if they protrude significantly inside the uterine cavity with a size not exceeding 4 cm in diameter (see Chapter 4). A uterine septum will be divided if it separates two distinct uterine cavities within one uterus corpus. A mucosal synechia would be treated if good restoration of the uterine cavity can be expected. A diagnosis of endometritis leads to treatment by a prolonged antibiotic treatment, and it is advised to check the result with a control hysteroscopy before considering the condition as being healed.

All these pathologies should be treated before a first course of IVF. The indications are even more evidence-based if there have been prior failures.

Laparoscopy

Diagnosis

Laparoscopy is not an out-patient procedure. It requires general anesthesia in the majority of cases. Complications occur in 2–3% of patients and can sometimes be life-threatening.

There are alternative techniques in order to investigate the female pelvis using the transvaginal route. Even though it can be considered as less invasive than the classical transparietal laparoscopy, its diagnostic performance, together with the poor therapeutic possibilities in case of anomalies detected, have not encouraged its widespread use as a routine investigation.

In the infertility work-up laparoscopy should not be considered as a first-line investigation. It should be performed when pelvic disease and tubal factor infertility are suspected (chronic pelvic pain, history of pelvic inflammatory disease or sexually transmitted infection, prior tubal pregnancy, history of pelvic surgery, in particular if concerning the reproductive organs: uterus, tubes, ovaries), or if a basic infertility work-up investigation is abnormal (abnormal ultrasonography, positive chlamydia serology, abnormal hysterosalpingography).

There are more uncertainties in case of "unexplained infertility". Many authors accept this classification if and only if, a thorough evaluation has been done, including a laparoscopy. When selecting the patients on the criterion of unexplained infertility, the probability of finding endometriotic lesions is as high as 40%, and in another 10% of the patients, another pelvic anomality (pelvic inflammatory disease, tubal adhesions) would be found. But the question is not what you can find but rather what you can do with the diagnosis. Performance of assisted procreation is such that trying to improve spontaneous fertility of the couple is often not profitable enough. It can be a waste of time, unless there is a significant improvement of ART results to be expected. Unfortunately, this is not usually the case for most of the conditions that are diagnosed in the context of unexplained infertility.

Treatment

There are conditions that indicate laparoscopic treatment prior to IVF. More and more RCTs demonstrate that treating the patient before IVF will improve the results of assisted procreation. This is the case for hydrosalpinges. Depending on the type of hydrosalpinx and other factors a prior salpingectomy may be indicated (Chapter 11) [10].

For endometriosis, indications are more complex. The improvement in IVF results after surgery depends on the type of the lesions to be treated and on the severity of the disease [11, 12] (Chapter 10).

For myomas, a majority of studies report no significant improvement after myomectomy [13, 14]. Surgical indications on myomas should not be influenced by the fact that the patient will undergo ART.

None of these conditions are likely to be discovered by systematic pre-IVF laparoscopy. All would be revealed by clinical symptoms, or an abnormal ultrasonography or hysterography, or laparoscopy would have been indicated because of specific risk factors. Indications for a laparoscopic treatment do not differ before IVF from what they would have been without use of IVF.

Indications for pre-IVF laparoscopy

1. Laparoscopy is avoided in case of definitely known cause of infertility (in particular male infertility) without suspicious clinical symptoms and normal pelvic imaging.
2. Laparoscopy is indicated if risk factors, history of the patient, pelvic examination, or abnormal imaging suggests pelvic disease.
3. Laparoscopy is indicated if there is a pathologic pelvis necessitating treatment before IVF: e.g., hydrosalpinges, severe endometriosis, endometriotic cysts. This indication is reinforced if there have been prior ART failures.

Conclusion

Hysteroscopy and laparoscopy are part of the global management of the patient. None of these investigations should be routine. However, their diagnosis and therapeutic performances are such that it would be unwise to systematically ignore them once the patient has been entered in an ART programme.

Although there are no RCTs to give evidence-based recommendations, a proper assessment of clinical situations results in an individually based recommendation. Using this approach, a reasonable optimization of ART can be expected, affecting both the efficiency of each ART cycle but also the cumulative pregnancy rate of the patient [15].

References

1. Nawroth F, Foth D, Schmidt T. Minihysteroscopy as routine diagnostic procedure in women with primary infertility. *J Am Assoc Gynecol Laparosc* 2003;**10**:396–98.
2. Lorusso F, Ceci O, Bettocchi S, *et al.* Office hysteroscopy in an in vitro fertilization program. *Gynecol Endocrinol* 2008;**24**:465–9.
3. Doldi N, Persico P, Di Sebastiano F *et al.* Pathologic findings in hysteroscopy before in vitro fertilization-embryo transfer. *Gynecol Endocrinol* 2005; **21**:235–7.
4. Karayalcin R, Ozcan S, Moraloglu O, Ozyer S, Mollamahmutoglu L, Batioglu S. Results of 2500 office-based diagnostic hysteroscopies before IVF. *Reprod BioMed Online* 2010;**20**:689–93.
5. Hinckley M, Milki A. 1000 office-based hysteroscopies prior to in vitro fertilization: feasibility and findings. *JSLS* 2004;**8**: 103–7.
6. Hatemi FM, Kasius JC, Timmermasn A. Prevalence of unsuspected uterine cavity abnormalities diagnosed by office hysteroscopy prior to in vitro fertilization. *Hum Reprod* 2010;**25**:1959–65.

7. El-Mazny A, Abou-Salem N, El-Sherbiny W, Saber W. Outpatient hysteroscopy: a routine investigation before assisted reproductive techniques? *Fertil Steril* 2011; **95**: 272–6.

8. Perez-Medina T, Bajo-Arenas J, Salazar F, *et al.* Endometrial polyps and their implication in the pregnancy rates of patients undergoing intrauterine insemination: a prospective, randomized study. *Hum Reprod* 2005;**20**:1632–5.

9. Bosteels J, Weyers S, Puttemans P, *et al.* The effectiveness of hysteroscopy in improving pregnancy rates in subfertile women without other gynaecological syptoms: a systematic review. *Hum Reprod Update* 2010;**16**: 1–11.

10. Déchaud H, Daurès JP, Arnal F, Humeau C, Hédon B. Does previous salpingectomy improve implantation and pregnancy rates in patients with severe tubal factor infertility who are undergoing in vitro fertilization? A pilot prospective randomized study. *Fertil Steril* 1998;**69**:1020–5.

11. Surrey E, Schoolcraft W. Does surgical management of endometriosis within 6 months of an IVF-ET cycle improve outcome? *J Assist Reprod Gen* 2003;**20**:365–70.

12. Littman E, Giudice L, Lathi R, *et al.* Role of laparoscopic treatment of endometriosis in patients with failed in vitro fertilization cycles. *Fertil Steril* 2005;**84**: 1574–8.

13. Surrey E, Minjarez D, Stevens J, Schoolcraft W. Effect of myomectomy on the outcome of assisted reproductive technologies *Fertil Steril* 2005;**83**:1473–9.

14. Klatsky P, Lane D, Ryan I, Fujimoto V. The effect of fibroids without cavity involvment on ART outcomes independent of ovarian age. *Hum Reprod* 2007;**22**: 521–6.

15. Audibert F, Hedon B, Arnal F, *et al.* Therapeutic strategies in tubal infertility with distal pathology. *Hum Reprod* 1991;**6**: 1439–42.

Chapter 4

The management of fibroids and polyps

Ben Kroon and Roger Hart

Background

Evidence suggests that pathology which distorts the endometrial cavity may impact implantation and the success of fertility treatments. Fibroids and polyps are the most common conditions that impact on the endometrial cavity, and as such are the subject of much investigative interest. Despite numerous publications, the association between both polyps and fibroids and infertility is unclear. Contentious also is the question of whether treatment of these conditions will improve fertility outcomes or IVF success rates. While surgical removal of the lesion may seem biologically attractive, post-operative morbidity such as endometrial scarring and myometrial damage may in fact contribute negatively to fertility. What follows is an outline of the current evidence regarding the effect of fibroids and polyps on fertility, and the effect of various treatment for these pathologies on fertility outcomes. Further, it will provide a proposed treatment algorithm to assist reproductive health specialists with management decisions.

Fibroids

Fibroids (leiomyomata) are the most common uterine tumour found in women of reproductive age. Classical presentations include menorrhagia and/or pelvic pressure symptoms, however women may present solely with delayed fertility. The effect of fibroids on fertility is the subject of much disagreement, largely because there is little high quality evidence from which to draw conclusions. Unfortunately, interpretation of the literature is made difficult because of the heterogeneity of not only the tumours themselves, but also the characteristics of the available studies. Most have small sample sizes and are retrospective, with varying control groups. In addition there is frequently either inadequate or inconsistent assessment of the uterine cavity, which is a prerequisite for accurate fibroid classification. In the face of these difficulties, Pritts *et al.* [1] and Sunkara *et al.* [2] have recently published reviews of the effect of fibroids and myomectomy on fertility, and the effect of fibroids on IVF, respectively. Pritts *et al.* considered the effect of fibroids in all locations and included studies of spontaneous or assisted conception, while Sunkara *et al.* considered specifically studies looking at the effect of intramural fibroids on IVF conceptions.

To enable discussion of fibroids it is imperative to use consistent terminology. No generally accepted definition exists, but the most commonly used is that proposed by the European Society of Hysteroscopy [3]. It defines a submucosal fibroid (SM) as one that deforms the

How to Improve Your ART Success Rates, ed. Gab Kovacs. Published by Cambridge

uterine cavity. Submucosal fibroids may be subdivided into Type 0 (pedunculated), type 1 (with extension <50% into the wall), and type 2 (sessile with extension ≥50% into the wall). An intramural (IM) fibroid does not deform the cavity and has less than 50% protruding from the wall, while subserosal (SS) fibroids have more than 50% protruding from the myometrium. Clearly this classification does not account for location within the uterus (such as peri-ostial or cervical fibroids), or the proximity of a fibroid to the endometrium, both factors potentially impacting upon fertility. Future classification systems will hopefully address these discrepancies. Fibroids are hypothesized to affect fertility outcomes by a number of mechanisms:

- Anatomical distortion of the cervix, uterine cavity or tubal ostia may affect sperm migration and/or hinder ovum retrieval and transport by the fallopian tube
- Promotion of abnormal uterine contractility
- Alteration of endometrial blood supply in the area of the fibroid
- Localized endometrial inflammation
- Release of vasoactive substances.

The effect of fibroids on fertility and IVF outcomes

Subserosal fibroids

The limited evidence available suggests that SS fibroids do not have a significant effect on fertility [1].

Intramural fibroids

The majority of studies looking at the effect of IM fibroids either inadequately or inconsistently evaluated the uterine cavity, rendering interpretation difficult. If suboptimal assessment was undertaken, it is possible that IM fibroids may have been mistaken for those with a submucosal component, contributing to a potential misinterpretation of the true effect of such tumours.

Pritts *et al.* found a reduction in clinical pregnancy rate (CPR) (RR 0.81, 95% CI 0.70–0.94), implantation rate (IR) (RR 0.68, 95% CI 0.59–0.80) and live birth rate/ongoing pregnancy rate (LBR/OPR) (RR 0.70, 95% CI 0.58–0.85) in women with IM fibroids. There was also an increase in miscarriage rate (MR) (RR 1.75, 95% CI 1.23–2.49). However, when only studies with adequate cavity assessment were included, the effect on CPR, LBR, and MR lacked significance, bringing into question the validity of the overall clinical conclusions.

Sunkara *et al.* agreed with the finding that IM fibroids reduced the CPR (RR 0.85, 95% CI 0.77–0.94) and LBR (RR 0.79, 95% CI 0.70–0.88) in IVF cycles undertaken in women with IM fibroids. In this population Sunkara *et al.* reported a non-significant reduction in IR (RR 0.87, 95% CI 0.73–1.03) and a trend towards an increase in MR (RR 1.24, 95% CI 0.99–1.57).

In light of these findings, we can infer that the presence of IM fibroids in women trying to conceive *may* be associated with reduced CPR, IR and LBR/OPR and an increase in MR; however, considerable uncertainty remains because of the quality of the available literature.

Submucosal fibroids

Because of the proximity of the fibroid to the endometrial cavity, it is intuitively more likely that SM fibroids would influence fertility outcomes, and this is borne out in the literature.

Pritts *et al.* reported a significant reduction in CPR (RR 0.36, 95% CI 0.18–0.74), IR (RR 0.28, 95% CI 0.12–0.65) and LBR/OPR (RR 0.32, 95% CI 0.12–0.85) in women with SM fibroids. The MR was correspondingly increased (RR 1.68, 95% CI 1.3–2.05). While not restricted to mode of conception, the Pritts review includes papers where the study group were women undergoing IVF treatments.

The effect of fibroid size upon fertility outcomes was evaluated in a number of studies reported on in the review by Pritts *et al.* It appears that fibroid size did not significantly correlate with fertility outcome, although there is limited information on this. The effect of fibroid number upon fertility outcomes has also not been adequately addressed.

Management of fibroids

When faced with a couple with unexplained infertility where the woman has a fibroid uterus, the management is clearly influenced by associated clinical symptoms. Where heavy menstrual loss, pressure symptoms, or clinical suspicion of leiomyosarcoma exist, treatment may be unavoidable. In asymptomatic cases treatment can be guided by the available evidence, based on fibroid location. It should be noted that for accurate determination of fibroid location, transvaginal ultrasound lacks sensitivity for the detection of SM fibroids. Where differentiation between submucosal and intramural fibroids is critical, sonohysterogram and hysteroscopy have better diagnostic accuracy. MRI is also highly reproducible and may exceed sonohysterography, transvaginal ultrasound, and hysteroscopy for the localization of fibroids.

If a decision is made that a fibroid warrants treatment, the management options are as follows.

Medical management

Gonadotropin-releasing hormone analogues (GnRHa) induce hypo-oestrogenaemia and a reduction in fibroid volume. When used pre-operatively GnRHa improve pre-operative haemoglobin, reduce uterine volume and fibroid size and reduce intra-operative blood loss, potentially allowing for a more conservative operative approach. Danazol, Mifepristone, aromatase inhibitors, and selective oestrogen and progestogen receptor modulators have also shown benefit in reducing fibroid volume, although their use in women presenting with infertility is unclear. In general, medical management of fibroids delays efforts to conceive and, apart from the specific indication for GnRHa above, is not recommended for the management of infertility associated with fibroids. There is no proven role for medical management of fibroids as an adjunct to improve IVF success.

Surgical management – the effect of myomectomy on fertility outcomes

As discussed above, SM and possibly IM fibroids have a negative effect on fertility and IVF outcomes, but it does not necessarily follow that myomectomy will improve success, as the influence of uterine scar formation on embryo implantation is unknown. The effect of myomectomy has again been well summarized by Pritts *et al.* Myomectomy for IM fibroids did not have a significant effect upon CPR (RR 3.77, 95% CI 0.47–30.14), MR (RR 0.76, 95% CI 0.30–1.94) or LBR/OPR (RR 1.67, 95% CI 0.75–3.72) when compared to controls with fibroids in situ.

When comparing women who underwent myomectomy for SM fibroids to those in whom fibroids were left in situ, Pritts *et al.* report an increase in CPR (RR 2.03, 95% CI 1.08–3.83), but no significant influence on MR (RR 0.77, 95% CI 0.36–1.66) or OPR/LBR (RR 2.65, 95% CI 0.92–7.66). In those studies that addressed myomectomy for SM fibroids where controls were infertile women with no fibroids, Pritts *et al.* found no significant difference in fertility between myomectomy and control groups, indicating that the procedure of hysteroscopic myomectomy itself has no detrimental effect upon implantation.

In conclusion, there is insufficient evidence to determine whether myomectomy for IM fibroids improves fertility outcomes; however, the limited available evidence suggests that hysteroscopic myomectomy for SM fibroids is not detrimental and is likely to improve fertility outcomes. It must be noted again that the quality of this evidence is poor and is not specific to women undergoing IVF cycles. The effect of fibroid size, number, and location within the uterus may impact on the usefulness of myomectomy, but there is inadequate evidence to comment on this.

For those patients offered myomectomy, a hysteroscopic approach is the treatment of choice for SM fibroids.

Abdominal myomectomy remains the routine approach for most surgeons faced with multiple or large fibroids. For surgeons with the appropriate skill set, a laparoscopic approach is appropriate in many situations. When compared with open myomectomy, laparoscopic myomectomy is associated with a reduced post-operative haemoglobin fall, reduced operative blood loss, a quicker recovery, reduced postoperative pain, and fewer overall complications, but with a longer operating time. More recent innovative approaches to the surgical management of fibroids include either temporary or permanent occlusion of the uterine artery. Such techniques are based on the theory that fibroids are exquisitely susceptible to ischaemia because of their tenuous blood supply, while normal myometrium is more resilient. These approaches are not sufficiently proven and should not be used in the management of fibroids in women desiring future fertility unless in the setting of clinical trials.

Alternative treatments

An alternative technique for managing fibroids is uterine artery embolization (UAE). This involves radiologically guided embolization of the uterine arteries with the intent of causing ischaemic injury to the fibroid. Normal myometrium generally recovers, while the fibroid necroses. While the results in terms of fibroid size and symptom reduction make this treatment attractive, the effect on reproductive outcomes is thus far poorly documented. Potential risks include premature ovarian failure due to inadvertent passage of embolic particles into the utero-ovarian anastomoses, and the risk of endometrial damage and synechia resulting from small diameter non-resorbable particles causing endometrial vascular ischaemia. Pregnancy complications such as higher rates of spontaneous miscarriage, preterm delivery, abnormal placentation, caesarean section, and post-partum haemorrhage have also been reported. In view of these reproductive outcomes, UAE is not recommended unless in the setting of clinical trials.

In addition to UAE, contemporary experimental techniques for managing fibroids without myomectomy include magnetic resonance-guided focused ultrasound surgery (MRgFUS), fibroid myolysis, and radiofrequency thermal ablation (RFA). The lack of information on fertility outcomes should preclude their use in women desiring future fertility unless in the setting of trials.

How do I improve IVF outcomes if my patient has fibroids?

Infertility clinicians must be aware that the evidence guiding management for women with fibroids is poor. Subserosal fibroids do not appear to have a significant effect on fertility outcomes and thus removal is usually undertaken for symptomatic reasons only. Intramural

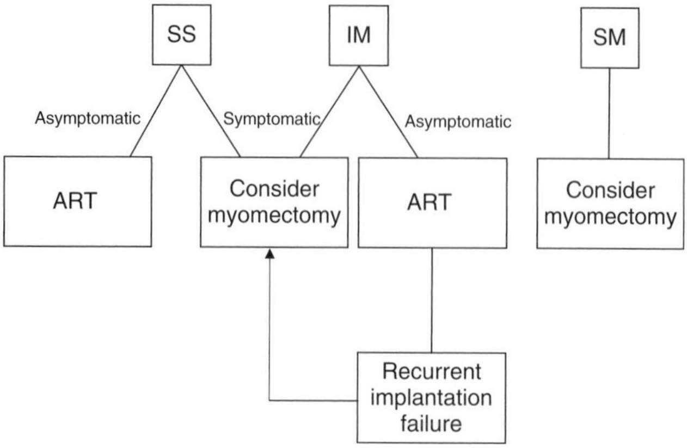

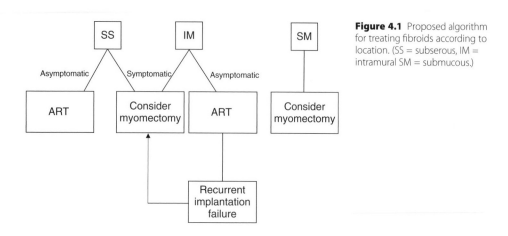

Figure 4.1 Proposed algorithm for treating fibroids according to location. (SS = subserous, IM = intramural SM = submucous.)

fibroids may be associated with reduced fertility and an increased miscarriage rate, but there is insufficient evidence to inform whether myomectomy for IM fibroids improves rates of spontaneous or assisted conception. Submucosal fibroids are associated with reduced fertility and an increased miscarriage rate, and hysteroscopic myomectomy appears likely to improve fertility outcomes. It is not clear whether multiple or larger fibroids have a different effect on fertility, and what the relative usefulness of myomectomy in these situations is.

Figure 4.1 is a proposed management algorithm for women presenting with infertility where uterine fibroids are present and no alternative cause is found.

Polyps and infertility

Endometrial polyps in the infertile population are generally benign, localized overgrowths of endometrium. They may be asymptomatic or present with abnormal menstrual bleeding. Polyps are hypothesized to contribute to reduced fertility by presenting an abnormal site for embryo implantation, mechanically impairing sperm transport, by causing irregular endometrial bleeding, creating an inflammatory response, or by causing increased endometrial secretion of glycodelin (a glycoprotein implicated in impaired fertilization and implantation).

As with fibroids, polyps may be detected by transvaginal ultrasound, hysterosalpingogram, saline infusion sonohysteroscopy, and hysteroscopy. Hysteroscopy is the gold standard investigation as it allows for real-time visualization and concurrent polypectomy if desired. Polypectomy may be achieved by a number of techniques including "blind" avulsion or curettage, but most precisely by transcervical resection. Unlike myomectomy which usually involves uterine muscle damage and repair, polypectomy generally leaves the basal endometrium intact, and hence complications such as synechiae are rare.

The association between polyps, polypectomy, and infertility is poorly described. It is unknown whether polyps are more common in the infertile population than their fertile counterparts.

In a recent systematic review of papers addressing the treatment of endometrial polyps, Lieng *et al.* [4] detail the findings of one randomized controlled trial (RCT) (215 women), three retrospective controlled studies (161 women), and a further seven case series (559 women) which report the effect of polypectomy on infertility. The sole RCT [5] randomized infertile women with an ultrasound diagnosis of endometrial polyps to hysteroscopic polypectomy (107) or to a control group who underwent diagnostic hysteroscopy with polyp biopsy (108). Following hysteroscopy both groups received four cycles of gonadotropin hyperstimulation with insemination (IUI). Those women receiving polypectomy had a significantly higher clinical pregnancy rate after four cycles (63%) than the control group (28%) (RR = 2.3; 95% CI 1.6–3.2). This suggests a benefit from polypectomy in women planned for IUI. The remaining evidence regarding polypectomy is poor, as most reports are retrospective observational studies lacking in a control group. High quality evidence addressing polypectomy prior to IVF or the issue of multiple or different sized polyps, is not available.

Conclusion

Overall studies are divided in their interpretation of the effect of polyps and polypectomy on fertility; however, the results of the single RCT suggest that polypectomy should be performed in infertile women, or those commencing fertility treatment. Hysteroscopic polypectomy is a relatively low cost and low risk procedure which may potentially improve fertility outcomes.

References

1. Pritts EA, Parker WH, Olive DL. Fibroids and infertility: an updated systematic review of the evidence. *Fertil and Steril* 2009;**91**:1215–23.
2. Sunkara S, Khairy M, El-Toukhy T *et al.* The effect of intramural fibroids without uterine cavity involvement on the outcome of IVF treatment: a systematic review and meta-analysis. *Hum Reprod* 2010;**25**: 418–29.
3. Wamsteker K, De Kruif J. Transcervical hysteroscopic resection of SM fibroids for abnormal uterine bleeding: results regarding the degree of IM extension. *Obstet Gynecol* 1993;**82**:736–40.
4. Lieng M, Itra O, Qvigstad E. Treatment of endometrial polyps: a systematic review. *Acta Obstet Gynecol* 2010;**89**:992–1002.
5. Perez-Medina T, Bajo-Arenas J, Salazar F *et al.* Endometrial polyps and their implication in the pregnancy rates of patients undergoing intrauterine insemination: a prospective, randomized study. *Hum Reprod* 2005;**20**:1632–5.

Chapter 5

Immunological screening in women undergoing IVF

Dominique M. Butawan and William H. Kutteh

Introduction

Approximately 12% of couples desiring children suffer from infertility. Despite thorough investigation, the cause of infertility remains unexplained in at least 10% of these couples. Since Gleicher's original description of the reproductive autoimmune failure syndrome in 1989, numerous studies have been performed in an attempt to identify specific immune factors or antibodies associated with pregnancy loss and infertility. Autoimmunity refers to an immune reaction of the body against substances normally present in the body.

Implantation is one of the most important aspects of pregnancy that these studies have targeted. Implantation represents a critical developmental process in that it requires the interaction of immunologically and genetically distinct tissues. The immune system may influence pregnancy success or failure during any of the critical steps of implantation.

Human preimplantation embryos express major histocompatability antigens theoretically capable of inducing an immune response. There is a possibility that maternal immune responses may play a role in the failure of implantation.

Autoimmune factors potentially related to pregnancy failure

Recent studies have investigated the role of autoimmune factors in implantation in women undergoing fertility treatment. The most commonly studied antibodies include antiphospholipid antibodies, antithyroid antibodies, antinuclear antibodies, antigliadin antibodies, antiovarian antibodies, and antisperm antibodies (Table 5.1).

Antiphospholipid antibodies

Antiphospholipid antibodies (APA) have been found in 15–20% of patients with recurrent pregnancy loss and in 15–20% of patients with unexplained infertility or recurrent implantation failure. These numbers are significantly higher then the frequency of APA found in control populations of women, which ranges from 2 to 5%. It has been postulated that these APA impair cytotrophoblast invasion and their differentiation into syncytiotrophoblasts, thus, impairing blastocyst implantation. In order for a patient to be diagnosed with antiphospholipid syndrome at least one of the clinical criteria and one of the laboratory criteria must be met as follows:

How to Improve Your ART Success Rates, ed. Gab Kovacs. Published by Cambridge

Table 5.1 Association of auto-antibodies with IVF patients

Autoantibody	Frequency in infertile women	Infertility association	Known associations
Antiphospholipid	Increased	Unproven	Recurrent pregnancy loss
Antithyroid	Slightly increased	Unproven	Thyroiditis; Miscarriage
Antigliadin	Slightly increased	Unproven	Celiac disease
Antisperm	No difference	Unproven	Fertilization failure
Antinuclear	Slightly increased	Unproven	Autoimmune disease
Antiovarian	Slightly increased	Unproven	Ovarian failure

Clinical criteria

1) Vascular thrombosis: One or more episodes of arterial, venous or small vessel thrombosis in any tissue or organ
2) Morbidity in pregnancy:
   (a) One or more unexplained deaths of a morphologically normal fetus at or beyond the 10th week of gestation
   (b) One or more premature births of a morphologically normal neonate prior to the 34th week of gestation secondary to eclampsia or severe pre-eclampsia or recognized features of placental insufficency
   (c) Three or more unexplained consecutive spontaneous miscarriages before the 10th week of gestation

Laboratory criteria (two or more occasions ≥12 weeks apart)

1) Lupus anticoagulant
2) Anticardiolipin antibodies of medium to high titers**
3) Anti-β2-glycoprotein in medium to high titers**

In this case, medium to high titers means more than 40 units of IgG or IgM antibody or greater than 99% of normal.

Antiphospholipid antibodies interact with the maternal–fetal interface and are associated with recurrent spontaneous miscarriage as well as pre-eclampsia, intrauterine growth restriction, and fetal demise. The involvement of APA with pregnancy is thought to be more of an autoimmune factor than a thrombophilic factor based on histological studies showing a lack of intravascular or intervillous blood clots in placentas obtained following spontaneous miscarriage. Potential mechanisms link APA with decreased release of human chorionic gonadotropin (hCG) from human placental explants, prevention of in vitro trophoblast migration and invasion, inhibition of trophoblast cell adhesion molecules and activation of complement on the trophoblast surface inducing an inflammatory response [1].

Antiphopholipid antibodies have been found in 15% of patients with recurrent first trimester loss. Treatment of these patients with unfractionated heparin and low-dose aspirin has been shown to improve live birth rates in most studies; however, treatment of patients with low molecular weight heparin and aspirin has not consistently shown the same benefit.

Moreover, recent studies have not shown a benefit of treatment using heparin in women with unexplained recurrent pregnancy loss.

Several published reports indicate that positive APA are found more frequently in patients undergoing IVF or who have failed IVF. However, positive APA have not been associated with decreased pregnancy rates in women undergoing IVF [1] and treatment with heparin and aspirin of women undergoing IVF who concurrently test positive for APA does not improve pregnancy or implantation rates [2]. The American Society of Reproductive Medicine states that assessment of APA is not indicated among couples undergoing IVF based on prospective studies looking at IVF outcomes among APA-positive and -negative subjects who were free from any treatment (intravenous immunoglobulin, heparin, aspirin). Although the prevalence of APA is higher among women undergoing IVF, their presence does not appear to influence the outcome of pregnancy, miscarriage, or live birth rate.

Antithyroid antibodies

Antithyroid antibodies (ATA), specifically thyroglobulin and thyroid peroxidase antibodies, are commonly found in patients with Graves disease, postpartum thyroiditis, and Hashimoto's thyroiditis. The prevalence of ATA has been reported in 15–20% of normal pregnant women and women undergoing assisted reproductive techniques compared to 20–25% in women with recurrent miscarriage and 45% of pregnant women with a diagnosis of hypothyroidism.

Multiple studies have investigated the role of thyroid autoimmunity in infertility, but the interpretation of the evidence as a whole is difficult, secondary to variations in study design. Some studies have shown a significantly increased relative risk for thyroid autoimmunity among endometriosis and polycystic ovarian syndrome compared to age-matched controls, suggesting that multi-factorial causes as opposed to isolated thyroid autoimmunity may be responsible for infertility. It has been suggested that ATA may be responsible for the increased incidence of infertility because thyroid hormone receptors have been described in human oocytes where they assist in the stimulation of granulosa cell function and trophoblastic differentiation.

The prevalence of ATA may be slightly higher in women experiencing IVF failure when compared to their counterparts. This finding is consistent with a recent review of the literature that stated that ATA are associated with increased risk of miscarriage but not clinical pregnancy and delivery rates in women undergoing IVF [3]. The reason behind this finding is unclear but may indicate an underlying autoimmune process that directly affects embryo implantation or ATA may reflect an overt thyroid dysfunction leading to the inability of the thyroid to meet the increased demands of pregnancy. Screening for thyroid dysfunction in patients experiencing multiple miscarriages may help to identify patients that may benefit from an inexpensive therapy and thus, reduce their chance for miscarriage. There are insufficient data to recommend screening asymptomatic infertile women for autoimmune thyroid dysfunction [4].

Antinuclear antibodies

Antinuclear antibodies (ANA) are a group of antibodies that target nuclear and cytoplasmic antigens that are essential to cell function through playing a role in transcription, translation, and cell cycle regulation. A positive ANA titer may be nonspecific or may be associated with multiple autoimmune disorders such as systemic lupus erythematosus. The role of ANA in infertility is largely undetermined. Some studies have suggested that ANA is associated with implantation failure secondary to an endometriosis-induced autoimmune reaction.

Antigliadin antibodies

Celiac disease is an intestinal inflammatory disease that is ultimately triggered by gluten in the diet. Patients often present with gastrointestinal symptoms such as diarrhea, abdominal pain, and bloating. In women with celiac disease, immune responses to gliadin fractions promote an inflammatory reaction in the intestines that can be diagnosed by biopsy. Pathology reveals infiltration of the lamina propria and the epithelium with inflammatory cells and villous atrophy. Recent studies have suggested that women with celiac disease may be at increased risk for miscarriages and possibly infertility. Autoimmune testing for antigliadin antibodies, anti-tissue transaminase IgA, and IgA antiendomysium antibody has been suggested by some to screen for subclinical celiac disease. However, a positive response to a gluten-free diet (avoiding wheat, rye, and barley) is also considered diagnostic of celiac disease. Until further studies are available, routine screening in women without symptoms of celiac disease is not recommended. In those women with symptoms of celiac disease, it would be appropriate to advocate a gluten-free diet.

Antiovarian antibodies

Antiovarian antibodies (AOA) include antibodies against a heterogeneous group of antigens, including molecular targets in the zona pellucida, theca interna, granulosa cells, ooplasm, and heat shock protein 90-β. Studies have suggested numerous associations of AOA with infertility, such as reduced fertilization rates and pregnancy rates, inhibited response to gonadotropin stimulation, altered egg and embryo development, and possibly implantation failures. Data are still inadequate to provide a solid link between AOA and infertility but their presence may be linked to ovarian hypofunction.

Antisperm antibodies

Sperm contain antigens that are foreign to both male and female immune systems. Production of antisperm antibodies (ASA) may be induced in the seminal plasma, in male or female serum, or in the cervical mucus when sperm are exposed to the immune system. Antisperm antibodies have been identified in 10% to 15% of men with infertility and in 15% to 20% of women with unexplained infertility. The prevalence and presumed significance reported depends on the population, source of the specimen (serum, cervical mucus, semen), and method of testing. These antibodies are postulated to interfere with the fecundity process through various mechanisms, such as interference with sperm transport within the female genital tract, alteration of sperm capacitation or acrosomal reaction, interference with fertilization, or inhibition of implantation of the early embryo. The best studies suggest that possible sites where sperm-bound ASA might interfere with fertilization include sperm binding to zona pellucida, sperm penetration of the zona pellucida, zona reaction, gamete fusion, embryo cleavage, and embryo development. However, these data are not strong enough to recommend generalized screening for ASA in the infertile population.

Thrombophilias

A thrombophilia is defined as a hereditary or acquired condition that predisposes affected individuals to thrombotic events. A hypercoaguable state includes inherited and acquired

Table 5.2 Common acquired and inherited thrombophilias

Thrombophilia	Inheritance	Prevalence	Non-pregnant DVT risk
Factor V Leiden G1691A mutation	Autosomal dominant	2–15%	3–8×
Factor II G20210A mutation (prothrombin mutation)	Autosomal dominant	2–3%	3×
MTHFR C677T mutation	Autosomal recessive	10–25%	2.5–4×
Antithrombin deficiency	Autosomal dominant	0.02%	25–50×
Protein C deficiency	Autosomal dominant	0.2–0.3%	10–15×
Protein S deficiency	Autosomal dominant	0.1–0.2%	2×
Activated protein C resistance	Acquired	10%	2×
Hyperhomocysteinemia	Acquired	10–15%	2–4×
Antiphospholipid antibodies	Acquired	5%	2×
Elevated factor VIII	X-linked	5–15%	5×

MTHFR: methylenetetrahydrofolate reductase; DVT: deep vein thrombosis.

disorders that lead to pathologic, thrombotic tendency or risk of thrombosis, which is also known as a prothrombotic state (Table 5.2).

Thrombophilias have been thought to cause a state of hypercoagulation at the implantation site impeding the connection between maternal and fetal blood flow, ultimately resulting in miscarriage. Some studies have argued that placental thrombosis cannot account for early implantation failure since intervillous circulation is not established until late first trimester. On the other hand, women with recurrent pregnancy loss may have a prothrombotic condition and have higher thrombin-antithrombin complexes. Excess thromboxane production has been reported at 4–7 weeks with lower levels of prostacyclin than in women without a history of recurrent loss.

Screening for thrombophilias in women who are infertile or in those with implantation failure remains controversial and should not routinely be performed in women undergoing IVF. The American College of Obstetricians and Gynecologists recommends only screening patients with a personal history of venous thromboembolism in the absence of other risk factors and in patients with a first degree relative who has a history of a high-risk thrombophilia or a venous thromboembolism prior to 50 years of age, not associated with other risk factors [5].

Conclusion

Failed implantation as a result of early embryo demise is thought to play a tremendous role in pregnancy failure. It was recently reported that the presence of antiphospholipid antibodies, antinuclear antibodies, and/or antithyroid antibodies does not affect the pregnancy outcome in donor oocyte recipients. This suggests that pregnancy loss and infertility may be secondary to other causes such as embryonic defects, defects in uterine receptivity, or multifactorial causes.

Unfortunately the majority of available data on the role of immunity in infertility is hindered by small or poorly conducted studies. This limits the ability to form definitive recommendations for the screening and treatment of autoimmunity in the infertile population. While the existence of two immunologically distinct organisms during pregnancy suggests an essential role of the immune system in fertility, additional studies are needed to suggest treatments and recommendations for immune modulation and screening in patients with infertility (Table 5.1). Similarly, additional studies are necessary before routine screening for thrombophilias can be recommended in women with infertility or implantation failure.

Funding

Frank Ling Research Grant in Obstetrics and Gynecology.

References

1. Buckingham KL, Chamley LW. A critical assessment of the role of antiphospholipid antibodies in infertility. *J Reprod Immunol* 2009;**80**:132–45.
2. The Practice Committee of the American Society for Reproductive Medicine. Antiphospholipid antibodies do not affect IVF success. *Fertil Steril* 2008;**90**:5172–3.
3. Toulis KA, Goulis DG, Ventis CA, *et al.* Risk of spontaneous miscarriage in euthroid women with thyroid autoimmunity undergoing IVF: a meta-analysis. *Europ J Endocrin* 2010;**162**:643–52.
4. Nardo LG, Granne I, Stewart J; Policy & Practice Committee of the British Fertility Society. Medical adjuncts in IVF: evidence for clinical practice. *Hum Fertil (Camb)* 2009;**12**:1–13.
5. Lockwood C, Wendel G. Inherited thrombophilias in pregnancy. American College of Obstetricians and Gynecologists Practice Bulletin Number 113. *Obstet Gynecol* 2010;**116**:212–22.

Chapter 6

Natural killer cell analysis

Gavin Sacks

Introduction

In reproductive medicine, natural killer (NK) cell analysis is at once a marketing dream and an academic nightmare. This chapter aims to help clinicians counsel patients effectively and contemplate a progressive approach to this new and still unproven topic. The lack of large trials and proven pathological mechanisms should not deter clinicians from trying to understand what is actually being tested, what it may mean, and how it may guide adjuvant therapy to improve IVF success rates.

NK cell biology

NK cells do not require activation in order to kill cells that are missing "self" markers of major histocompatibility complex (MHC) class I, as in cells affected by intracellular infection or cancer. Hence NK cells, part of the innate and evolutionary older branch of the immune system, have a primary function of 'immune surveillance'. Since placental cells do not express classic MHC class I proteins (probably to avoid attack by maternal T cells) they are vulnerable to attack by NK cells instead.

NK cells are lymphocytes with a $CD3^{-}CD56^{+}$ phenotypic profile. Two main subtypes exist. $CD56^{+Bright}$ express high density CD56, are $CD16^{-}$ and produce cytokines (IFN-γ, TNF-β, IL-10, and GM-CSF). $CD56^{+Dim}$ express low density CD56, are $CD16^{+}$, have limited cytokine output, and are primarily responsible for NK cell cytotoxicity. These two subtypes also express different activating receptors (CD69) and inhibiting receptors (killer immunoglobulin-like receptors (KIR) and CD94).

NK cells are distributed widely in all tissues, but are especially concentrated in the uterus. Uterine (u)NK cell numbers increase enormously from 10% of stromal cells in the proliferative phase to 20% in the late-secretory phase, and >30% in early pregnancy. Thus uNK cells appear to regulate trophoblast (placental cell) invasion, although their precise function in reproduction is still not known. Ninety per cent of uNK cells are the $CD56^{+Bright}$ phenotype. They have never been shown to be cytotoxic to trophoblast cells in vivo, and in vitro require co-culture with interleukin (IL)-2 to induce cytotoxicity (not surprisingly, IL-2 is not usually present at the maternal–fetal interface). In the absence of implantation, uNK cells undergo apoptosis thus heralding menstruation. It is likely that the majority of uNK cells are recruited directly from the peripheral blood pool of NK cells every month, and recent studies have suggested correlation between uNK and blood (b)NK cell numbers.

How to Improve Your ART Success Rates, ed. Gab Kovacs. Published by Cambridge

However, the precise relationship between bNK cells and uNK cells is unclear, especially since over 90% of bNK cells are $CD56^{+Dim}$ while over 90% of uNK cells are $CD56^{+Bright}$. In other words, the overwhelming majority of uNK cells represents <10% of the bNK cell population.

Methods of assessment

Much of the controversy surrounding NK cell analysis is largely the result of poor study design, over-interpretation of results, and lack of understanding of the complexities of the laboratory methods used. In most published studies the 'patient' group is very heterogenous, often including women with both recurrent miscarriage and repeated IVF failure (which themselves can have varied definitions). Controls are difficult to recruit (some studies have no control group), and even more difficult to define. It is entirely plausible, for example, that a previously 'fertile' woman used as a control may have developed secondary reproductive failure.

Uterine NK cells

The assessment of uNK cells is normally done by immunohistochemistry, the subjectiveness and limitations of which are rarely appreciated. First of all, it is only possible to count $CD56^{+}$ cells, without any measurement of subtype or level of activation. Thus for example, high levels of $CD56^{+Bright}$ may reflect a very different immunological environment to high levels of $CD56^{+Dim}$. Secondly, the endometrium is a complex glandular histological structure, and counting cells in one area gives wildly different results to counting in another. It takes a considerable effort for a pathologist to develop a reliable and consistent method of counting. Most tests for uNK cells are performed at the time of the 'implantation window'. But uNK cell numbers vary enormously on a daily basis, and interpretation of cell levels needs to be appropriate for that exact day of the cycle with respect to ovulation. Few laboratories will have sufficient data to be able to do that.

Blood NK cells

The main criticism for analysis of bNK cells is that they are mainly of different phenotype to the majority of uNK cells, and therefore cannot bear any useful relationship to uNK cell numbers, and in any case are far from the site of embryo implantation. But endometrial biopsy is an invasive and painful procedure, and the prospect of a blood test assessment of immunological dysfunction has significant appeal. Although the majority (90%) of uNK and bNK cells are of different phenotype, it is simply not known how changes in the ratio of subtypes may affect implantation. Thus, it is hypothesized that higher levels of activated $CD56^{+Dim}$ bNK cells may lead to an altered phenotype ratio in the endometrium due to monthly recruitment [1]. Alternatively, it is also possible that bNK cell activity represents a marker for some other (as yet undefined) immunological disorder. This marker may be non-specific – in the same way as a raised white blood cell count or C-reactive protein level indicates the likelihood of infection somewhere in the body.

A number of assays have been used for the analysis of bNK cells, including the proportion of bNK cells out of all lymphocytes, concentration, surface markers of activation, and in vitro assays of biological activity. These methods are not necessarily correlated, and results may be potentially affected by venepuncture conditions and transport to the laboratory, protocols for preparation and labelling, and the gating of cell populations in flow cytometry analysis.

Although population studies demonstrate a wide reference range for bNK cells (3–31%), the corrected range for females is 5–20% (and this includes women with reproductive failure). There are also numerous other physiological variables that could affect bNK cell levels, including acute stress and exercise (increased), the menstrual cycle, and IVF stimulation (differential effects on different tests performed).

NK cell analysis in reproductive failure

Peripheral blood NK cell analysis in reproductive failure was first described in 1996 by Alan Beer's group in Chicago. In a poorly controlled study it was famously claimed that high levels could be defined by bNK cell numbers >12%, and that no women with bNK levels over 18% had a successful pregnancy outcome, unless treated with immunoglobulin therapy. Other groups have since shown that in women with unexplained reproductive failure, bNK cells have higher preconceptual activity and cytotoxicity (^{51}chromium-release assay), higher expression of the surface activation marker CD69, and lower expression of the inhibitory marker CD94. Women with raised NK cell activity have about a four-fold increase risk of miscarriage with karyotypically normal fetuses. In early pregnancy (including after IVF), lower levels of bNK cell cytotoxicity are significantly associated with live birth. One study showed that bNK cell cytotoxicity is higher in women with primary than those with secondary recurrent miscarriage.

In women with unexplained infertility, high bNK cell activity is associated with significantly lower conception rates over a 2-year follow up. In the IVF setting, it has been claimed that lower bNK cell cytotoxicity on the day of embryo transfer is significantly associated with live birth. And another study used a receiver operating characteristic analysis to show that women with raised CD69 expression on bNK cells had a significantly reduced implantation rate (13.1 versus 28.2%), pregnancy rate (23.1 versus 48.3%) and live birth rate (7.7 versus 40.2%), and manifested a higher miscarriage rate (66.7 versus 16.7%).

Given the invasive nature of uNK cell testing, there are fewer such studies in women with reproductive failure. However, numerous studies have similarly demonstrated that women with unexplained recurrent miscarriage or repeated IVF failure have 'high' uNK cell levels [2]. Perhaps most significantly, it has been shown that preconceptual numbers are increased in women who subsequently have karyotypically normal miscarriages. And a critical study using flow cytometry rather than immunohistochemistry showed that women with unexplained recurrent miscarriage have increased uNK cells of the $CD56^{+Dim}$ subtype. This supports the hypothesis that increased or activated bNK cells (primarily $CD56^{+Dim}$ cells) alter the uNK cell subtype population, which may be in turn detrimental to successful implantation.

In Sydney, we have showed that high levels of bNK cells are strongly correlated with high levels of uNK cells, and for bNK cells the strongest discriminating factors (for women with reproductive failure versus controls) are: (1) the number of bNK cells expressed as a percentage of lymphocytes (normal <18%) and (2) the concentration of activated $CD56^{+Dim}$ bNK cells (determined with the CD69 marker; normal $<12 \times 106$/l)[3]. The assessment of uNK cells is obviously more invasive and is potentially useful if: (1) further confirmation is wanted or (2) bNK cell levels are low or borderline.

Ultimately though, it boils down to whether it is worth measuring NK cells anyway. Is there effective treatment? And does that treatment improve IVF success rates?

Targeted immune therapy

Immune therapy to try to improve IVF success rates (and reduce miscarriage rates) has a long and chequered history. This is partly due to the legacy of Peter Medawar's classic 1950s paper in which pregnancy immunology was compared with a tissue transplant, and hence the need for maternal immune suppression. More recent work has significantly refined that hypothesis, with some elements of the maternal immune system suppressed and others activated. It is clear that NK cells are a critical part in the maternal recognition of a conceptus and establishment of the maternal–fetal interface. Animals with depleted NK cells do not have successful pregnancies. Implantation and pregnancy in general are inflammatory states, and it is hypothesized that the absence of inflammation can be just as detrimental as an excessive inflammatory state.

Most women having IVF do not require additional immune suppressive therapy (trials from 15–20 years ago did not show benefit). Some more recent trials have shown that immune therapy improves IVF success rates in women with repeated IVF failure, suggesting that there may be a subgroup of women who do benefit from immune therapy [4]. So, can NK cell testing identify that subgroup who have excessive immunological activity leading to a poor endometrial environment (e.g., abnormal local cytokine profile) and lower success rates? Can such women be targeted for immune therapy?

A randomized controlled trial to assess the effectiveness of immune therapy in women with high NK cell activity is urgently needed. A number of observational studies since Beer's 1996 paper have suggested benefit, although their interpretation is prone to possible bias. They have also all involved women with unexplained repeated reproductive failure (rather than first time IVF couples for example), and tended to include a mix of women with repeated IVF failure and miscarriage. Considerable care is essential to assess the methods of NK analysis, and treatment protocols are highly variable, often including multiple therapy with intravenous immunoglobulin (IVIG), aspirin, heparin, and dexamethasone. Given these constraints though, it has been shown that both uNK and bNK cell numbers and activity can be suppressed by IVIG and by prednisolone. It has also been shown that in women with repeated IVF failure with high NK cell activity, treatment produces significantly better pregnancy rates [5].

Immune therapy is currently crude and non-specific. Options include prednisolone, dexamethasone, IVIG, intralipid, and anti-TNF-alpha. Heparin and even progesterone provide milder immune suppressive effects and should be considered given their safety and cost. There is no NK specific drug and, given our current understanding of pregnancy immunology, no particular therapy is obviously preferable (immune therapies have never been compared in a single trial). Therapies should be regarded as experimental, with determining factors including cost, potential harm to mother and fetus, and availability.

Conclusion

Interest in NK cell analysis has so far primarily been for patients with otherwise *unexplained* reproductive failure. It has been used as a means of exploring possibilities that are, by definition, at the frontiers of knowledge. In the absence of a randomized controlled trial on the effectiveness of NK cell testing and treatment, we simply do not yet know who (if anyone) benefits.

We must be cautious in assuming that everyone with 'unexplained infertility' must have an 'overactive' immune system. In Sydney 15–25% of women with unexplained repeated reproductive failure have high NK cell levels (although a normal NK result does not exclude the possibility of an immune disorder). We must also remember that high NK cell levels may not be the cause of the problem – they may simply be associated with it. On the other hand, treatment with immune therapy (on an empirical basis) is not necessarily confined to women with high NK cells. So, what is the place of NK cell testing in women about to start IVF?

NK cell testing offers the *potential* to target immune therapy to women who are more likely to benefit from it, and so may improve success rates. And NK testing may be beneficial in other ways too. Many women appreciate the concept of looking for a cause of their infertility. It gives them confidence that their doctor is thinking and individualizing their problem rather than simply booking IVF cycles. By acknowledging the importance of the immune system it may reduce stress, and can give some patients the hope they need to keep trying.

Methodology is critical. Any test must be thoroughly validated and, in the absence of better quality evidence, NK testing for targeted immune therapy should be done in the context of a trial. Patients should be advised of the experimental nature of the approach and considerable caution should be undertaken to avoid the situation where marketing preceeds the evidence. In that way, it is incumbent on us to push this frontier of reproductive medicine, rather than simply turn our back on it. Our patients expect nothing less.

References

1. Lachapelle MH, Miron P, Hemmings R, Roy DC. Endometrial T, B, and NK cells in patients with recurrent spontaneous abortion. Altered profile and pregnancy outcome. *J Immunol* 1996;**156**:4027–34.
2. Tuckerman E, Mariee N, Prakash A, Li TC, Laird S. Uterine natural killer cells in peri-implantation endometrium from women with repeated implantation failure after IVF. *J Reprod Immunol* 2010;**87**:60–6.
3. King K, Smith S, Chapman M, Sacks G. Detailed analysis of peripheral blood natural killer cells in women with recurrent miscarriage. *Hum Reprod* 2010;**25**:52–8.
4. Clark DA, Coulam CB, Stricker RB. Is intravenous immunoglobulins (IVIG) efficacious in early pregnancy failure? A critical review and meta-analysis for patients who fail in vitro fertilization and embryo transfer (IVF). *J Assist Reprod Genet* 2006;**23**:1–13.
5. Heilmann L, Schorsch M, Hahn T. CD3-CD56+CD16+ natural killer cells and improvement of pregnancy outcome in IVF/ICSI failure after additional IVIG-treatment. *Am J Reprod Immunol* 2010; **63**:263–5.

Chapter 7

How to improve your IVF success rate: Weight control

Anne Clark

It is estimated that 30–50% of men and women in the reproductive age group are now overweight or obese, particularly in the developed world. As increased weight is associated with reduced fertility in both men and women, it is a major issue when it comes to maximizing successful outcomes in IVF treatment cycles [1]. In addition, increased weight is also associated with increased treatment costs as higher doses of gonadotropins are required, the follicular response is poorer and the miscarriage rate is 30–50% higher [1, 2]. However, the lack of success of hundreds of diets and the billions of dollars spent fruitlessly on weight reduction programmes is testament to the solution not being an easy one. Just instructing fertility patients to lose weight is unlikely to succeed and in fact the added pressure can lead to a further escalation in weight [2].

Adipose tissue is now recognized as the largest endocrine organ in the human body, with effects on glucose homeostasis, steroid production, the immune system, haematopoesis, and reproductive function [3]. Its ability to convert androgens to oestrogens, due to the presence of P450 aromatase, is just one example that impacts on reproduction. As adipose tissue increases insulin resistance also increases, resulting in hyperandrogenism and disordered ovulation in women and changes in sperm parameters in men. The discovery of adipokines, adipose tissue endocrine products, in recent years has seen increased research to understand the role of adipose tissue in reproduction.

However, increased weight per se is not as important as the distribution of the adipose tissue. Upper body fat and a waist-hip ratio <0.8, i.e., an 'apple' shape, is associated with greater metabolic and reproductive dysfunction than lower body fat, i.e., a 'pear' shape.

Scarcity of body fat also has a significant adverse impact on reproductive function but to a much lesser extent than a similar excess of body fat. It is also much less common and will not be discussed further. Weight control through lifestyle intervention and psychological support is the ideal treatment plan.

Most studies consider overweight or obesity in the female partner is associated with reduced success after an assisted reproduction procedure. Others report differences only when marked obesity (body mass index (BMI) >35 kg/m^2) is present. However, a flaw with most studies is they only focus on the woman and the woman's weight, and do not take into account the variable of her partner's BMI and the impact that could have on his sperm and the likelihood of success in an IVF cycle. Being overweight or obese tends to cluster in couples and not all sperm are created equal!

How to Improve Your ART Success Rates, ed. Gab Kovacs. Published by Cambridge University Press.

So what to do with the patient who has too much adipose tissue? It is now accepted wisdom that lifestyle intervention should be the initial treatment approach for the overweight or obese infertile patient prior to any other fertility treatment. Ideally, dietary changes should be combined with regular physical activity and attention to psychological interventions, particularly stress management and behavior modification [4]. Studies have shown that women only require modest reductions in weight (5 to 7 kg) to significantly reduce insulin sensitivity with associated improvement in pregnancy rates, both spontaneous and following fertility treatments, and a significant reduction in miscarriage rates [2]. However, though this is a time when couples are truly motivated to make lifestyle changes the amount of time and professional support required means lifestyle intervention is often underutilized or difficult to achieve as a therapeutic strategy.

Use of pharmacological agents

Combining lifestyle modification with the pharmacological anti-obesity treatments orlistat and sibutramine, however, has been shown to result in improved outcomes in terms of weight loss.

Orlistat

Orlistat is a gastric and pancreatic lipase inhibitor that reduces absorption of dietary fat [5]. It has been in clinical use for over ten years. A Cochrane review shows that the addition of orlistat causes 2.9% more weight loss compared with diet and lifestyle changes alone. Levels of fat-soluble vitamins A, D and E can be lowered by orlistat treatments. Low vitamin D levels, in particular, are associated with lower fertility in both men and women, higher miscarriage rates, and most importantly, if the woman remains low in vitamin D during pregnancy, an increased risk for the resulting child to develop multiple sclerosis or schizophrenia as an adult (see Table 7.1). Therefore it is critical that vitamin D levels are monitored and supplemented if necessary prior to pregnancy occurring.

Sibutramine

Sibutramine is a centrally acting serotonin and noradrenalin re-uptake inhibitor that promotes weight loss by enhancing satiety. A Cochrane meta-analysis shows patients on sibutramine lose an average 4.35% more weight compared to placebo. Though no adverse effects on the fetus have been observed after sibutramine use in the first trimester it is recommended that if pregnancy is not desired, an effective contraception should be used as normal ovulation can resume after even a minimal weight loss, particular in polycystic ovarian syndrome (PCOS) patients [2].

Bariatric surgery

The lack of success of traditional weight-reduction treatments involving hypocaloric diets and exercise has lead to an increasing use of bariatric surgery. Bariatric procedures were first developed in the mid-1950s and over the past six decades have undergone numerous modifications. The priority is to make them as safe as possible and less disruptive to normal human anatomy thus causing fewer postoperative nutritional deficiencies and complications while simultaneously achieving maximum weight loss [5]. Following the surgery, ovulation

Table 7.1 Impact of nutritional deficiencies and sperm DNA damage on fertility and pregnancy outcomes

	Women[1]			Men[2]
	Iodine deficiency	**Vitamin D deficiency**	**Raised homocysteine levels**	**Increased sperm DNA damage**
% New patients affected at FertilityFirst	57%	30%	19%	53%
Cause of infertility	Yes	Yes	Yes	Yes
Cause of long-term adverse health effects for children	Yes – Irreversible reduction in IQ of up to 10 points, linked to autism	Yes – Increased risk of multiple sclerosis, schizophrenia and diabetes	Yes – Increased risk of congenital malformations and asthma	Yes – Increased risk of congenital malformations, Down's Syndrome, childhood cancers, autism etc
Increased miscarriage rate	Yes	Yes	Yes	Yes
Pregnancy complications increased	Yes	Yes	Yes	Not studied to date
Pregnancy-induced hypertension	Yes	Yes	Yes	
Placental abruption	–	–	Yes	
Intra-uterine growth retardation	–	Yes	Yes	
Prematurity	–	Yes	Yes	
Low birth weight	Yes	Yes	Yes	
Still birth	Yes	–	Yes	Not studied to date

[1] $n = 4385$; [2] $n = 3672$.

can be restored postoperatively within a few months, often suddenly and unexpectedly as lifestyle modification programs have also found [2]. Monitoring for nutritional deficiencies is crucial but there are no agreed guidelines for the management of nutrition pre or during pregnancy in women after bariatric surgery. Most centers recommend monitoring of iron, vitamin B_{12}, folate, calcium, and soluble vitamin levels and adequate replacement according to the type of bariatric surgery undergone previously [5].

The timing of conception after any weight loss program remains a controversial issue. Women who are overweight or obese are more predisposed to pregnancy complications including pre-eclampsia, gestational diabetes, caesarean section, and a higher risk of a macrosomic baby. However, as knowledge of epigenetic intrauterine effects increase, care also needs to be taken that too much weight loss does not occur too close to conception. Otherwise the resultant child can be programmed for birth into a 'famine' environment, with increased risks of intrauterine growth restriction, preterm labour and a 'Barker Hypothesis' outcome in adult life.

Certainly, if rapid weight loss occurs, such as after bariatric surgery or a very low kilo joule diet, conception should be delayed for one to two years after the former and probably three to six months after the latter.

A major issue in many fertility management plans is that though the woman is only half the couple, she gets most of the attention and the male partner is asked to contribute little to the success of the treatment beyond a semen sample. And yet we have evidence that obesity and overweight also has a significant effect on male reproductive function, with oligozoospermia and aesthenozoospermia increasing with increasing BMI, worsening from overweight to obese men, as a result of reduced levels of testosterone and increased levels of oestradiol. More importantly, as a man's weight increases so does the likelihood of increased sperm DNA damage, with consequent adverse effects not just decreasing fertilization rates, but increasing the risk of miscarriage and the increased risk of adverse outcomes for childhood diseases and/or cancer in the resulting child (Table 7.1). It is known that approximately 50% of men with normal semen parameters attending a fertility clinic will have raised levels of sperm DNA damage and increasing to 70% of those with abnormal semen parameters. If this is not corrected the chances of pregnancy, including after IVF, are significantly reduced.

Therefore, any strategy of lifestyle modification needs to apply equally to both partners. If both partners are obese, their chances of having to wait more than a year for the woman to get pregnant is 2.7 times higher than those of a couple of ideal weight. For non-obese but overweight couples, the probability of having to wait more than one year for a pregnancy was 1.4 times higher. This has to impact on the success of any IVF treatment cycle.

Further, the dietary patterns that have lead to a person's increased weight can also be associated with nutritional deficiencies that impact on getting pregnant and staying pregnant, including after IVF treatment cycles. If these nutritional deficiencies continue into pregnancy they can also adversely impact on the child's long-term health and brain development. Table 7.1 shows impact on getting pregnant and a successful outcome and the percentage of patients attending my own clinic who were deficient in iodine and vitamin D and had raised homocysteine levels as a result of folate and/or B vitamin deficiencies. Correcting these prior to starting treatment improves the chances of a healthy ongoing pregnancy.

Recent research is showing that adiponectin, one of the main adipokines produced by adipose tissue, has a positive effect on insulin-resistance and higher levels are associated with better success rates in IVF cycles [5]. Lower levels are reported in women with endometriosis and women with PCOS, particularly obese PCOS women. Adiponectin levels in follicular fluid were found to be higher in women who received recombinant LH [6] perhaps contributing to the improved pregnancy rates reported after its addition in some IVF cycles.

To conclude, both thinness and obesity have a negative impact on reproduction. Therefore, weight control and/or reduction for many couples about to embark on IVF is a critical component to their chances of success, not just for getting pregnant but staying pregnant and having a healthy child. Weight control and/or reduction will improve their chances of success as well as benefiting their long-term health and longevity as parents. It is also important to treat weight control as a couple issue, not just a woman's issue. Just as being overweight or obese tends to cluster in couples so does the adverse impact on fertility. Attention also needs to be paid to addressing any nutritional deficiencies to maximize IVF success and timing treatment appropriately after any significant weight loss to avoid adverse epigenetic effects on the resulting child.

References

1. Bellver J, Ayllon Y, Ferrando M, *et al.* Female obesity impairs in vitro fertilization outcome without affecting embryo quality. *Fertil Steril* 2009;**93**:447–54.
2. Clark AM, Thornley B, Tomlinson L, Galletley C, Norman RJ. Weight loss in obese infertile women results in improvement in reproductive outcome for all forms of fertility treatment. *Hum Reprod* 1998;**13**:1502–5.
3. Bohler H, Mokshagundam S, Winters S. Adipose tissue and reproduction in women. *Fertil Steril* 2010;**94**:795–825.
4. Pasquali R, Gambineri A. Approaches to lifestyle management. In: *Current Management of Polycystic Ovary Syndrome.* London: Royal College of Obstetricians and Gynaecologists 2010; pp. 105–115.
5. Miras AD, le Roux W. Management of obesity in polycystic ovary syndrome, including anti-obesity drugs and bariatric surgery. In: *Current Management of Polycystic Ovary Syndrome.* London: Royal College of Obstetricians and Gynaecologists 2010; pp. 105–115.
6. Bersinger NA, Birkhauser MH, Wunder DM. Adiponectin as a marker of success in intracytoplasmic sperm injection/embryo transfer cycles. *Gynecol Endocrinol* 2006;**22**:479–83.
7. Gutman G, Barak V, Maslovitz S, *et al.* Recombinant luteinizing hormone induces increased production of ovarian follicular insulin sensitivity. *Fertil Steril* 2008;**91**:1837–41.

Chapter 8

Do vitamins and natural supplements improve pregnancy rates?

Lisa J. Moran and Robert J. Norman

Maternal and perinatal outcomes of assisted reproductive technology (ART) can be improved greatly by adoption of optimal nutritional and lifestyle practices for both males and females. Lifestyle practices potentially associated with adverse perinatal outcomes include being underweight or overweight, smoking, excessive alcohol or caffeine intake, excessive exercise, inadequate micronutrient intake, and increased psychological stress. Additional nutritional factors with potential effects on pregnancy or birth outcomes include folate (neural tube defects [NTD], reduced sperm count), iodine (infant cognitive development, pregnancy loss), zinc (pregnancy complications, pre-eclampsia, growth retardation, congenital abnormalities, impaired sperm maturation), vitamin D and/or calcium intake, magnesium, selenium, copper and calcium (pre-term delivery, pre-eclampsia or abnormalities in fetal development), and iron (intrauterine growth restriction and anaemia). There is also increasing interest in the effects of natural therapies on perinatal and obstetric outcomes. Of these, maternal vitamin, mineral or natural therapy supplementation prior to ART may potentially improve ART outcomes and pregnancy rates.

Issues to consider include which are the most important micronutrients to supplement with and the efficacy, safety, and cost-effectiveness of single micronutrient supplementation compared to supplementation with combined multivitamins and natural therapies. Nutritional interventions pre or during pregnancy should aim to optimize the health of both the mother and the baby. The clinical endpoints of interest include both pregnancy rates and adverse perinatal and obstetric pregnancy outcomes such as low birth weight, preterm birth, miscarriage, congenital abnormalities, and pre-eclampsia. Assisted reproductive techniques may be associated with a low birth weight and a higher risk of multiple gestation, and multiple gestation is associated with adverse obstetric and perinatal outcomes such as pregnancy complications, hypertension, and pre-eclampsia, low birth weight, and intrauterine growth retardation, pre-term birth or miscarriage, and deleterious long-term health. The literature on improving these outcomes in non-ART births is therefore relevant to assess.

Folic acid

Guidelines for micronutrient intake before conception and during pregnancy predominantly focus on folic acid. Folic acid (vitamin B9) is well researched with regards to prevention of NTD and other congenital abnormalities. Clinical recommendations for Australia advise a

How to Improve Your ART Success Rates, ed. Gab Kovacs. Published by Cambridge

dietary intake of 600 μg/day during pregnancy (estimated average requirement 520 μg/day, upper limit of intake 1000 μg/day) with additional daily supplementation of 0.5 mg for at least one month prior to conception and during the first three months of pregnancy for preventing NTD. Higher doses are recommended for women at high risk of NTD (personal or family history of NTD, women with diabetes or women taking antiepileptic medications or folic acid antagonists). Other conditions can confer additional risk for NTD including variants in genes responsible for homocysteine metabolism such as methylenetetrahydrofolate reductase. While additional supplementation is likely warranted in these women, this has not yet been studied. There is more limited research examining effects of folate supplementation on other perinatal and obstetric adverse outcomes in ART and non-ART pregnancies. An update of a Cochrane review concluded that high doses (5 mg/day) of folic acid during pregnancy (< 30 weeks gestation) was associated with a reduced risk of low birth weight (<2500 g) (RR 0.73, 95% CI 0.53–0.99) although no differences were observed for mean birth weight, placental weight, or gestational age [1]. Folic acid supplementation pre and during pregnancy (Level I Evidence) is therefore recommended for reducing NTD but there is limited evidence as to additional perinatal or obstetric benefits.

Iodine

Additional micronutrients having sufficient evidence to warrant supplementation pre or during pregnancy include iodine. Iodine deficiency is present in both developing countries and some developed countries. Iodine deficiency during pregnancy or breastfeeding leads to increased risk of miscarriage, premature labour, and fetal neurological damage with even mild to moderate maternal hypothyroidism increasing the risk of intellectual deficit. Supplementation data in mildly iodine-deficient populations relate to effects on childhood neurocognitive development. A recent trial in Andalusia, Southern Spain compared neuropsychological outcomes in 133 mothers supplemented with 300 μg/day potassium iodine/day for the first trimester of pregnancy compared to 61 receiving no iodine supplements [2]. The control group consisted of selected women who were not prescribed an iodine-enriched supplement in pregnancy, introducing methodological weakness. Children (aged 5.5–12.4 months) of supplemented mothers had more favourable outcomes on cognitive and psychomotor development as measured by the Psychomotor Development Index and Behavior Rating Scale. While there is a lack of good quality data assessing the effect of iodine supplementation on perinatal and obstetric outcomes in developed countries (Level III Evidence), the association of iodine status on fetal neuropsychological development and current deficiencies in the populations of both developed and developing countries warrant intervention. In March 2010 the National Health and Medical Research Council of Australia recommended iodine supplementation of 150 μg/day pre and during pregnancy and breastfeeding with women with pre-existing thyroid conditions to receive specialist medical advice. This is in addition to the recommendations for dietary intake of 220 μg/day (estimated average requirement 160 μg/day, upper limit 1100 μg/day). There is limited evidence specifically on the potential beneficial effects of this supplementation on any additional perinatal and obstetric outcomes.

Vitamin D

Other micronutrients of importance to ensure adequate nutrition include vitamin D because of its role in calcium absorption and the association between maternal and child vitamin D deficiency and poor fetal and infant skeletal growth and mineralization and rickets. A recent

US Government evidence review noted a limited number of randomized controlled trials assessing vitamin D supplementation in pregnancy. The identified trials reported on supplementation during the third trimester of pregnancy with one trial reporting no differences in birth weight or birth length for doses of 1000 IU/day and a second trial reporting increased birth weight (190 g) for vitamin D supplementation of 1.2 million IU in total over pregnancy (Level II Evidence). The authors noted limited and conflicting data and methodological issues and heterogeneity including differences in population vitamin D sufficiency, variations in the dosage, and lack of description of randomization or blinding [3]. Current Australian guidelines for vitamin D intake during pregnancy recommend an acceptable intake of 5 μg/day or 200 IU/day (upper limit of 80 μg/day or 3200 IU/day), ensuring adequate levels through appropriate sun exposure and screening women with dark skin or who get little sun exposure for vitamin D deficiency, and supplementing where necessary.

Other vitamins

Due to the potential beneficial effects of a range of micronutrients on perinatal and obstetric outcomes, there has been increasing controversy as to whether multivitamin supplementation should be recommended before and during pregnancy and whether this confers any additional benefits compared to use of folate in isolation. There remain concerns such as additional cost of multivitamins compared to use of clinically recommended micronutrients in isolation such as folate and iodine, interactive effects of multivitamins affecting absorption, and potential adverse effects from excessive intake of some multivitamins which may be particularly relevant in a nutrient replete population. A Cochrane review reported multivitamin supplementation resulted in a statistically significant decrease in the number of low birth weight babies (RR 0.93, 95% CI 0.76–0.91), small for gestational age babies (RR 0.92, 95% CI 0.86–0.99) and maternal anaemia (RR 0.61, 95% CI 0.52–0.71) in nine trials with 15 378 women [4] (Level I Evidence). No evidence of effect was reported for preterm birth (RR 0.92, 95% CI 0.82–1.04) or perinatal mortality (RR 1.05, 95% CI 0.90–1.23). When the multivitamin trials were compared to iron-folic supplementation in isolation, the effects on perinatal and maternal outcomes were no longer significant. This suggests the protective perinatal and obstetric outcomes were a result of the iron and folate supplementation with no further benefit conferred by additional multivitamins.

However, this subgroup analysis contained fewer studies (maximum of five). It was also not possible to determine the dose and optimal micronutrient supplementation composition (ranging from 3 to 15 micronutrients including vitamin A, beta carotene, vitamin D, vitamin E, vitamin C, vitamin K, vitamin B1, vitamin B2, niacin, riboflavin, vitamin B6, vitamin B12, folic acid, iron, zinc, copper, selenium, iodine, magnesium, phosphorus), the timing of supplementation commencement (ranging from early pregnancy to 36 weeks), and the optimal duration of supplementation (ranging from delivery to 12 weeks post-delivery) due to wide variability between the studies for these features. These trials were predominantly in low or middle income countries, raising the issue of comparability with high income countries where nutritional adequacy may be more likely. The authors concluded that this review provided insufficient evidence to support policy change to multivitamin supplementation. Some recent updates suggest that multivitamin supplement can confer an additional benefit to the folate supplements. While this offers promising support of the growing importance of micronutrient sufficiency on perinatal and obstetric outcomes, the applicability to ART-births in developed countries is currently limited.

Natural therapies

Additional interest has been raised in the potential beneficial effect of natural supplements on spontaneous and ART pregnancies. One small study examined the effect of a nutritional supplement containing chasteberry, green tea extract, L-arginine, vitamins including E, B6, B12, and folate, and minerals including zinc, magnesium, iron, and selenium on progesterone levels, basal body temperatures, menstrual cycle length, pregnancy rate, and side-effects in 93 women who had tried to unsuccessfully conceive for 6–36 months [5]. Supplement use was associated with a trend towards increased mid-luteal progesterone, higher pregnancy rate (26% versus 10% $p = 0.01$) and no serious adverse effects (Level II Evidence). However, there is currently no high quality evidence to support their use before or during pregnancy for optimizing perinatal or obstetric outcomes. The safety of any natural therapy component also needs to be rigorously assessed prior to recommendation of its use pre or during pregnancy.

Vitamins and minerals in men

There is emerging evidence on the positive effects of ensuring adequate micronutrient intake for males before pregnancy to optimize reproductive health. Nutritional factors with potential adverse effects on male infertility include deficiencies in folate (reduced sperm count), zinc (impaired sperm maturation), and vitamin C or E (increased sperm DNA oxidation). A Cochrane Review is currently underway examining the effects of antioxidants on sperm quality and the results will be awaited with great interest. With regards to other micronutrients, a double-blind randomized controlled trial investigated combined zinc sulphate (66 mg/day) and folic acid (5 mg/day) supplementation over 26 weeks in 47 fertile and 40 subfertile males. Sperm concentration was significantly increased in subfertile males while no other parameters were affected in either group and sperm concentration did not alter in fertile males [6] (Level II Evidence). This is an extension from previous research where a positive effect only of combined zinc and folate on sperm concentration was noted and no individual effect of zinc or folate in isolation. These studies reported variable improvements in sperm concentration (from 18–74%), and no concurrent changes in markers of zinc nutrient status or endocrine parameters, indicating further research is warranted on the mechanisms of effect. However, this research provides promising results on the positive effects of micronutrient supplementation on male subfertility which should be further investigated prior to clinical recommendations.

We conclude that there is evidence on the effects of folic acid and iodine supplementation preconception and during pregnancy on improving perinatal and child outcomes which can be applied to optimize healthy outcomes from ART pregnancies. There is limited evidence as to the effect of these micronutrients on improving pregnancy rates and obstetric outcomes. This is due to a lack of high quality data or lack of consensus on the number and combination of micronutrients or natural therapy components, dose, timing and duration of supplementation, safety and adverse effects of supplementation, and utility for populations of varying nutritional status. These issues warrant further attention. Areas for future research include optimal pre-conception micronutrient intakes for both men and women, whether optimal micronutrient intakes differ for ART and non-ART pregnancies, and whether efficacy of supplementation varies in nutrient replete versus deficient populations and developed versus developing countries.

References

1. Charles DH, Ness AR, Campbell D, *et al.* Folic acid supplements in pregnancy and birth outcome: re-analysis of a large randomised controlled trial and update of Cochrane review. *Paediatr Perinat Epidemiol* 2005;**19**:112–24.
2. Velasco I, Carreira M, Santiago P, *et al.* Effect of iodine prophylaxis during pregnancy on neurocognitive development of children during the first two years of life. *J Clin Endocrinol Metab* 2009;**94**:3234–41.
3. Chung M, Balk EM, Brendel M, *et al.* Vitamin D and calcium: a systematic review of health outcomes. *Evid Rep Technol Assess* (Full Rep) 2009:1–420.
4. Haider BA, Bhutta ZA. Multiple-micronutrient supplementation for women during pregnancy. *Cochrane Database Syst Rev* 2006:CD004905.
5. Westphal LM, Polan ML, Trant AS. Double-blind, placebo-controlled study of Fertilityblend: a nutritional supplement for improving fertility in women. *Clin Exp Obstet Gynecol* 2006;**33**:205–8.
6. Ebisch IM, Pierik FH, De Jong FH, Thomas CM, Steegers-Theunissen RP. Does folic acid and zinc sulphate intervention affect endocrine parameters and sperm characteristics in men? *Int J Androl* 2006;**29**:339–45.

Chapter 9

Polycystic ovary patients – is there a role for metformin?

Chris Brewer and Adam Balen

The polycystic ovary syndrome (PCOS) is a common endocrinopathy affecting women of reproductive age, the condition is estimated to have a prevalence of between 5 and 10%. The clinical presentation of PCOS is a heterogeneous collection of clinical, biochemical, and sonographic features including: menstrual cycle disturbance, hirsuitism, acne, alopecia, obesity, elevated luteinizing hormone (LH), hyperandrogenaemia, hyperinsulinaemia, insulin resistance, and morphologically polycystic ovaries. Several phenotypes of PCOS exist forming a spectrum of a disorder ranging from a mild to severe disturbance; however, a recent consensus meeting of experts (ASRM/ESHRE, Rotterdam 2003) clarified the diagnostic criteria, PCOS being diagnosed if at least two of the following three criteria are met, in the absence of other pathology [1–4]:

1. Oligo- and/or anovulation
2. Clinical or biochemical evidence of hyperandrogenism
3. Ultrasound evidence of polycystic ovaries (12 or more antral follicles 2–9 mm and/or ovarian volume greater than 10 cm^3)

The pathophysiology of PCOS is multifactorial and polygenic. The underlying pathophysiological determinants of the clinical features of PCOS are a disturbance in ovarian and systemic biochemistry/endocrinology. Hyperandrogenaemia and hyperinsulinaemia/insulin resistance are at the heart of the disorder. Insulin resistance is thought to arise from aberrant phosphorylation of tyrosine and serine residues on the insulin receptor and increased insulin resistance leads to a compensatory hyperinsulinaemia. The ovary is the source of excess androgen, arising from disordered control of steroidogenesis, arising from an exaggerated response to LH by theca cells and augmented by the effect of insulin binding to IGF-1 receptors. Hyperinsulinaemia also results in reduced production of sex-hormone binding globulin leading to a rise in circulating bio-available androgen. Elevated insulin levels lead to decreased hepatic production of insulin-like growth factor binding protein-1 (IGFBP-1), this in turn leads to a greater bioavailability of IGF-1 and -2, the IGF-1/2 are important regulators of ovarian follicular maturation and steroidogenesis [1–4]. Dysregulated and excessive ovarian androgen production leads to an uncoupling from normal folliculogenesis, with associated poor follicle maturation and increased follicular atresia.

Anovulatory subfertility is common among women with PCOS (up to 80%), indeed PCOS accounts for 80–90% of cases of WHO group II anovulatory subfertility. Ovulation induction is the first line treatment for subfertile women with PCOS. However, in vitro fertilization is an

How to Improve Your ART Success Rates, ed. Gab Kovacs. Published by Cambridge University Press.

effective treatment for women with PCOS who remain refractory to standard ovulation induction or who have co-existing pathology, such as tubal disease or male factors. Women with PCOS present a challenge when undergoing in vitro fertilization because they may respond sensitively to stimulation. It has been well documented that women with PCOS undergoing IVF treatment develop more follicles in response to stimulation and have significantly more oocytes recovered per cycle, albeit with a higher proportion of immature oocytes, when compared with women with normal ovaries. Similarly serum levels of estradiol are significantly higher among women with PCOS undergoing IVF treatment. As such, they are at particular risk of complications during IVF treatment, especially ovarian hyperstimulation syndrome (OHSS). Mild OHSS is common and is said to occur in up to 33% of in vitro fertilization cycles. The reported incidence of moderate to severe OHSS in patients with PCOS undergoing IVF treatment is in the region of 10–18%, this compares to 0.3–5% in non-PCOS patients undergoing IVF treatment [1–4].

As insulin resistance and hyperinsulinaemia contribute significantly to the pathophysiological process in PCOS, it would be rational to assume therefore that pharmacological agents that modulate insulin sensitivity should improve the symptoms of PCOS. Insulin sensitizing agents that have been used in PCOS include metformin, rosiglitazone, pioglitazone, and D-chiro-inositol. Metformin, an oral biguanide, is the most widely used and investigated agent and has better safety data. The use of metformin was first reported in 1994 and was observed to reduce body weight, improve menstrual cyclicity and fertility. Metformin appears to act through systemic alleviation of insulin excess and through direct ovarian effects. Metformin reduces hepatic gluconeogenesis leading to decreased insulin secretion; it increases peripheral glucose utilization and increases insulin sensitivity. Metformin has also been observed to have a direct effect upon theca and granulosa cells mediated through receptor kinase modulation. Metformin may reduce hyperandrogenaemia and may reverse the abnormalities of gonadotropin secretion seen in women with PCOS.

Once lauded as the panacea for PCOS, current evidence suggests a more restricted role for metformin. A recent systematic review of insulin sensitizing agents concluded that metformin as a first-line agent was less effective than clomiphene, owing to lower ovulation and pregnancy rates (OR = 0.63, 95% CI 0.43–0.92). Whilst adjunctive treatment (metformin and clomiphene) was associated with higher ovulation (pooled OR = 3.46, 95% CI 1.97–6.07) and clinical pregnancy rates (CPR) (pooled OR = 1.48, 95% CI 1.12–1.95) this did not translate to higher live birth rates (pooled OR = 1.05, 95% CI 0.75–1.47), and as such its use in ovulation induction is limited. Those patients who had previously demonstrated clomiphene resistance did however benefit from adjunctive metformin. Interestingly, sub-analysis by body mass index (BMI) revealed metformin (in comparison with clomiphene) to be more effective in the non-obese (CPR, OR 3.47, 95% CI 1.52–7.40) than in the obese (CPR, OR 0.34, 0.21–0.55), with the overall analysis favouring clomiphene [4]. Insulin resistance has been observed to be a positive predictor of response to metformin. Indeed, hyperinsulinaemic lean women with PCOS have been observed to display a higher ovulation rate with metformin.

Metformin has been widely used and investigated as an adjunct to controlled ovarian hyperstimulation in IVF. When assessing metformin's role as an adjunct to IVF treatment for women with PCOS, one must consider two important points:

(1) Does metformin enhance the efficacy of IVF treatment?
   - Live birth rate (LBR) is the most important measure of this.

(2) Does metformin enhance the safety profile of IVF treatment?
- Incidence of moderate-severe OHSS after treatment is the most important measure of this for patients with PCOS who are at particular risk of developing OHSS.

Five randomized controlled trials have evaluated the role of metformin as an adjunct to IVF (see Table 9.1)[5–9], in four trials metformin was used in the context of the long gonadotropin releasing hormone (GnRH) agonist down-regulation protocol with recombinant follicle stimulating hormone (FSH) [5–8]; in one trial metformin was used in a short GnRH antagonist protocol with recombinant FSH [9]. In these studies metformin was commenced before treatment but the duration of and dose of metformin therapy varied among the trials; clearly this variation makes comparisons and conclusions drawn through meta-analysis a little tentative. The metformin regimens ranged from 500 mg twice daily to 850 mg thrice daily, and was taken for up to 16 weeks prior to treatment and mostly was continued up to the day of the human chorionic gonadotropin (hCG) trigger. Only two trials reported a priori power/sample size calculations to justify the number of participants [5; 7] and it should be noted that these calculations were not based upon the clinically relevant parameters noted above, one trial on fertilization rate [5] and the other on serum estradiol concentration on the day of hCG trigger [7]. None of the trials assessed live birth rate (LBR) or OHSS incidence as the main outcome measures. In all of the trials the diagnosis and inclusion of women with PCOS was based on the current Rotterdam consensus criteria (ESHRE/ASRM 2003).

Live birth rate

The larger of the two trials [5] reporting live birth rates detected a significant improvement in LBRs among those women who had taken metformin, 32.7% in the metformin arm and only 12.2% in the placebo arm ($p = 0.027$). The LBR in the placebo was comparatively very low and perhaps lower than the baseline rate one might expect in patients with PCOS [5]. Kjotrod *et al.* did not detect any differences in LBR overall (metformin 31% versus placebo 32% ($p = 0.7$)); however, in the sub-group analysis (BMI<28) there was an improvement in LBR with metformin although this was not statistically significant, metformin 43% versus placebo 15% ($p = 0.12$)[7]. It is worth noting that the average BMI in Tang *et al.* [5] was 27.9 and 26.9 in the metformin and placebo groups respectively; as such these findings concur with the findings of Kjotrod *et al.* insomuch as that metformin may improve LBR among lean PCOS women undergoing IVF [7]. The pooled data of these two trials demonstrated that women taking placebo were less likely than those taking metformin to have a live birth, the 95% CI did however cross unity (OR 0.49, 95% CI 0.17–1.38, $p = 0.18$) [1].

Clinical pregnancy rate

Tang *et al.* observed a significant increase in CPR among those women who had taken metformin, metformin 38.5% versus placebo 16.3% ($p = 0.023$)[5]. The other trials reporting CPR did not demonstrate a significant increase with metformin [6–8], as with LBR Kjotrod *et al.* observed a non-significant increase among the lean PCOS taking metformin (57% versus 23%) [7]. Pooled data analysis found the CPR to be significantly higher among those who took metformin compared to placebo (placebo versus metformin OR 0.53, 0.32–0.89, $p = 0.017$) [1]. Onalan *et al.* included patients who had had assisted hatching, and when this data is included the trend to improved CPR with metformin remained but was no longer

Table 9.1 Five randomized controlled trials have evaluated the role of metformin as an adjunct to IVF

Trial	Participants	Intervention	Comparison	Study design	Protocol	Age	BMI (kg/m^2)	Fertilization rate (%)	Clinical pregnancy rate (%)	Live birth rate (%)	OHSS rate (%)
Tang *et al.* [5] *n* = 94 (101 cycles) Metformin = 52 Placebo = 49	PCOS[1]	850 mg metformin PO BD from start of GnRHa until oocyte retrieval	Placebo	Double blind randomized controlled trial	Long GnRHa & rFSH	Metformin = 31.3 Placebo = 31.1	Metformin = 27.9 Placebo = 26.9	Metformin = 52.9 Placebo = 54.9 *p* = 0.641	Metformin = 38.5 Placebo = 16.3 *p* = 0.023 CPR/cycle	Metformin = 32.7 Placebo = 12.2 *p* = 0.027 LBR/cycle	Metformin = 3.8 Placebo = 20.4 *p* = 0.023 (severe OHSS with hospitalization)
Kjotrod *et al.* [7] *n* = 73 Metformin = BMI<28 = 18 BMI>28 = 19 Placebo = BMI<28 = 15 BMI>28 = 21	PCO morphology +oligomenorrhoea +one of: testosterone >2.0 nmol/l SHBG<30 nmol/l LH:FSH ratio>2 Fasting insulin c-peptide>1 nmol/l Hirsuitism	500 mg PO BD metformin for at least 16 weeks prior to treatment ending on day of hCG trigger	Placebo	Double blind randomized controlled trial Stratification by BMI.	Long GnRHa & rFSH	Metformin = BMI<28 = 29 BMI>28 = 28.9 Placebo = BMI<28 = 30.7 BMI>28 = 29.9		All = Metformin = 53 Placebo = 55 *p* = 0.5 BMI<28 = Metformin = 50 Placebo = 54 *p* = 0.4 BMI>28 = Metformin = 54 Placebo = 55 *p* = 0.55	All = Metformin = 48 Placebo = 48 *p* = 0.8 BMI<28 = Metformin = 57 Placebo = 23 *p* = 0.12 BMI>28 = Metformin = 41 Placebo = 58 *p* = 0.5	All = Metformin = 31 Placebo = 32 *p* = 0.7 BMI<28 = Metformin = 43 Placebo = 15 *p* = 0.12 BMI>28 = Metformin = 35 Placebo = 47 *p* = 0.5	All = Metformin = 3.2 Placebo = 12.5 *p* = 0.3 BMI<28 = Metformin = 0 Placebo = 23 *p* = 0.13 BMI>28 = Metformin = 5.9 Placebo = 5.3 *p* = 0.9
Onalan *et al.* [6] *n* = 108 Metformin = 53 Placebo = 55	Oligomenorrheoa +at least one of: Hyperandrogenism Hirsuitism (FG score>7) Testosterone > 3.15 nmol/l	850 mg PO metformin for 8 weeks prior to treatment BMI<28 = BD BMI>28 = TDS	Placebo	Double blind randomized controlled trial	Long GnRHa & rFSH Assisted hatching if: □ Age>35y □ Thick zona □ Abnormal zona □ Fragmentation □ Slow embryonic development	Metformin = 29.3 Placebo = 29.8	Metformin = 25 Placebo = 23.5	Metformin = 73.6 Placebo = 71.7 *p* = 0.56	Metformin = 30.2 Placebo = 40 *p* = 0.6	Not reported	Not reported

Trial	Participants	Intervention	Comparison	Study design	Protocol	Age	BMI (kg/m^2)	Fertilization rate (%)	Clinical pregnancy rate (%)	Live birth rate (%)	OHSS rate (%)
Fedorcsak *et al.* [8] $n = 17$ (entered study) $n = 9$ (completed cross over)	PCOS[1] Insulin resistance	500 mg metformin PO TDS for 3 weeks prior to GnRHa until day of hCG trigger	Internal control as cross over	Open label cross over trial	Long GnRHa & rFSH	31	31.5	Metformin = 49.8 Placebo = 59.7	Metformin = 33.3 Placebo = 22.2	Not reported	Metformin = 0 Placebo = 0
Doldi *et al.* [9] $n = 40$ Metformin = 20 Placebo = 20	PCOS[1]	1.5 g Metformin/ day for 8 weeks prior to treatment until day of oocyte retrieval	No metformin	Open label randomized controlled trial	Short GnRH antagonist & rFSH	Not reported	Not reported	Not reported	Not reported	Not reported	Metformin = 5 Placebo = 15 $p<0.05$

[1]Diagnosis made according to Rotterdam ASRM/ESHRE consensus criteria (2003).
A recent meta-analysis has combined the results of these trials and has attempted to establish the efficacy of metformin as an adjunct to IVF in women with PCOS [1] (see Table 9.2).

Table 9.2 A recent meta-analysis to establish the efficacy of metformin as an adjunct to in vitro fertilization (IVF) in women with polycystic ovary syndrome (PCOS)

Summary of meta-analysis			
Live birth rate (per woman)	Placebo vs metformin	OR 0.49 (95% CI 0.17–1.38, $p = 0.18$)	Favours metformin
Clinical pregnancy rate (per woman)	Placebo vs metformin	OR 0.53 (95% CI 0.32–0.89, $p = 0.017$)	Favours metformin
Miscarriage rate (per woman)	Metformin vs placebo	OR 0.84 (95% CI 0.40–1.75, $p = 0.64$)	Favours metformin
OHSS rate	Metformin vs placebo	OR 0.24 (95% CI 0.12–0.47, $p = 0.000044$)	Favours metformin

Source: reference [1].
OR, odds ratio; CI, confidence interval; OHSS, ovarian hyperstimulation syndrome.

statistically significant as the 95% CI crossed unity (OR 0.71, 95% CI 0.39–1.28, P = 0.25)[1]. Metformin treatment was associated with a non-significant reduction in miscarriage rates (OR 0.84, 95% CI 0.4–1.75, $p = 0.64$)[1].

Ovarian hyperstimulation syndrome

Metformin treatment was associated with a reduction in the incidence of OHSS. Pooling of the data from trials reporting OHSS incidence demonstrated that metformin significantly reduces the incidence of OHSS following the long GnRH agonist down-regulation protocol (OR 0.27, 95% CI 0.16–0.47, $p = 0.000044$) [1]. The trial of adjunctive metformin use with the short GnRH antagonist protocol observed a reduction in the incidence of OHSS in the metformin arm, metformin 5% versus placebo 15% [9]. This was reported as being statistically significant; however, the validity of the statistical test used by the authors is questionable and the difference is not significant when an appropriate test of categorical data is applied.

The short GnRH antagonist protocol has been associated with a reduction in the incidence of OHSS when compared with the long GnRH agonist down-regulation protocol, as such the scope for reduction in OHSS may be less and could explain the difference observed in statistical significance. It is pertinent to note that Doldi *et al.* was a small trial of only 40 patients and was not appropriately powered to detect any differences in OHSS incidence [9]. This issue is currently being addressed by an adequately powered prospective randomized control trial being conducted by our group (ISRCTN 21199799).

Metformin has been observed to significantly reduce serum testosterone concentration (1.96 nmol/l versus 2.52 nmol/l $p = 0.269$) and reduce the free androgen index (2.43 versus 3.34) on the day of hCG administration. In this study it was observed that the free androgen index (FAI) correlated negatively with the day 12 post-embryo transfer serum β-hCG levels, additionally it was observed that FAI was significantly lower in conception cycles [5]. The exact mechanism of how metformin exerts its effect remains to be fully elucidated; however, through alleviation of hyperandrogenism and insulin resistance at the ovarian level one can speculate that folliculogenesis might be improved. Metformin may improve follicular growth and development and as such improve the developmental potential of the embryo. It is interesting to note that Tang *et al.* observed no difference in average embryo score of the transferred embryos despite observing an improvement in CPR and LBR [5], therefore one might speculate that metformin induces changes that confer a metabolomic advantage to the oocytes and embryos enhancing their developmental potential; however, this requires further investigation and clarification.

Tang *et al.* also observed that the serum vascular endothelial growth factor (VEGF) and serum estradiol concentrations on the day of hCG administration were significantly reduced among those who had taken metformin. Significantly elevated estradiol on the day of hCG trigger is associated with an increased risk of OHSS, likewise VEGF is implicated in the pathogenesis of OHSS and elevated serum VEGF is associated with an increased risk of developing OHSS [5]. Attenuation of such risk factors may be the mechanism through which metformin reduces the OHSS incidence. Insulin induces VEGF expression; therefore, metformin may reduce VEGF expression by ameliorating the hyperinsulinaemia/insulin resistance associated with PCOS.

In summary, the current evidence would support the use of metformin as an adjunct to IVF treatment, particularly in the context of the long agonist protocol. The role of metformin as an adjunct to the short antagonist protocol requires further clarification. Metformin is an inexpensive drug with a good safety profile in healthy patients, such as those undergoing IVF treatment. Metformin may be associated with unpleasant gastrointestinal side-effects in up to 10% of cases; however, none of the trials reported poor compliance with therapy. Whilst metformin may not necessarily improve the 'take home baby rate' after IVF, it has been observed to improve the safety of IVF treatment by reducing the incidence of moderate-severe OHSS in those patients who are at particular risk. As clinicians we are mandated to provide treatment that is both efficacious and safe, as such we advocate the use of metformin as an adjunct to IVF treatment for women with PCOS.

References

1. Tso LO, Costello MF, Albuquerque LE, Andriolo RB, Freitas V. Metformin treatment before and during IVF or ICSI in women with polycystic ovary syndrome. *Cochrane Database Syst Rev* 2009: CD006105.
2. Costello MF, Chapman M, Conway U. A systematic review and meta-analysis of randomized controlled trials on metformin co-administration during gonadotrophin ovulation induction or IVF in women with polycystic ovary syndrome. *Hum Reprod* 2006;**21**:1387–99.
3. Moll E, van der Veen F, van Wely M. The role of metformin in polycystic ovary syndrome: a systematic review. *Hum Reprod Update* 2007;**13**:527–37.
4. Tang T, Lord JM, Norman RJ, Yasmin E, Balen AH. Insulin-sensitising drugs (metformin, rosiglitazone, pioglitazone, D-chiro-inositol) for women with polycystic ovary syndrome, oligo amenorrhoea and subfertility. *Cochrane Database Syst Rev* 2009:CD003053.
5. Tang T, Glanville J, Orsi N, Barth JH, Balen AH. The use of metformin for women with PCOS undergoing IVF treatment. *Hum Reprod* 2006;**21**:1416–25.
6. Onalan G, Pabuccu R, Goktolga U, *et al.* Metformin treatment in patients with polycystic ovary syndrome undergoing in vitro fertilization: a prospective randomized trial. *Fertil Steril* 2005;**84**:798–801.
7. Kjotrod SB, von During V, Carlsen SM. Metformin treatment before IVF/ICSI in women with polycystic ovary syndrome; a prospective, randomized, double blind study. *Hum Reprod* 2004;**19**:1315–22.

8. Fedorcsak P, Dale PO, Storeng R, Abyholm T, Tanbo T. The effect of metformin on ovarian stimulation and in vitro fertilization in insulin-resistant women with polycystic ovary syndrome: an open-label randomized cross-over trial. *Gynecol Endocrinol* 2003;**17**:207–14.

9. Doldi N, Persico P, Di Sebastiano F, Marsiglio E, Ferrari A. Gonadotropin-releasing hormone antagonist and metformin for treatment of polycystic ovary syndrome patients undergoing in vitro fertilization-embryo transfer. *Gynecol Endocrinol* 2006;**22**:235–8.

Chapter 10

How to improve your IVF pregnancy rate: Treatments for endometriosis

G. David Adamson and Mary E. Abusief

Introduction

Studies have suggested 30–50% of patients with endometriosis have infertility. While the exact pathophysiological mechanisms causing infertility in women with endometriosis remain unknown, hypotheses include distortion of pelvic anatomy, abnormal peritoneal, hormonal and cellular function, ovulatory and endocrine abnormalities, and impaired implantation. Optimizing fertility in women with endometriosis can be challenging. This chapter will review options including observation, ovarian suppression, ovarian stimulation, surgery, and assisted reproductive technologies.

Symptoms and diagnosis

Symptoms of endometriosis are variable. While some women are completely asymptomatic, others have a variety of symptoms including severe dysmenorrhea, dyspareunia, chronic pelvic pain, ovulatory pain, cyclic bowel and bladder complaints, and infertility. Because there is considerable overlap with these symptoms and other etiologies for pelvic pain (such as irritable bowel syndrome and interstitial cystitis) and infertility, there is often a delay in diagnosis, especially for patients with early disease. Physical examination can be normal or patients may have findings suggestive of the disease including a non-mobile uterus, pelvic tenderness, uterosacral ligament nodularity or adnexal mass. Ultrasound may be helpful in identifying the presence of endometriomas but cannot identify endometriotic peritoneal implants. Laparoscopy remains the gold standard for diagnosis of endometriosis. Careful evaluation of pelvic and abdominal peritoneum and organs and visual findings of endometriosis implants is sufficient for diagnosis. Histological confirmation is ideal but a negative biopsy does not exclude presence of the disease.

Staging

Staging endometriosis is an important step in the care of women with the disease. Staging enables clinicians to approach the diagnosis with uniformity, specificity and allow for standardized comparisons. Various staging systems for endometriosis have been developed over the years, all of which have deficits. In 1979, the American Fertility Society (AFS) (now the

How to Improve Your ART Success Rates, ed. Gab Kovacs. Published by Cambridge University Press.

American Society for Reproductive Medicine, or ASRM) developed a staging system that was revised in 1985 and is currently the most widely utilized system [1]. Despite its usefulness as a classification tool, the AFS system has fallen short in its ability to predict post-treatment outcomes. The newest and most comprehensive system for staging endometriosis is the endometriosis fertility index (EFI) [2]. Unlike the AFS system, which is limited in its ability to predict future reproductive function, the EFI is a validated clinical tool that can be used to predict pregnancy rates (PR) after surgical staging in patients who attempt non-IVF conception (Figure 10.1).

Observation

Fecundity rates in women with endometriosis are generally accepted to be lower than in women without the disease. In untreated women with infertility and endometriosis, monthly fecundity rates range from 2% to 10%, much lower than the expected 15–20% fecundity rate in normal couples.

Ovarian suppression

Medical therapy including ovarian suppression can be utilized to decrease symptoms of pain associated with endometriosis. However, very good and consistent evidence shows no benefit of ovarian suppression with respect to fecundity. Options for medical therapy include gonadotropin-releasing hormone agonists (GnRH-a) and antagonists, combination estrogen-progestin, progestin only, and danazol therapy. In studies comparing PR among women undergoing treatment with ovarian suppression versus no treatment or placebo, no differences in PR were observed. However, time to pregnancy is longer when ovarian suppression is used. Therefore, women with endometriosis whose primary problem is infertility should not be treated with ovarian suppression [3].

Surgery

The role of surgery in the treatment of endometriosis has historically been controversial. The first randomized controlled trial (RCT) that addressed the question of whether laparoscopic ablation of endometrial implants and adhesiolysis in patients with early stage endometriosis showed that treatment improved fertility compared to diagnostic laparoscopy alone [4]. A subsequent systematic review and meta-analysis favored surgical therapy as a means to increase fecundity [5]. For women with more advanced stage endometriosis, there is a dearth of evidence from controlled studies on the question of whether surgery improves fertility [6]. Observational studies demonstrate lower spontaneous conception rates in women with more advanced stage endometriosis. Further RCTs are needed to fully answer these questions. Based on our clinical experience and available data, all endometriosis and endometriomas should be resected and normal pelvic anatomy restored to the extent possible. If endometriomas greater than 4 cm in diameter are present laparoscopic cystectomy is superior to drainage and coagulation in improving fertility [6]. Combination medical and surgical treatment consisting of either preoperative or postoperative medical therapy has not been found to increase fecundity and may delay fertility treatments [3].

Controlled ovarian stimulation and intrauterine insemination

In patients with early stage endometriosis, treatment with intrauterine insemination (IUI) combined with ovarian stimulation improves PR over the use of IUI alone. A large RCT demonstrated that gonadotropin (GN)/IUI treatment improves monthly fecundity rate

ENDOMETRIOSIS FERTILITY INDEX (EFI)
SURGERY FORM
LEAST FUNCTION (LF) SCORE AT CONCLUSION OF SURGERY

Score		Description
4	=	Normal
3	=	Mild Dysfunction
2	=	Moderate Dysfunction
1	=	Severe Dysfunction
0	=	Absent or Nonfunctional

	Left		Right		
Fallopian tube	☐	+	☐		
Fimbria	☐	+	☐		
Ovary	☐	+	☐		
Lowest Score	☐	+	☐	=	☐
	Left		Right		LF Score

To calculate the LF score, add together the lowest score for the left side and the lowest score for the right side.If an ovary is absent on one side, the LF score is obtained by doubling the lowest score on the side with the ovary.

ENDOMETRIOSIS FERTILITY INDEX (EFI)

Historical Factors			Surgical Factors		
Factor	Description	Points	Factor	Description	Points
Age			LF Score	☐	
	If age is 35≤ years	2		If LF Score = 7 to 8 (high score)	3
	If age is 36 to 39 years	1		If LF Score = 4 to 6 (imoderate score)	2
	If age is ≥40 years	0		If LF Score = 1 to 3 (low score)	0
Years infertile			AFS Endometriosis Score		
	If years infertile is ≤ 3	2		If AFS Endometriosis Lesion Score is < 16	1
	If years infertile is > 3	0		If AFS Endometriosis Lesion Score is ≥ 16	0
Prior Pregnancy			AFS Total Score		
	If there is a history of a prior pregnancy	1		If AFS total Score is < 71	1
	If there is no history of prior pregnancy	0		If AFS total Score is ≥ 71	0
Total Historical Factors			Total Surgical Factors		

EFL = TOTAL HISTORICAL FACTORS + TOTAL SURGICAL FACTORS: ☐ Historical + ☐ Surgical = ☐ EFI Score

ESTIMATED PERCENT PREGNANT BY EFI SCORE

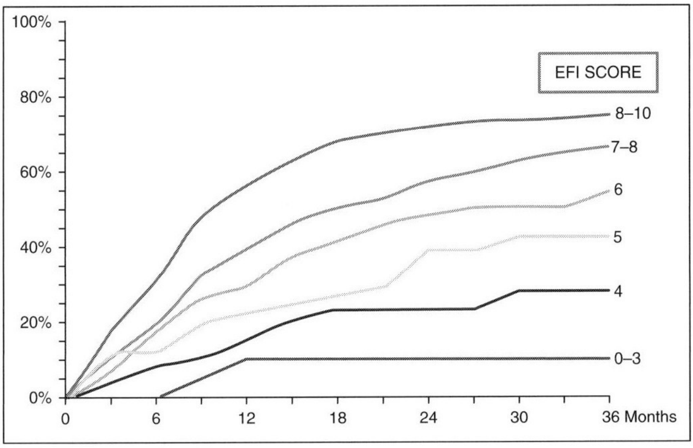

Figure 10.1 Endometriosis fertility index surgery form.

significantly over intracervical insemination alone, IUI alone, or GN/intracervical insemination. Another RCT in patients after surgical treatment of endometriosis demonstrated a significant increase in cycle fecundity after treatment with four cycles of clomiphene citrate/IUI versus timed intercourse. Multiple other studies have demonstrated the superiority of treatment with GN with or without IUI in patients with early stage endometriosis versus observation, IUI alone, or clomiphene citrate therapy/IUI [7].

In vitro fertilization

For women with endometriosis who have blocked or dysfunctional fallopian tubes, significant male factor, or no success with other therapies, IVF is indicated. Although it is generally accepted that IVF improves PR in patients with endometriosis versus expectant management, definitive data confirming this is available only from one small RCT [8]. Some studies have revealed that patients with minimal/mild endometriosis have a decrease in number of eggs retrieved and lower implantation and pregnancy rates as compared to those patients undergoing IVF for a diagnosis of tubal factor or unexplained infertility [9]. Severe endometriosis was associated with a greater impact than mild. Other studies have suggested reduced oocyte quality in women with moderate and severe disease [10]. It has also been reported that there might be a lower response to ovarian stimulation, possibly because of endometriotic cysts or prior ovarian surgery. Genetic, molecular and metabolic studies have implicated deregulation of select implantation genes as a factor affecting outcomes. However, no currently available data convincingly demonstrate that pre-IVF surgery or other treatment will change the influence, if any, of these potential markers on IVF with respect to fertilization, implantation, pregnancies, or live births.

Other reports have suggested no difference in pregnancy rates in patients with tubal disease and with different stages of endometriosis [11]. Large-scale international data registries also show no difference in pregnancy rates in patients with endometriosis, but these data may be limited by the lack of an endometriosis-specific patient registry. Some clinicians believe that extensive disease with an AFS score of greater or equal to 71 might be associated with reduced pregnancy rates, but no studies have had adequate statisfical power evaluate the impact of extensive disease. It is also not clear if there is a differential impact of peritoneal, ovarian, and adenomyotic disease. It is possible that IVF results might be lower in studies of patients who had laparoscopic retrieval because of adhesions and anatomic distortion, while pregnancy rates might not be lower with vaginal retrieval in which access to follicles is easier.

In patients with endometriosis, treatment with GnRHa for 3–6 months prior to IVF cycle start appears to increase ongoing PRs [12, 13]. Although IVF cycle stimulation with both GnRHa and GnRH antagonists appear to result in similar implantation and clinical PR, use of GnRHa may result in an increased number of MII oocytes and embryos. Treatment with IVF does not appear to increase risk for endometriosis recurrence in patients with later stage disease. Data from observational studies demonstrate that women undergoing IVF with early versus late stage endometriosis have better live birth rates. Currently, for women with stage III/IV endometriosis who fail to conceive following conservative surgery or because of advancing reproductive age, IVF is an effective alternative. However, some studies have shown a lower cumulative pregnancy rate over 4 cycles. IVF is the appropriate treatment for patients with compromised tubal function, male factor infertility or who have had a lack of success with previous treatments [14].

Surgical removal of endometriomas prior to IVF is controversial and very difficult to evaluate because of many confounding variables: unilateral versus bilateral disease, size and number of current endometriomas, recurrence of endometriomas, history of prior surgery and whether observed effects are due to previous presence of endometrioma and/or its surgical treatment. While one systematic review found no benefit of endometriosis removal in asymptomatic women undergoing IVF, another meta-analysis concluded that the presence of an endometrioma is associated with a decrease in number of retrieved oocytes but not embryo quality or outcome of pregnancy [15, 16]. Some studies have shown that laparoscopic endometriomectomy before IVF improves pregnancy rates while others have shown no benefit [14, 17, 18].

Excision of the cyst wall has generally been shown to be superior to drainage and coagulation. In one study of women with unilateral endometriomas not previously operated on there was a decreased response to GN therapy [16]. Decreased ovarian reserve and response culminating in decreased number of oocytes retrieved has generally been reported in patients with previous ovarian surgery but these outcomes have not been associated with lower pregnancy rates in any well-controlled studies. Nevertheless, most clinicians believe the potential benefit from endometrioma removal has to be weighed against the risk for removal of normal ovarian tissue and a subsequent further decrease in ovarian response.

Laparoscopic excision of recurrent endometriomas showed that the re-operation group had increased use of IVF and a higher frequency of irregular menses and high FSH. Pregnancy rates were 41% in the control group (one endometriomectomy operation) versus 32% in the re-operated group, but this difference was not statistically different [19]. Removal of endometriomas has been controversial. While one expert has proposed that all endometriomas greater than 3 cm in size be removed prior to IVF (especially in patients with history of poor ovarian response to stimulation), other experts advise removal of endometriomas only greater than 4 cm in size. The latter group also emphasized the need to counsel patients about the risk of post-operative decline in ovarian function and that candidates for ovarian re-operation should be carefully selected. One expert's recommendation for endometrioma surgery is that large endometriomas (> 3 cm) should be treated before IVF, especially if ovarian response is poor [17]. Others have subsequently recommended laparoscopic treatment for endometriomas > 4 cm, but emphasized the need to explain the risk of poor ovarian response post-operatively and that a decision to operate needs to be very carefully considered if the patient has had previous ovarian surgery [14, 18].

Conclusion

In summary, in patients with clinically suspected mild endometriosis who have acceptable sperm quality, ovarian stimulation with clomiphene citrate and IUI for three to four cycles can be utilized for first line treatment. Patients who are suspected to have moderate to severe endometriosis, or who fail first line therapy should undergo laparoscopy. Surgery well performed is effective treatment for all stages of endometriosis and endometriomas for infertility and also for pain, if present. The EFI can be used to determine the prognosis for patients after surgery. Good prognosis patients, under 35 years, can attempt on their own or with ovarian stimulation combined with IUI for up to 15–18 months, the duration determined by their clinical situation and response to treatment. Poorer prognosis patients, based on the EFI, can proceed sooner to IVF. If pregnancy does not occur, repeat surgery has limited benefit for infertility but may have some benefit for pain control. Pre-IVF ovarian suppression for severe or extensive endometriosis is reasonable. Pre-IVF surgery for large (3–4 cm) endometriomas may be beneficial in selected patients.

References

1. Revised American Fertility Society classification of endometriosis: 1985. *Fertil Steril* 1985;**43**:351–2.
2. Adamson GD, Pasta DJ. Endometriosis fertility index: the new, validated endometriosis staging system. *Fertil Steril* 2009;**94**:1609–15.
3. Adamson GD, Pasta DJ. Surgical treatment of endometriosis-associated infertility: meta-analysis compared with survival analysis. *Am J Obstet Gynecol* 1994;**171**:1488–504; discussion 504–5.
4. Marcoux S, Maheux R, Berube S. Laparoscopic surgery in infertile women with minimal or mild endometriosis. Canadian Collaborative Group on Endometriosis. *N Engl J Med* 1997;**337**:217–22.
5. Jacobson TZ, Barlow DH, Koninckx PR, Olive D, Farquhar C. Laparoscopic surgery for subfertility associated with endometriosis. *Cochrane Database Syst Rev* 2002:CD001398.
6. Chapron C, Vercellini P, Barakat H, *et al.* Management of ovarian endometriomas. *Hum Reprod Update* 2002;**8**:591–7.
7. Deaton JL, Gibson M, Blackmer KM, *et al.* A randomized, controlled trial of clomiphene citrate and intrauterine insemination in couples with unexplained infertility or surgically corrected endometriosis. *Fertil Steril* 1990;**44**:1083–8.
8. Soliman S, Daya S, Collins J, Jarrell J. A randomized trial of in vitro fertilization versus conventional treatment for infertility. *Fertil Steril* 1993;**59**:1239–44.
9. Barnhart K, Dunsmoor-Su R, Coutifaris C. Effect of endometriosis on in vitro fertilization. *Fertil Steril* 2002;**77**:1148–55.
10. Garrido N, Navarro J, Garcia-Velasco J, *et al.* The endometrium versus embryonic quality in endometriosis-related infertility. *Hum Reprod Update* 2002;**8**: 95–103.
11. Olivennes F, Feldberg D, Liu HC, *et al.* Endometriosis: a stage by stage analysis – the role of in vitro fertilization. *Fertil Steril* 1995;**64**:392–8.
12. Surrey ES, Silverberg KM, Surrey MW, Schoolcraft WB. Effect of prolonged gonadotropin-releasing hormone agonist therapy on the outcome of in vitro fertilization-embryo transfer in patients with endometriosis. *Fertil Steril* 2002;**78**:699–704.
13. Sallam HN, Garcia-Velasco JA, Dias S, Arici A. Long-term pituitary down-regulation before in vitro fertilization (IVF) for women with endometriosis. *Cochrane Database Syst Rev* 2006: CD004635.
14. Kennedy S, Bergqvist A, Chapron C, *et al.* ESHRE guideline for the diagnosis and treatment of endometriosis. *Hum Reprod* 2005;**20**:2698–704.
15. Gupta S, Agarwal A, Agarwal R, Loret de Mola JR. Impact of ovarian endometrioma on assisted reproduction outcomes. *Reprod Biomed Online* 2006;**13**:349–60.
16. Somigliana E, Vercellini P, Vigano P, Ragni G, Crosignani PG. Should endometriomas be treated before IVF-ICSI cycles? *Hum Reprod Update* 2006;**12**:57–64.
17. Canis M, Pouly JL, Tamburro S, *et al.* Ovarian response during IVF-embryo transfer cycles after laparoscopic ovarian cystectomy for endometriotic cysts of >3 cm in diameter. *Hum Reprod* 2001;**16**: 2583–6.
18. Hart R, Hickey M, Maouris P, Buckett W, Garry R. Excisional surgery versus ablative surgery for ovarian endometriomata: a Cochrane Review. *Hum Reprod* 2005;**20**:3000–7.
19. Esinler I, Bozdag G, Aybar F, Bayar U, Yarali H. Outcome of in vitro fertilization/intracytoplasmic sperm injection after laparoscopic cystectomy for endometriomas. *Fertil Steril* 2006;**85**:1730–5.

Chapter 11

Management of hydrosalpinges

S. F. van Voorst and N. P. Johnson

The paradox of hydrosalpinges and IVF

In vitro fertilization was primarily developed to treat tubal infertility, a logical rationale to circumvent abnormally functioning tubes. However, comparison of IVF success rates of patients receiving IVF for tubal subfertility with results of patients receiving IVF for other reasons, showed that women with hydrosalpinges had lower implantation rates and a two-fold risk of early pregnancy loss. As tubal disease is present in 10–30% of IVF patients, and hydrosalpinges may reduce IVF success rates up to 50% this is important in clinical practice. Approriate management of hydrosalpinges is an important key in improving IVF success rates.

How hydrosalpinges affect IVF success rates

Several theories explain how hydrosalpinges might have a negative effect on IVF outcome. The hydrosalpinx fluid itself seems to have a key role, exerting a possible effect at three different levels; on the oocytes, the transferred embryo, and on the implantation process. Oocytes and transferred embryos may be exposed to toxic factors, or to the lack of factors important in embryonic development, in the hydrosalpinx fluid. The fluid hinders implantation mechanically by disturbing endometrial interaction with the transferred embryo. Hydrosalpinx fluid might also simply exert a wash out effect on the newly implanted embryo: directly by leakage of fluid through the uterine cavity and indirectly by altering endometrial peristalsis.

These suggested pathophysiologic mechanisms resulted in a concept for treatment: interventions aim to minimize exposure of recruited oocytes and transferred embryos to the hazardous hydrosalpinx fluid to optimize IVF results.

Treatment options prior to IVF to improve IVF success rates

Ideally the primary goal in the management of tubal factor infertility should be to achieve pregnancy in the most efficient manner – a one-step approach would be preferable above a two-step approach.

Thus reconstructive surgery merits consideration. Reconstructive surgery may cure infertility allowing maybe even subsequent spontaneous conception. The problem with reconstructive surgery is that it only seems efficient in a select group of patients, but evidence to identify this group is sparse. Factors likely to be prognostic are the extent of tubal pathology: the presence of functional mucosa seems the most positive prognostic sign.

How to Improve Your ART Success Rates, ed. Gab Kovacs. Published by Cambridge University Press.

However, histopathological evaluation of the hydrosalpinx tubes reveals that the occurrence of healthy mucosa is rare. In addition, the presence of coexisting disease and the skill of the surgeon are important. As reconstructive surgery is performed on fewer and fewer patients, it is important that the surgeon has maintained skill and case numbers to be able to assure results. Furthermore it is important that the patient has time to await the beneficial effect, therefore younger patients seem more eligible to undergo tubal reconstructive surgery. The place of reconstructive surgery is debated as IVF success rates, possibly combined with complementary surgery in case of hydrosalpinges, continue to improve. As it is not known which patient group profits most from tubal reconstructive surgery and as there is no evidence showing that this one step approach is more efficient than IVF with or without a surgical intervention to ameliorate IVF success rates, the case for reconstructive surgery is ever dwindling.

The two-step approach may consist of medical or surgical treatment prior to the IVF cycle. Of course a two-step approach means a 'double intervention' for the patient and a time delay to IVF. The two-step approach is supported by a growing body of evidence, the burden and risks of interventions are minimized by the the advancing approaches for gynaecological surgery.

Medical treatment prior to IVF

As acute or chronic infection may be an underlying pathophysiologic mechanism of the hydrosalpinges that can explain the lower IVF success rates in women with hydrosalpinges, antibiotic treatment around the period of the oocyte retrieval has been proposed as an intervention that could improve IVF success rates. Somewhat soft evidence in support of this comprises two retrospective studies in which women with hydrosalpinges were treated with doxycycline and whose results of IVF were similar to women with no hydrosalpinges undergoing IVF. The advantage of course is the conservative nature of the treatment. However more evidence is needed, in the form of randomized controlled trials (RCTs), to establish the potential positive effect.

Salpingectomy

Removal of the tubes, preferably laparoscopically rather than by laparotomy, permanently removes any leakage of hydrosalpinx fluid into the uterine cavity. Besides the beneficial effect on IVF outcomes, advantages are optimization of oocyte retrieval conditions: ovaries are easier to access and as chronically infected tissue prone to abscess formation or torsion is removed, the risk of infection is likely to be lower during and after the IVF cycle. Additionally removal of the diseased tube reduces the risk of chronic pelvic pain in the future. The disadvantages of salpingectomy are the permanent character with a psychological burden (any possibility of conceiving spontaneously is removed with bilateral salpingectomy) and it has been proposed that ovarian function may be impaired due to reduction of ovarian blood flow after salpingectomy, although there is no evidence that this leads to lower pregnancy rates. Nonetheless the mesosalpinx should be transected as close as possible to the fallopian tube and diathermy used as sparingly as possible for haemostasis at laparoscopic salpingectomy. The procedure is feasible in the majority of patients but may be difficult where major adhesions are present. Adverse effects of salpingectomy that have been reported in case reports are the increased risk of interstitial pregnancies, ovarian pregnancy, cornual fistulae, or cornual rupture.

Tubal occlusion

Proximal tubal occlusion is a less invasive yet permanent way to prevent leakage of hydrosalpinx fluid into the uterine cavity. Proximal occlusion is likely to reduce the chance of ectopic pregnancy to a similar degree as salpingectomy. Different methods and approaches for tubal occlusion are available – clipping (such as with Filschie clips or microinserts by a laparoscopic approach), electrocautery, and, depending on the occlusion technique, a hysteroscopic approach may be possible, such as the application of the newer techniques for sterilization (Essure, Adiana, Ovabloc) to achieve occlusion of hydrosalpinges. Whilst promising in rationale, these hysteroscopic occlusion techniques have yet to be fully evaluated in randomized control trials that examine clinically important outcomes in IVF. A possible drawback of these techniques is that the effect of these foreign bodies in the pregnant uterus are unknown – they may mimic the effect of an IUD, preterm labour being a possible concern. The advantage of occlusion firstly is the less invasive character and a shorter hospital stay. Secondly the procedures may have a shorter operative learning curve and the techniques are easier to perform for women with extensive adhesions than salpingectomy. The disadvantage is that the potentially inflammatory tubes remain, along with the risk of abcess formation, torsion and long term chronic pelvic pain.

Salpingostomy

Salpingostomy by a laparoscopic or laparotomy approach, aims to create a new ostium of the fallopian tube with well-everted fimbrial mucosa, in the case of distal tubal occlusion. A disadvantage is that reocclusion may occur. The major advantage of salpingostomy is that the chance of spontaneous subsequent pregnancies is potentiated (although this outcome is dependent on the status of the tubal mucosa). However threadbare evidence comprises case series and one prospective cohort study, there being no RCTs available. Pregnancy rates of 20–43% are reported. There are no trials comparing salpingostomy alone to IVF.

Aspiration

Hydrosalpinx fluid can be aspirated under transvaginal ultrasound guidance at any stage in the IVF process, including the stage of oocyte retrieval. Particularly in the situation where the finding of a hydrosalpinx is unsuspected, this treatment seems an option where the opportunity for other surgical treatments has passed. Evidence consists of mainly retrospective trials and case series, which are conflicting. The results of the one RCT seem promising (see below). Drawbacks are that the hydrosalpinges may reoccur within an unknown timespan (often within a few days) and that there is a potential risk of infection at the crucial time of oocyte retrieval. The latter might be preventable by administration of antibiotics. Furthermore it has been sugested that aspiration might further damage the fallopian tube and increase yet further the risk of ectopic pregnancy.

Efficacy of different surgical treatments in the management of hydrosalpinges

The patient burden, surgical risks, and drawbacks of each specific treatment necessitate the best available evidence for a two-step approach in the management of tubal factor infertility. A Cochrane systematic review of RCTs was updated in 2009 to assess and compare the value of surgical treatments for tubal disease prior to IVF [1].

All RCTs comparing a surgical treatment for tubal disease prior to IVF with a control group (either a treatment or no treatment) were considered eligible for inclusion. The studied outcomes were live birth, ongoing pregnancy, viable-, clinical- and biochemical pregnancy, ectopic pregnancy rate, miscarriage rate, multiple pregnancy rate, surgical complication rate and ovarian response to IVF. Trials were sought according to methodology of the Cochrane Menstrual Disorders and Subfertility Group. Two reviewers independently performed study selection, data extraction, and assessed trial quality. Statistical analyses were performed in accordance with Cochrane Handbook guidelines. Peto odds ratios were calculated where pooling was justified and where heterogeneity was absent.

Five RCTs analyzing a total of 676 women were included. Of the included trials, two assessed the effectiveness of laparoscopic salpingectomy compared to no salpingectomy for women with hydrosalpinges prior to IVF [2, 3], two trials compared effectivness of laparoscopic tubal occlusion with laparoscopic salpingectomy and no intervention [4, 5], and one trial assessed ultrasound guided aspiration of hydrosalpinges during the IVF cycle [6].

Details of the study characteristics are more fully described in the publication of the Cochrane review [1]. Study size varied between 60 and 204 patients. Patients had uni- or bilateral hydrosalpinges diagnosed at laparoscopy or hysterosalpingography in four trials, in the aspiration trial hydrosalpinges were also diagnosed during the IVF cycle itself by ultrasound. Results included in the analysis were the results of the first IVF cycle patients had ever undergone. Important patient demographics were similar in the intervention and control groups. The surgical intervention was performed 2–3 months prior to the IVF cycle, except for in the aspiration trial (aspiration was performed at time of oocyte retrieval). The intervention was performed uni- or bilaterally depending on whether the hydrosalpinges were uni- or bilateral. In the aspiration trial antibiotics were administered when the ultrasound guided drainage was performed. Study quality was generally good.

Results are presented in Figure 11.1. None of the included trials reported on the primary outcome: live birth. The odds of ongoing pregnancy (Peto OR 2.14, 95% CI 1.23–3.73) and of clinical pregnancy (Peto OR 2.31, 95% CI 1.48–3.62), however, were increased with laparoscopic salpingectomy for hydrosalpinges prior to IVF. Laparoscopic occlusion of the fallopian tube versus no intervention did not increase the odds of ongoing pregnancy significantly, although the confidence intervals were wide owing to the small numbers where ongoing pregnancy was assessed (Peto OR 7.24, 95% CI 0.87–59.57) but clinical pregnancy (Peto OR 4.66, 95% CI 2.47–10.01) had sufficient power to show a significant increase.

Comparison of tubal occlusion to salpingectomy did not show a significant advantage of either surgical procedure in terms of ongoing pregnancy (Peto OR 1.65, 95% CI 0.74–3.71) or clinical pregnancy (Peto OR 1.28, 95% CI 0.76–2.14). Efficacy of ultrasound guided aspiration was reported in a single RCT, which did not show a significant increase in the odds of clinical pregnancy and confidence intervals were wide (Peto OR 1.97, 95% CI 0.62–6.29).

Throughout the different comparisons no significant differences were found in the odds of ectopic pregnancy, miscarriage, and surgical complications as data were underpowered. The mean number of oocytes retrieved in patient groups treated with salpingectomy were similar to the numbers of oocytes retrieved in control groups.

In conclusion, this systematic review of RCTs further supports laparoscopic salpingectomy and presents laparoscopic tubal occlusion as an alternative as the odds of clinical pregnancy are improved and comparison of results with laparoscopic salpingectomy fail to show a difference in effectiveness. Further evidence is needed to assess the value of ultrasound

Study or subgroup	Treatment Events	Treatment Total	Control Events	Control Total	Weight	Odds ratio M-H, fixed, 95% CI
1.1.1 Salpinjectomy versus no surgical treatment - outcome: ongoing pregnancy rate						
Kontoravdis 2006	17	50	2	15	11.3%	3.35 [0.68, 16.58]
Dechaud 1998	13	30	6	30	19.0%	3.06 [0.97, 9.66]
Strandell 1999	31	116	15	88	69.7%	1.77 [0.89, 3.54]
Subtotal (95% CI)		**196**		**133**	**100.0%**	**2.20 [1.26, 3.82]**
Total events	61		23			
Heterogeneity: $Chi^2 = 0.95$, df = 2 ($P = 0.62$); $I^2 = 0\%$						
Test for overall effect: $Z = 2.79$ ($P = 0.005$)						
1.1.2 Tubal occlusion versus no surgical treatment - outcome: ongoing pregnancy rate						
Kontoravdis 2006	17	50	1	15	100.0%	7.21 [0.87, 59.57]
Subtotal (95% CI)		**50**		**15**	**100.0%**	**7.21 [0.87, 59.57]**
Total events	17		1			
Heterogeneity: Not applicable						
Test for overall effect: $Z = 1.83$ ($P = 0.07$)						
1.1.3 Tubal occlusion versus no surgical treatment - outcome: clinical pregnancy rate						
Kontoravdis 2006	20	50	2	15	26.1%	4.33 [0.88, 21.30]
Moshin 2006	31	78	8	66	73.9%	4.78 [2.01, 11.38]
Subtotal (95% CI)		**128**		**84**	**100.0%**	**4.66 [2.17, 10.01]**
Total events	51		10			
Heterogeneity: $Chi^2 = 0.01$, df = 1 ($P = 0.92$); $I^2 = 0\%$						
Test for overall effect: $Z = 3.95$ ($P = 0.0001$)						
1.1.4 Aspiration versus no surgical treatment - outcome: clinical pregnancy rate						
Hammadieh 2008	10	32	6	32	100.0%	1.97 [0.62, 6.29]
Subtotal (95% CI)		**32**		**32**	**100.0%**	**1.97 [0.62, 6.29]**
Total events	10		6			
Heterogeneity: Not applicable						
Test for overall effect: $Z = 1.14$ ($P = 0.25$)						
1.1.5 Tubal occlusion versus salpingectomy - outcome: ongoing pregnancy rate						
Kontoravdis 2006	23	50	17	50	100.0%	1.65 [0.74, 3.71]
Subtotal (95% CI)		**50**		**50**	**100.0%**	**1.65 [0.74, 3.71]**
Total events	23		17			
Heterogeneity: Not applicable						
Test for overall effect: $Z = 1.22$ ($P = 0.22$)						
1.1.6 Tubal occlusion versus salpingectomy - outcome: clinical pregnancy rate						
Kontoravdis 2006	26	50	20	50	38.0%	1.65 [0.74, 3.59]
Moshin 2006	31	78	23	60	62.0%	1.06 [0.53, 2.12]
Subtotal (95% CI)		**128**		**110**	**100.0%**	**1.28 [0.76, 2.14]**
Total events	57		43			
Heterogeneity: $Chi^2 = 0.63$, df = 1 ($P = 0.43$); $I^2 = 0\%$						
Test for overall effect: $Z = 0.92$ ($P = 0.36$)						

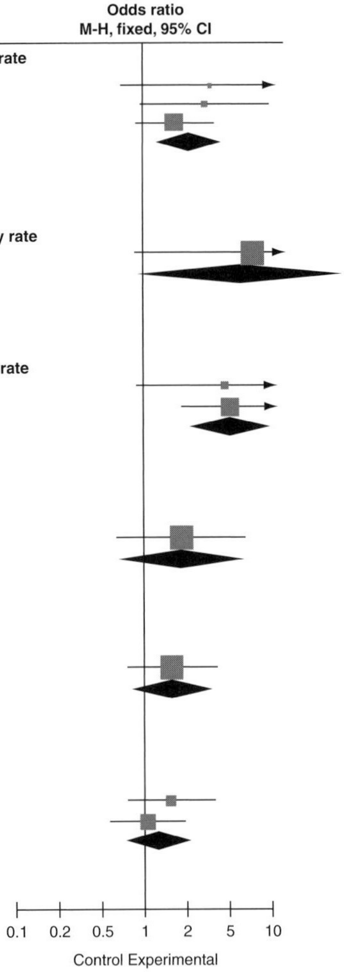

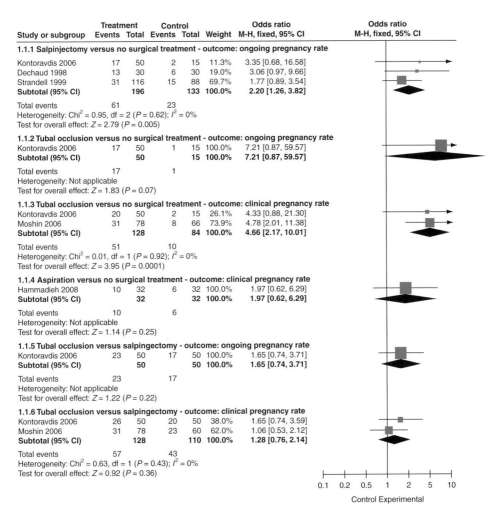

Figure 11.1 Forest plots exhibiting the efficacy of surgical interventions prior to IVF. Sections 1.1.1.–1.1.4 compare surgical interventions to no interventions. Sections 1.1.5 and 1.1.6 compare tubal occlusion (control) to salpingectomy (experimental).

This summary of surgical treatment for tubal disease in women due to undergo IVF by Johnson N, van Voorst S, Sowter MC, Strandell A, Mol BWJ, Cochrane Database of Systematic Reviews 2010, Issue 1. Art. No.: CD002125. DOI: 10.1002/14651858.CD002125.pub3 is reproduced with permission. Copyright Cochrane Collaboration.

guided aspiration of hydrosalpinges. Larger trials with more power are necessary to draw conclusions on adverse effects.

Discussion

Although the body of evidence is growing for all treatments for hydrosalpinges, many questions remain. Whilst the evidence base guides practice in most cases, a treatment plan should be formulated on an individual patient basis.

Firstly, a one-step approach might be preferable for younger women with hydrosalpinges suitable for tubal reconstructive surgery, although a substantial risk of ectopic pregnancy remains. More research is however necessary to formulate criteria to do so and comparative data are necessary to compare efficacy with IVF approaches.

Other patients with hydrosalpinges should be offered a surgical intervention prior to IVF. Laparoscopic salpingectomy or laparoscopic occlusion performed unilaterally in case of a unilateral hydrosalpinx, and bilaterally in case of a bilateral hydrosalpinx, are the first choice treatments. The choice for salpingectomy or occlusion may be made based on patients factors (extent of tubal pathology, comorbidity, psychological burden) or clinician factors (primarily surgical skill). Further research should evaluate the effect of different occlusion techniques. More evidence, in the form of RCTs, is necessary to assess the beneficial effect of antibiotic treatment and ultrasound guided aspiration of the hydrosalpinges.

Further research should focus on which extent of tubal pathology benefits the most from which surgical treatment, which time scheme should be applied regarding the time to the IVF treatment, and in case of a unilateral hydrosalpinx should patients await spontaneous conception after surgery, or should they undergo IVF?

Summary and conclusion

1. The presence of hydrosalpinges adversely affect the success rate of IVF.
2. Salpingectomy and tubal occlusion performed prior to the IVF treatment improve subsequent pregnancy rates and are recommended as first line treatments to improve IVF success rates.
3. There are many questions to be addressed before comprehensive treatment algorithms can be established for women with hydrosalpinges, particularly the place of antibiotic treatment, aspiration of hydrosalpinx fluid prior to or during IVF, restorative surgery as opposed to IVF approaches, even restorative surgery followed, if required, by definitive surgery and IVF. Until these questions are addressed the choice for which treatment should be made based on patient and clinician factors.

References

1. Johnson N, van Voorst S, Sowter MC, *et al.* Surgical treatment for tubal disease in women due to undergo in vitro fertilisation. *Cochrane Database Syst Rev* 2010: CD002125.
2. Dechaud H, Daures JP, Amal F, *et al.* Does previous salpingectomy improve implantation and pregnancy rates in patients with severe tubal factor infertility who are undergoing in vitro fertilization? A pilot prospective randomized study. *Fertil Steril* 1998;**69**:1020–5.
3. Strandell A, Lindhard A, Waldenstrom U, *et al.* Hydrosalpinx and IVF outcome: a prospective randomized multicentre trial in Scandinavia on salpingectomy prior to IVF. *Hum Reprod* 1999;**14**:2762–9.
4. Kontoravdis A, Makrakis E, Pantos K, *et al.* Proximal tubal occlusion and salpingectomy result in similar inprovements in in vitro fertilisation outcome in patients with hydrosalpinx. *Fertil Steril* 2006;**86**:1642–8.
5. Moshin V, Hotineanu A. Reproductive outcome of the proximal tubal occlusion prior to IVF in patients with hydrosalpinx. *Hum Reprod* 2006;**21** (suppl. 1):i193–i194.
6. Hammadieh N, Coomerasamy A, Bolarinde O, *et al.* Ultrasound-guided hydrosalpinx apsiration during oocyte collection improves outcome in IVF – a randomized controlled trial. *Hum Reprod* 2008;**23**:1113–7.

Chapter 12

Intrauterine insemination – who should be treated and what are the expectations?

Willem Ombelet

Introduction

Intrauterine insemination (IUI) aims to bypass the cervical-mucus barrier and to increase the number of motile spermatozoa with a high proportion of normal forms at the site of fertilization, as close as possible to the oocytes. Washing procedures are needed to remove prostaglandins, infectious agents, non-motile spermatozoa, leucocytes, immature germ cells, and antigenic proteins. This may enhance sperm quality by decreasing the release of lymphokines and/or cytokines and also a reduction in the formation of free oxygen radicals. The final result is an improved fertilizing capacity of the sperm sample in vitro and in vivo.

Despite the extensive literature on the subject of artificial homologous insemination, controversy remains about the effectiveness of this very popular treatment procedure [1, 2]. In this chapter an attempt is made to find out who should be treated and what we can expect from intrauterine inseminations.

Compared to IVF, IUI is a simple and non-invasive technique which can be performed without expensive infrastructure with a good success rate within three or four cycles. It is a safe and easy treatment procedure with minimal risks and monitoring. All these factors are also responsible for a high couple compliancy for IUI compared to IVF.

IUI for whom: effectiveness of IUI

Despite the fact that IUI is one of the most frequently used treatments in reproductive medicine, a structured review [1] showed that the number of studies assessing its effectiveness is limited and that most of these studies have small sample sizes. This results in imprecise effect estimates, as demonstrated by the non-significant effects and large confidence intervals observed when reviewing the literature. Also, many studies do not adhere to present quality standards for design, conduct, and report of clinical trials. Therefore it was concluded that there is an urgent need for more RCTs in which IUI is compared to expectant management or IVF. This conclusion was also made by the ESHRE Capri Workshop Group in 2009 [2]. More reviews on the effectiveness of IUI have been published in the Cochrane library for the indications cervical factor subfertility, unexplained subfertility, and male subfertility [3, 4, 5]. In all Cochrane reviews the major concern about IUI is the uncontrolled increase in multiple pregnancy rates when ovarian stimulation is used.

How to Improve Your ART Success Rates, ed. Gab Kovacs. Published by Cambridge University Press.

Cervical factor subfertility

In case of cervical hostility, it seems logical to perform IUI. Bypassing the hostile cervix should increase the probability of conception. In a Cochrane review it was concluded that there is no evidence from the published studies that intrauterine insemination is an effective treatment for cervical hostility [3]. It seems that cervical factor subfertility is a very uncommon reason of subfertility and IUI should not be seen as a useful therapy in these cases. According to Cohlen, natural cycle IUI should be preferred for cervical hostility [1].

Unexplained infertility

In case of unexplained infertility the treatment is often empiric. A meta-analysis comparing IUI and timed intercourse (TI) in natural cycles showed no difference in results, therefore IUI in natural cycles seems ineffective in case of unexplained infertility. When controlled ovarian hyperstimulation (COH) is used, IUI increases the live birth rate compared to IUI alone [4]. The likelihood of pregnancy was also increased for treatment with IUI compared to TI both in stimulated cycles. It was shown in different studies that three cycles of COH-IUI in couples with unexplained infertility was just as effective as one IVF cycle in achieving pregnancy, but IUI was less invasive and less expensive than IVF.

Male factor subfertility

In a Cochrane review, Cohlen *et al.* [5] concluded that IUI is superior to TI, both in natural cycles and in cycles with COH (natural cycles-IUI versus TI: OR 2.43, COH-IUI versus TI: OR 2.14). According to this review, IUI in natural cycles should be the treatment of choice in case of moderate to severe male subfertility providing an inseminating motile count (IMC) of more than 1 million can be obtained after sperm preparation and in the absence of a triple sperm defect. In another Cochrane review, it was shown that there was insufficient evidence of effectiveness to recommend or advise against IUI with or without COH above TI, or vice versa [6]. Large, high quality randomized controlled trials, comparing IUI with or without COH with pregnancy rate per couple as the main outcome of interest are lacking.

Risks and complications of IUI

If controlled ovarian stimulation is used, the major complication remains the high incidence of multiple pregnancies, Multiples are responsible for considerable mortality, morbidity, and costs. US data from 2004 show that ovulation induction outside of IVF was estimated to be responsible for 28 912 twins and 1654 higher order multiples, of which 371 were quadruplet and even higher orders. These represent 22% of all twin and 40% of all triplet and 71% of all quadruplet and higher order babies born that year. In Europe, the number of cycles performed is still increasing. In 2001, 15 countries performed 52 939 IUI cycles, in 2004 19 countries performed almost twice as many cycles. Pregnancy rates per insemination have remained well above 12%, but so have the multiple pregnancy rates. Twin rates and triplet rates were 10% and 1% respectively in 2005.

Careful monitoring remains essential and cancellation of the insemination procedure, escape IVF, and follicular aspiration before IUI are reasonable options. Transvaginal ultrasound-guided aspiration of supernumerary ovarian follicles increases both the efficacy and the safety of

COH-IUI with gonadotropins. This method represents an alternative for conversion of over-stimulated cycles to IVF (escape IVF). On the other hand, the use of natural cycle IUI, clomiphene citrate, or minimal dose regimen with gonadotropins are valuable options to prevent the unacceptable high multiple gestation rate described after ovarian hyperstimulation. Multifetal pregnancy reduction should be considered as a last resort.

These options also decrease the risk for ovarian hyperstimulation syndrome (OHSS) to almost zero.

Cost of ART-related services

Intrauterine insemination seems to be a cost-effective approach compared to IVF if: (1) at least one tube is patent, (2) if more than 1 million motile spermatozoa can be found after sperm washing, and (3) if the multiple pregnancy rate can be reduced to a reasonable percentage, this means as low or lower than the multiple pregnancy rate in IVF programmes. Studies performed in the Netherlands, the UK and the USA clearly showed that stimulated IUI for unexplained and moderate male factor infertility is a cost-effective approach when compared to IVF.

Intrauterine insemination as a first line treatment: what can be expected

In the selection of couples to be treated with IUI or IVF/intracytoplasmic sperm injection (ICSI), it would be interesting to establish cut-off values of semen parameters above which IUI is a real alternative for IVF/ICSI in male subfertility. According to the literature, IMC and sperm morphology are the most valuable sperm parameters to predict IUI outcome. A trend towards increasing conception rates with increasing IMC was reported, but the cut-off value above which IUI seems to be successful however varies between 0.3 and 20 million. According to a number of meta-analyses 5% normal forms (according to strict Tygerberg criteria) and 1 million motile spermatozoa after sperm preparation (IMC) are believed to be potential cut-off values to predict the success rate after IUI treatment, although prospective randomized studies are lacking. In our experience a cut-off value of 1 million (IMC) is a valuable tool to select patients for IUI, even with morphology scores below 5%.

Using this cut-off value the cumulative ongoing pregnancy rate after three IUI cycles using clomiphene citrate or low dose gonadotropins or recombinant follicle stimulating hormone (recFSH) seems to be comparable with one IVF-cycle (25–30%). But clinical practice can be very contradictory to common scientific knowledge. Most IVF centers worldwide still do not perform IUI as a first-line procedure, even if tubes are patent and more than 1 million motile spermatozoa can be found after sperm washing. Excellent counseling based on evidence and taking into account cost-effectiveness both for the couple and the society is mandatory and crucial.

Age and IUI success

According to a review by De Brucker and Tournaye [1] above the age of 37, success rates decline, but despite this fact, women up to 40 years, may be encouraged to continue IUI treatment, in case of donor insemination even up to 42 years of age. Overall, superovulation with IUI yields better results than unstimulated IUI, but not in women over 37 years who may rather benefit from natural cycle IUI. When the female partner is older than 35 years, a synergistic adverse effect of paternal age has been reported.

Other factors influencing IUI success

Theoretically, improved chances for conception may be expected when two consecutive inseminations are performed in the same IUI cycle since ovulation of oocytes does not occur in a synchronized pattern but rather in waves of release after human chorionic gonadotropin (hCG) administration. Based on the results of two trials, double IUI showed no significant benefit over single IUI although it seems that a large randomized controlled trial of single IUI versus double IUI is mandatory. A trilaminar image rather than the exact endometrial thickness and/or doppler measurement of the spiral and uterine arteries provide a favourable prediction of pregnancy in IUI although treatment should not be cancelled because of inadequate endometrial thickness. According to a Cochrane review there is insufficient evidence to recommend any specific sperm washing technique. Results from studies comparing semen parameters may suggest a preference for gradient technique, but firm conclusions cannot be drawn due to a lack of large high quality randomized controlled trials. Whether the addition of substances in the sperm preparation such as pentoxyphylline, antioxidants, etc. may improve the results remains unclear and certainly unproven. A significantly higher pregnancy rate has been reported in a subpopulation of couples without male factor subfertility when platelet-activating factor was added during semen processing for IUI.

The catheter type does not affect the outcome after IUI and it also seems that looking for the optimal time of abstinence is not very important in IUI programs.

Conclusion

I believe that the future of IUI will depend on our ability to maintain the multiple pregnancy rates at an acceptable level and this will undoubtedly be the most important challenge in the near future. In most cases of cervical hostility, unexplained and moderate male infertility, expectant management and timed intercourse in natural cycles are the first choice option. When unsuccessful, IUI can be promoted as the best first-line treatment in most cases of subfertility provided at least one tube is patent and an IMC of more than 1 million can be obtained after sperm preparation. In this selected group of patients it is unwise to start with assisted reproductive techniques such as IVF and ICSI since these techniques are more invasive and less cost-effective.

References

1. Artificial Insemination: an update (Eds Ombelet W & Tournaye H). *Facts, Views & Vision in ObGyn* 2010;**2**:1–67. www.fvvo.eu

2. ESHRE Capri Workshop Group. Intrauterine insemination. *Hum Reprod Update* 2009;**15**: 265–77.

3. Helmerhorst FM, van Vliet HA, Gornas T, *et al.* Intrauterine insemination versus timed intercourse for cervical hostility in subfertile couples. *Cochrane Database Syst Rev* 2005: CD002809.

4. Verhulst SM, Cohlen BJ, Hughes E, *et al.* Intra-uterine insemination for unexplained subfertility. *Cochrane Database Syst Rev* 2006:CD001838.

5. Cohlen BJ, Vandekerckhove P, te Velde ER, *et al.* Timed intercourse versus intra-uterine insemination with or without ovarian hyperstimulation for subfertility in men. *Cochrane Database Syst Rev* 2000;**2**: CD000360.

6. Bensdorp AJ, Cohlen BJ, Heineman MJ, *et al.* Intra-uterine insemination for male subfertility. *Cochrane Database Syst Rev* 2007:CD000360.

Chapter 13

What superovulation protocol is best?

Anthony J. Rutherford

Introduction

Although Louise Brown, the world's first baby conceived through in vitro fertilization came from an oocyte from a natural menstrual cycle, stimulation to induce multi-follicular development has become an integral part of IVF treatment. The concept of having a choice of embryos available for transfer and selecting the best to replace is established practice in most programs throughout the world. Initial superovulation protocols relied on the use of urinary gonadotropins either alone or in combination with oral anti-oestrogens such as clomifene or tamoxifen. In these protocols the pituitary gland remained functional, which necessitated frequent serum monitoring to detect a potential spontaneous luteinizing hormone (LH) surge. If an LH surge was detected the oocyte collections required rescheduling, or if the surge was too premature or inadequate, the treatment cycle was cancelled. Porter and Craft were the first to report the use of a gonadotropin-releasing hormone agonist (GnRH) in an IVF cycle, which abolished this risk. GnRH agonists were introduced into clinical practice in the late 1980s with dramatic effect, substantially increasing the clinical pregnancy rate and reducing the number of cancelled cycles. A decade later, GnRH antagonists were introduced into clinical practice, producing a much simpler, shorter, patient-friendly approach. A combination of GnRH antagonist and agonist protocols are in use in IVF centers today. This chapter will briefly outline the physiology of superovulation, and deal with how these stimulation protocols have evolved over the past 25 years, to allow the clinician to make evidence-based judgements on which protocol to use in individual patient groups.

Physiological considerations

Primary follicles grow over a period of 80–90 days into small antral follicles around 2–4 mm, which are present throughout the menstrual cycle and are sensitive to follicle stimulating hormone (FSH). In a normal cycle the dominant follicle is recruited from a group of 10–20 antral follicles that respond to the rise in FSH that begins at the interface between two consecutive menstrual cycles. Initially, several follicles may overcome their FSH threshold for stimulation and start to grow in this FSH window, which lasts a median of around six days. As FSH levels start to fall due to the negative inhibition of the pituitary gland from rising oestradiol and inhibin B, the most sensitive follicle continues to develop while others enter a pathway towards atresia. In most women the dominant follicle is evident from cycle day 7 at around 10 mm in diameter, having developed more FSH receptors than its peers, and in

How to Improve Your ART Success Rates, ed. Gab Kovacs. Published by Cambridge University Press.

addition LH receptors, enabling it to continue to grow despite falling FSH levels. During this early development background levels of LH stimulate androgen substrate in theca cells to promote granulosa cell-mediated oestradiol production.

All IVF stimulation protocols attempt to widen the FSH window allowing more of the cohort of antral follicles to overcome their FSH threshold, a process known as recruitment, then continue to support their development through to maturity.

GnRH agonists bind avidly to the LH releasing hormone (LHRH) surface receptors on the pituitary gonadotroph cells, before the drug–receptor complex is internalized, causing the release of all stored gonadotropins. Unlike native LHRH, the pituitary receptors remain avidly bound to the GnRH agonist within the cell, and over a period of around 11 days the pituitary cells lose a significant proportion of their cell surface receptors – a process known as desensitization, or down regulation. GnRH agonists can be administered by nasal spray, daily subcutaneous injection or by a monthly depot preparation. In contrast, GnRH antagonists, simply bind to the pituitary gonadotroph cell surface receptors, blocking their function. This allows the pituitary to recover more quickly when the antagonist is discontinued.

Stimulation protocols

Which gonadotrophins to use?

Exogenous FSH can be sourced from urinary and recombinant preparations (see Table 13.1). Both sources provide highly purified gonadotropins. Urinary gonadotropins are generally although not exclusively, combined with limited LH activity, provided by human chorionic gonadotropin (hCG). Recombinant LH and hCG are also available. There has been tremendous debate as to whether the choice of gonadotropin preparation makes a difference in clinical practice [1]. Although earlier studies indicated that the use of a preparation containing LH activity provided significantly more 'top quality' embryos and a higher ongoing pregnancy rate, the most recent meta analysis, published in 2010, involving over 4040 patients in 16 studies, reached the conclusion that there is no significant difference in clinical pregnancy rates, whichever preparation is used [2]. However, most studies indicate that more oocytes are obtained with recombinant preparations [3]. Other practical considerations are that the varying degrees of pituitary suppression seen with GnRH agonist preparations may influence the low levels of endogenous LH required to provide androgen substrate. When using depot agonists, which cause the most profound suppression, it may be prudent to use preparations containing LH activity. Furthermore, some studies have indicated the addition of LH in the late follicular phase may be helpful in women with low ovarian reserve (see Chapter 18).

Recently, investigators have tested the concept that as follicles achieve dominance they develop LH receptors and can continue to grow in response to exogenous LH activity. A pilot study was conducted in women using an antagonist protocol substituting recombinant FSH by 200 IU hCG when a minimum of six follicles > 12 mm, and oestradiol levels were greater than 600 ng/l. This resulted in significantly shorter duration and lower total dose of FSH use without compromising success rates with on-going pregnancy rates of 37% in the treatment group. Further, more detailed studies need to be performed to confirm these encouraging findings.

Advances in recombinant biology have allowed development of a new fusion FSH molecule, containing an alpha subunit and a beta subunit modified with the carboxy terminal peptide of an hCG beta subunit attached. This creates a long-acting FSH which has a two-fold increased elimination half-life. This new molecule known as Corifollitropin alfa (Schering-Plough) has a

Table 13.1 Currently available gonadotropins used in IVF practice

Recombinant gonadotropins	Trade names	Type
Follitropin alfa	Gonal F	FSH
Follitropin beta	Puregon	FSH
Lutropin alfa	Luveris	LH
Follitropin alfa & Lutropin alfa	Pergoveris	FSH & LH
Chorionic gonadotropin alfa	Ovitrelle	hCG
Corifollitropin alfa	?	FSH CTP
Urinary gonadotropins		
Menotropin	Merional Menopur	FSH 'LH' activity FSH 'LH' activity
Urofollitropin	Fostimon Bravelle	FSH FSH
Chorionic gonadotropin	Choragon Pregnyl	hCG hCG

similar pharmacodynamics profile as recombinant FSH (rFSH) and can initiate and sustain follicular growth for one week. Mathematical modelling indicates the dose of long-acting FSH is dependent on a woman's weight with a dose of 100 μg required for women under 60 kg, and 150 μg over this weight. The Engage trial (n = 1506) compared the use of Corifollitropin alfa to conventional recombinant FSH (Follitropin beta) in a fixed start antagonist protocol. Additional rFSH was added on day 8 until the criteria for hCG was reached. The duration of stimulation was similar in both groups, as was the number of oocytes retrieved and the ongoing pregnancy rate. One concern is the potential for ovarian hyperstimulation (OHSS) although in these carefully selected trial participants the overall rate of OHSS was similar in both groups.

Although most of the comparative studies looking at the differing gonadotropin preparations have employed GnRH agonist protocols, more recently GnRH antagonist studies have shown similar outcomes. Therefore it is reasonable to conclude that in most clinical scenarios clinician and patient choice should determine which preparation is employed.

How much gonadotropin to use?

Superovulation requires a dose of FSH sufficient to overcome the threshold value to allow multi-follicular development, which will vary between individuals. Inadequate response will reduce the chance of a successful outcome, whereas too much gonadotropin will risk the development of OHSS, the most significant side-effect of IVF treatment. The starting dose of FSH will vary between clinics and generally is within the range of 100–250 IU/day, with the dose increasing in older women. Dosing normograms have been constructed, which take into account factors known to influence successful stimulation, such as smoking, the antral follicle counts (AFC), a reduced ovarian volume, increasing age, and low ovarian Doppler studies. By individualizing the dose of FSH a more coordinated response was achieved with clinically significant higher pregnancy rates and fewer patients with OHSS. Body mass index is another important parameter to consider when deciding on the dose of FSH required as a woman with a higher BMI needs more FSH to achieve a similar degree of stimulation. More accurate markers of ovarian function are now available including anti-mullerian hormone (AMH) in conjunction with AFC to select the most appropriate dose. A recent meta-analysis indicated that the best starting dose in women younger than 39 with normal ovulatory function was 150 IU/L per day. This achieved the best compromise in terms of oocyte yield, clinical pregnancy and embryo cryopreservation rates while reducing rates of OHSS [2]. Although it is common practice to increase the FSH dose with increasing age this does not compensate for the age related decline in egg yield. In women with evidence of diminished ovarian reserve, there appears to be little benefit to be gained from increasing the FSH dose above 300 IU.

Based on ovulation induction protocols in women with polycystic ovary syndrome (PCOS), a step-down protocol for IVF stimulation has been proposed, starting with a higher FSH dose to recruit the initial cohort of follicles, then reducing the dose of FSH after five days, closing the FSH window, so stopping the recruitment of further small follicles as the cycle progresses, to reduce the risk of OHSS in vulnerable patients. Although theoretically sound, there is no hard evidence to support such an FSH regimen.

When to start stimulation?

The principle of superovulation is to keep the FSH window open to allow recruitment of a cohort of follicles. In GnRH agonist cycles, stimulation is started after pituitary suppression is evident, which can be determined biochemically from a low serum oestradiol, or on ultrasound by a thin endometrium and no evidence of ovarian activity. In women with a functional pituitary gland, as seen initially in all antagonist cycles, FSH is usually started from cycle day 2. However, it can be started as late as day 7 and still achieve multiple follicular development, although by day 7 the resulting follicle cohort is smaller. This important finding paved the way for a minimal approach to stimulation reducing the risk of OHSS, and of creating large numbers of superfluous oocytes and embryos.

Which is better – conventional or mild stimulation?

There is growing evidence that milder stimulation regimens are preferable to the conventional approach to stimulation on all accounts. Mild stimulation protocols do result in fewer oocytes with optimum implantation rates associated with five oocytes compared to ten oocytes with conventional stimulation. Two recent studies have demonstrated that although conventional higher dose regimens produce more oocytes, and may create more embryos, when these are analysed for common aneuploidies, similar numbers of euploid embryos are created using both approaches. The high concentration of steroids generated during routine stimulation does have a negative impact on uterine endometrial receptivity when compared to natural cycles. If mild stimulation is combined with single embryo transfer, this has shown to be more cost effective per live birth than conventional stimulation and replacing two embryos over a set time period. Finally milder stimulation is more patient friendly, requires fewer drugs, and is associated with a lower risk of complications such as OHSS.

When to give hCG?

Human chorionic gonadotropin, administered approximately 34–36 hours prior to egg collection, starts a cascade reaction, leading to resumption of the final maturation processes necessary to produce metaphase II oocytes, and ovulation. There is little evidence to suggest recombinant hCG (dose: 6500 IU Ovitrelle) is any more successful than urinary hCG (dose: 5000–10 000 IU). In women at significant risk of OHSS and using an antagonist cycle, a one-off dose of GnRH agonist has been used to stimulate a surge release of stored LH. While this may reduce the risk of OHSS, the subsequent pregnancy rates following this intervention are significantly lower in autologous embryo replacement cycles. However, this method has been successfully employed for egg donor cycles.

Which GnRH analogue to use?

Most current stimulation protocols employ agents to block the LH surge, either GnRH agonists or GnRH antagonists [4]. The most commonly employed agonist protocol involves a period of down regulation of between 10 and 14 days before starting stimulation, known as the long protocol. The agonist can be started either in the early follicular phase, or in the mid-luteal phase, equally effectively. The agonist is continued until the day of hCG. Similar ongoing pregnancy rates are achieved with all agonist preparations, although more gonadotropin is required with the deeper suppression seen with depot preparations.

GnRH antagonist protocols have commonly employed one of two approaches, a fixed start usually on day 6 or a more flexible approach when the lead follicle reaches 14 mm. Both approaches appear to be equally as effective. Starting the antagonist on the same day of stimulation also seems to be efficacious in high responding patients. One potential disadvantage of the antagonist protocol is the reliance on the natural cycle making workload planning difficult. This can be overcome by pre-treatment with the oral contraceptive pill, which can be used for varying lengths of time (Chapter 16). The oral contraceptive pill should be stopped five days prior to the start of stimulation.

A more detailed direct comparison between these two protocols is to be found in Chapter 15. In summary the latest meta-analysis demonstrates that although more oocytes are retrieved with GnRH agonists there is no difference in overall live birth rates when compared with antagonist cycles (OR 0.86, 95% CI 0.72–1.02). The agonist cycles are not deemed to be as patient friendly, requiring a longer period on medication, both analogue and length of FSH stimulation. In addition, there was a significant reduction in the incidence of hospital admission for OHSS using the antagonist approach (OR 0.46, 95% CI 0.26–0.82).

Protocols for specific indications

Fertility preservation

Patients that face losing ovarian function as a result of chemo- or radiotherapy often present at short notice in an attempt to preserve fertility by storing oocytes or embryos. Most IVF protocols are cycle dependent. In those that are already on the oral contraceptive pill, a modified antagonist protocol is probably the most time efficient regimen to use, with the dose of gonadotropin dependant on age. Radio- or chemotherapy can start following the oocyte recovery. This is discussed in detail in Chapter 45.

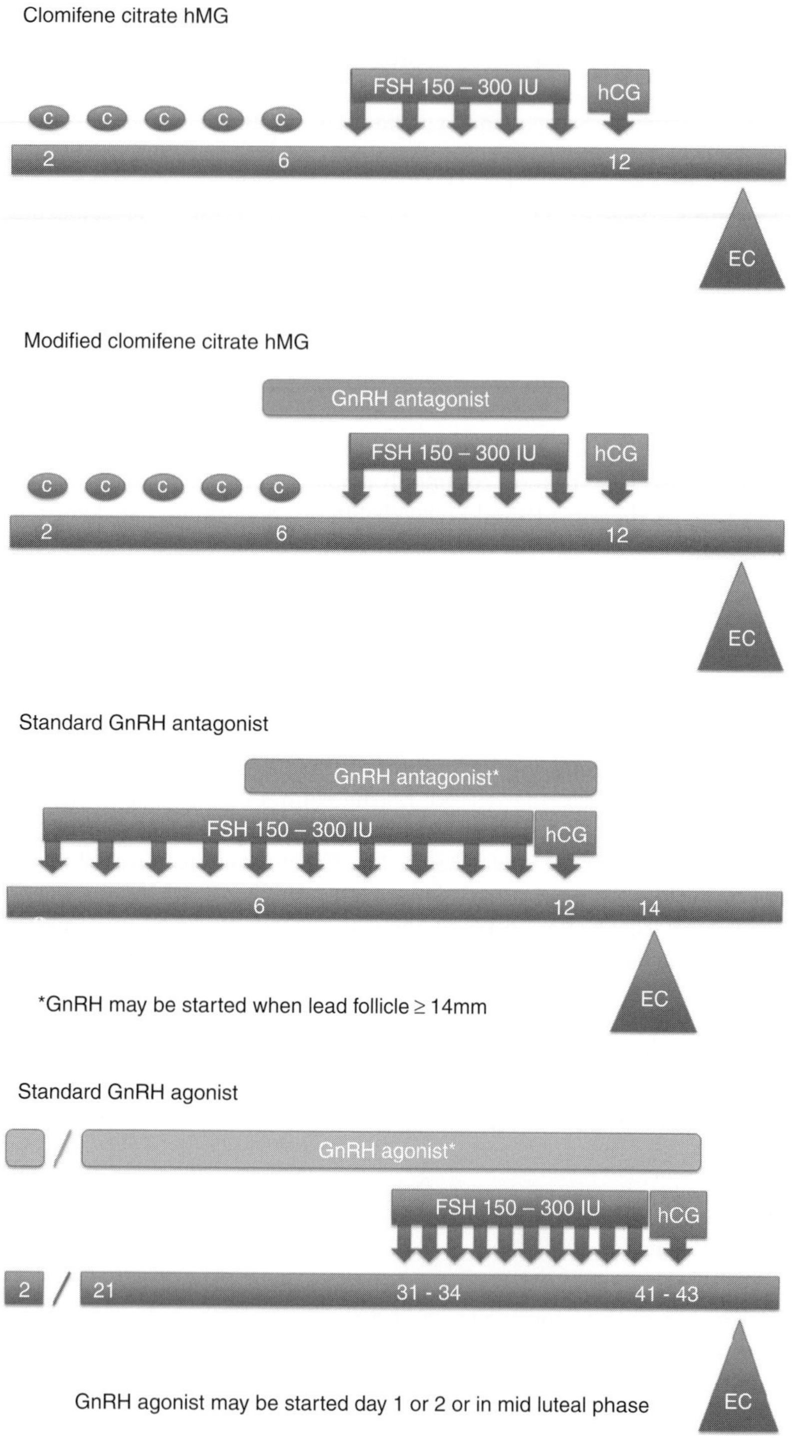

Figure 13.1 Comparison of regimens for controlled ovarian hyperstimulation.

Polycystic ovary syndrome

Polycystic ovaries present particular challenges for IVF stimulation with the main risk OHSS. The background incidence of severe OHSS requiring hospital admission varies between 1 and 2%, but is increased substantially in women with PCOS to around 5%. This is due to the large numbers of antral follicles with similar thresholds for FSH, which leads to multiple follicular development. Judicious use of FSH, with a much lower starting dose (100 IU) and close monitoring is required. The introduction of GnRH agonist protocols made a huge difference to IVF for women with PCOS, who were more likely to have a premature LH surge. Most of the studies performed comparing analogue IVF protocols specifically excluded women with PCOS, and although now there are a number of small comparative studies available they have not been powered sufficiently to reach firm conclusions. Nevertheless, as the risk of OHSS is significantly greater in women with PCOS, the use of an antagonist cycle would appear to be a sensible approach, starting the antagonist early in the cycle due to the potential exaggerated response. In addition, adjunct metformin seems to significantly reduce the risk of OHSS (see Chapter 9).

Severe endometriosis

Women with significant endometriosis have lower pregnancy rates than those with tubal factor infertility. Three small studies have shown that long-term administration of depot GnRH agonists for 3–6 months prior to stimulation will improve the chance of a clinical pregnancy. Further large-scale trials are required to confirm this benefit (See Chapter 10).

Poor responders

Those women with poor ovarian reserve, as judged by pre-treatment ovarian reserve testing or inadequate response to stimulation in previous IVF treatment remains a difficult issue to resolve. Although many treatments have been tried, few have proven to be successful, principally as the fundamental problem, failing ovarian function cannot be reversed. Indeed some have reverted to natural cycle IVF with modest results in younger women. Apart from the use of slightly higher doses of gonadotropins (no more than FSH 300 IU – see above), perhaps with some LH activity, a recent review has shown that *no* manipulation of the stimulation protocol has a significant impact on outcome, with the exception of additional growth hormone administered throughout the stimulation phase. However, the increased probability of a live birth (OR 5.22, CI 95% 1.09–24.99) is based on a number of small studies. In view of the considerable expense and questionable value adjunct growth hormone therapy should not be employed until better evidence exists to confirm benefit [5] (see Chapter 19).

Conclusion

Stimulation protocols for IVF have evolved substantially over the past 25 years, as have the medications available. Our understanding of the potential impact of superovulation on both ovarian and uterine physiology has changed as more complex techniques allow closer inspection of the endometrium and embryo. It is clear that simpler more patient-friendly stimulation is more cost effective with a better safety profile.

References

1. Lehert P, Schertz JC, Ezcurra D. Recombinant human follicle-stimulating hormone produces more oocytes with a lower total dose per cycle in assisted reproductive technologies compared with highly purified human menopausal gonadotrophin: a meta-analysis. *Reprod Biol Endocrinol* 2010;**8**:112.
2. Sterrenburg MD, Veltman-Verhulst SM, Eijkemans MJC, *et al.* Clinical outcomes in relation to the daily dose of recombinant follicle stimulating hormone for ovarian stimulation in in vitro fertilization in presumed normal responders younger than 39 years: a meta-analysis. *Hum Reprod* 2011;**17**:184–96.
3. Devroey P, Boostanfar R, Koper NP, *et al.* A double-blind, non-inferiority RCT comparing corifollitropin alfa and recombinant FSH during the first seven days of ovarian stimulation using a GnRH antagonist protocol. *Hum Reprod* 2009;**24**:3063–72.
4. Kolibianakis EM, Collins J, Tarlatzis BC, *et al.* Among patients treated for IVF with gonadotrophins and GnRH analogues, is the probability of live birth dependent on the type of analogue used? A systematic review and meta-analysis. *Hum Reprod Update* 2006;**12**:651–71.
5. Kyrou D, Kolibianakis EM, Venetis CA, *et al.* How to improve the probability of pregnancy in poor responders undergoing in vitro fertilization: a systematic review and meta-analysis. *Fertil Steril* 2009;**91**:749–66.

Chapter 14

FSH versus hMG: Gonadotropins are gonadotropins are gonadotropins

Hesham Al-Inany, Hamdy Azab and Walid El Sherbiny

Introduction

Gonadotropins are used widely to stimulate follicular development in infertile women. In the 1970s, urinary human menopausal gonadotropin (hMG) was the most widely used gonadotropin in infertility treatment, and contained follicle stimulating hormone (FSH) and luteinizing hormone (LH) in a 1:1 ratio, with many other urinary proteins. Some years later, highly specific monoclonal antibodies selectively binding to FSH molecules were developed, thus enabling the unbound urinary protein along with the LH to be removed, thus creating the highly purified FSH-HP [1]. Consequently, the FSH content and type is the same in all forms of FSH-containing urinary gonadotropin, and the only difference lies in the content of LH and urinary proteins. In the mid 1990s, recombinant FSH was introduced and this step was considered a landmark in the production of gonadotropins [2]. In the new millennium, HP-hMG with its LH-like activity derived from human chorionic gonadotropin (hCG) has been marketed, replacing the standard hMG. Recently, corifollitropin alfa, a long-standing single injection, has been approved for marketing.

The primary efficacy endpoint used to show the difference between different preparations of gonadotropins was the number of oocytes retrieved [3]. This endpoint was chosen because it is the direct goal of ovarian stimulation and the parameter that is most easily assessed. However, pregnancy rate is the ultimate goal of infertility treatment and take home baby rate is the ideal parameter for comparison [4].

To compare the effectiveness of recombinant follicle stimulating hormone (rFSH) with hMG, one should make this comparison for ovulation induction then for controlled ovarian hyperstimulation in IVF/ intracytoplasmic sperm injection (ICSI) cycles. In addition, it is now customary to freeze supernumerary embryos and to transfer frozen/thawed embryos if transfer of fresh embryos has failed. Hence, we will compare rFSH with hMG in cryothawed cycles. As cost plays an important factor for decision makers, cost effectiveness will be also considered.

Choice in women undergoing ovulation induction

In a randomized control trial (RCT), stimulation with HP-hMG was associated with ovulation rates similar to rFSH in anovulatory World Health Organization (WHO) Group II women. Luteinizing hormone activity modified follicular development so that fewer intermediate-sized follicles developed [5]. However, as the aim of ovulation induction is to develop one or two follicles, there is a lack of properly conducted RCTs comparing different gonadotropins in

How to Improve Your ART Success Rates, ed. Gab Kovacs. Published by Cambridge University Press.

ovulation induction. Thus there is insufficient evidence to claim superiority of one drug over the other except for hypogonadotropic hypogonadism (anovulatory WHO Group I women) where hMG should be used to compensate for the deficiency of FSH and LH [6].

hMG versus rFSH in IVF/ICSI cycles

Al-Inany *et al.* conducted a meta-analysis including 12 trials comparing HMG versus rFSH and found that the live-birth rate was significantly higher with hMG (OR 1.20, 95% CI 1.01–1.42) versus rFSH, but OHSS (ovarian hyperstimulation syndrome) rates (OR 1.21, 95% CI 0.78–1.86) were not significantly different. There were significantly fewer treatment days and total dose in the rFSH group compared with the hMG group [4].

To determine whether this improvement in pregnancy rates was due to introducing HP-hMG with LH-like activity to the market, Al-Inany *et al.* conducted another meta-analysis focusing on HP-hMG vs rFSH [4]. The probability of clinical pregnancy following HP-hMG administration was higher than rFSH and reached borderline significance (OR 1.21, 95% CI 1.00–1.45). Subgroup analysis comparing both drugs in IVF cycles demonstrated a statistically significant better ongoing pregnancy/live-birth rate in favor of HP-hMG (OR 1.31, 95% CI 1.02–1.68). On the other hand, there was almost an equal ongoing pregnancy/live-birth rate in ICSI cycles (OR 0.98, 95% CI 0.7–1.36). According to these data HP-hMG should be preferred over rFSH in women undergoing assisted reproduction if IVF is the intended method of fertilization.

A further meta-analysis showed a significant increase in live birth rate with hMG when compared with rFSH (RR 1.18, 95% CI 1.02–1.38, $p = 0.03$). The pooled risk difference (RD) for the outcome of live birth rate was 4% (95% CI 1–7%) for these study populations. There was also an increase in clinical pregnancy rates with hMG when compared with rFSH (RR 1.17, 95% CI 1.03–1.34). No significant differences were noted for gonadotropin use, spontaneous abortion, multiple pregnancy, cancellation, and OHSS rates [9].

Cost effectiveness

A cost-effectiveness study of hMG compared to rFSH in a developing country setting was conducted and demonstrated that hMG is more cost-effective than rFSH [10]. This was further supported by another study comparing the success rate and economic cost between HP-hMG and rFSH combining fresh and frozen IVF cycles (one fresh and up to two subsequent fresh or frozen cycles conditional on availability of cryopreserved embryos). The mean costs per IVF treatment for HP-hMG and rFSH were UK £5393 and £6269, respectively (number needed to treat to fund one additional treatment was seven; $p < 0.001$). With maternal and neonatal costs applied, the median cost per IVF baby delivered with HP-hMG was UK £11,157 and UK £14,227 with rFSH ($p < 0.001$). The cost saving using HP-hMG remained after varying model parameters in a probabilistic sensitivity analysis [11].

Comparison regarding cryothawed embryos

The effectiveness of frozen-embryo transfers (FET) following ovarian stimulation with hMG versus rFSH has not been well investigated except recently when meta-analysis of RCTs using the agonist long down-regulation protocol showed no evidence of significant difference between the uses of urinary gonadotropins or rFSH regarding live birth rate or ongoing pregnancy rates (OR 0.43; 95% CI 0.15–1.23).

hMG versus FSH in antagonist protocols

Bosch and colleagues in a randomized trial compared HP-hMG versus rFSH in antagonist cycles. No significant differences were observed between HP-hMG and rFSH in terms of the ongoing pregnancy rate per started cycle (35.0 versus 32.1%, respectively; $p = 0.61$).

Requena and colleagues compared ovarian stimulation using HP-hMG, rFSH, or a combination of both (rFSH + HP-hMG) with an antagonist protocol. An improved top-quality embryos/retrieved oocytes (TQE/RO) ratio was obtained together with a greater percentage of frozen embryos in the patients that incorporated HP-hMG to their stimulation protocol, however, no differences were found in the ongoing pregnancy rates between groups. Thus, it can be assumed that there is no significant difference regarding ongoing pregnancy rates between hMG and rFSH when utilized in antagonist protocols. There was no study comparing the cost of these two protocols.

Poor responders

In a RCT, a combination of rFSH and rLH was compared to rFSH in poor-responders. There was no significant difference between both groups regarding pregnancy rate and miscarriage rate or incidence of severe ovarian hyperstimulation syndrome [13]. In another study, 240 GnRH-antagonist cycles were initiated in poor responders. One hundred and fifty-three progressed to oocyte retrieval. Seventy-five patients received rFSH for ovarian stimulation, and 66 received hMG in combination with rFSH. In patients aged <40 years, there were no significant differences in amount and duration of treatment, number of oocytes retrieved, and number of embryos between treatment groups. In patients aged ≥40 years, significantly fewer oocytes were retrieved in groups who received exogenous LH in their stimulation, resulting in significantly fewer fertilized embryos. Implantation and clinical pregnancy rates did not differ by treatment group [14]. Thus, there is an evidence of no benefit of adding recombinant LH for women with poor response.

Corifollitropin alfa

Recently a long acting rFSH, corifollitropin alfa, has been proposed to be a suitable substitution for daily rFSH administration in women undergoing controlled ovarian stimulation in IVF/ICSI cycles. Due to its ability to initiate and sustain multiple follicular growth for an entire week, a single subcutaneous injection of ELONVA may replace the first seven injections of rFSH preparations. There was no randomized controlled trials comparing it to hMG but the recently conducted RCTs ENSURE demonstrated comparable efficacy to daily rFSH (OR 1.47, 95% CI 1.08–2.02) [15]. There was no claim of higher efficacy or safety compared to any other gonadotropins [16].

Gonadotropins for male subfertility

The treatment of idiopathic male infertility is empirical. hMG and rFSH have been used to improve sperm parameters in idiopathic male infertility with the goal of increasing pregnancy rates. Four RCTs with 278 participants were included in the analysis. None of the studies had an adequate sample size and they had variable follow-up periods. None of the studies reported live birth or miscarriage rates. Compared to placebo or no treatment, gonadotropins showed a significantly higher pregnancy rate per couple randomized within three months of completing therapy (OR 4.17, 95% CI 1.30–7.09). However, there are no RCTs comparing hMG to rFSH for idiopathic male factor.

References

1. Zafeiriou S, Loutradis D, Michalas S. The role of gonadotropins in follicular development and their use in ovulation induction protocols for assisted reproduction. *Eur J Contracept Reprod Health Care* 2000;**5**:157–67.
2. Out HJ, Driessen SGAJ, Mannaerts BMJL, *et al.* Recombinant follicle-stimulating hormone (follitropin beta, Puregon) yields higher pregnancy rates in in vitro fertilization than urinary gonadotropins. *Fertil Steril* 1997;**68**:138–42.
3. Out HJ Mannaerts BMJL, Driessen SGAJ, *et al.* Recombinant follicle stimulating hormone (rFSH;Puregon) in assisted reproduction: more oocytes, more pregnancies. Results from five comparative studies. *Hum Reprod Update* 1996;**2**:162–71.
4. Al-Inany H, Aboulghar M, Mansour R, Serour G. Meta-analysis of recombinant versus urinary-derived FSH: an update. *Hum Reprod* 2003;**18**:305–13.
5. Platteau P, Andersen AN, Balen A, *et al.* Similar ovulation rates, but different follicular development with highly purified menotrophin compared with recombinant FSH in WHO Group II anovulatory infertility: a randomized controlled study. *Hum Reprod* 2006;**21**:1798–804.
6. Krause BT, Ohlinger R, Haase A. Lutropin alpha, recombinant human luteinizing hormone, for the stimulation of follicular development in profoundly LH-deficient hypogonadotropic hypogonadal women: a review. *Biologics* 2009;**3**:337–47.
7. Al-Inany HG, Abou-Setta AM, Aboulghar MA, Mansour RT, Serour GI. Efficacy and safety of human menopausal gonadotrophins versus recombinant FSH: a meta-analysis. *Reprod Biomed Online* 2008;**16**:81–8.
8. Al-Inany HG, Abou-Setta AM, Aboulghar MA, Mansour RT, Serour GI. Highly purified hMG achieves better pregnancy rates in IVF cycles but not ICSI cycles compared with recombinant FSH: a meta-analysis. *Gynecol Endocrinol* 2009;**25**:372–8.
9. Coomarasamy A, Afnan M, Cheema D, *et al.* Urinary hMG versus recombinant FSH for controlled ovarian hyperstimulation following an agonist long down-regulation protocol in IVF or ICSI treatment: a systematic review and meta-analysis. *Hum Reprod* 2008;**23**:310–5.
10. Al-Inany HG, Abou-Setta AM, Aboulghar MA, Mansour RT, Serour GI. HMG versus rFSH for ovulation induction in developing countries: a cost-effectiveness analysis based on the results of a recent meta-analysis. *Reprod Biomed Online* 2006;**12**:163–9.
11. Wex-Wechowski J, Abou-Setta AM, Kildegaard Nielsen S, Kennedy R. HP-HMG versus rFSH in treatments combining fresh and frozen IVF cycles: success rates and economic evaluation. *Reprod Biomed Online* 2010;**21**:166–78.
12. Al-Inany HG, Van Gelder P. Effect of urinary versus recombinant FSH on clinical outcomes after frozen-thawed embryo transfers: a systematic review. *Reprod Biomed Online* 2010;**21**:151–8.
13. Barrenetxea G, Agirregoikoa JA, Jiménez MR, *et al.* Ovarian response and pregnancy outcome in poor-responder women: a randomized controlled trial on the effect of luteinizing hormone supplementation on in vitro fertilization cycles. *Fertil Steril* 2008;**89**:546–53.
14. Chung K, Krey L, Katz J, Noyes N. Evaluating the role of exogenous luteinizing hormone in poor responders undergoing in vitro fertilization with gonadotropin-releasing hormone antagonists. *Fertil Steril* 2005;**84**:313–8.
15. Devroey P, Boostanfar R, Koper NP, *et al.* A double-blind, non-inferiority RCT comparing corifollitropin alfa and recombinant FSH during the first seven days of ovarian stimulation using a GnRH antagonist protocol. *Hum Reprod* 2009;**24**:3063–72.

16. Fatemi HM, Oberyé J, Popovic-Todorovic B, *et al.* Corifollitropin alfa in a long GnRH agonist protocol: proof of concept trial. *Fertil Steril* 2010;**94**: 1922–4.

17. Attia AM, Al-Inany HG, Farquhar C, Proctor M. Gonadotrophins for idiopathic male factor subfertility. *Cochrane Database Syst Rev* 2007;**4**: CD005071.

Chapter 15

Agonists or antagonists for ovarian stimulation?

V. Vloeberghs, C. Blockeel and P. Devroey

Introduction

In the past 30 years, reproductive treatment has evolved in many ways. The first IVF baby was born in 1978 after IVF in a natural cycle, while today women are routinely treated with ovarian stimulation protocols inducing multi-follicular development and suppressing endogenous luteinizing hormone (LH) surge.

The availability of gonadotropins and gonadotropin-releasing hormone (GnRH) analogues has allowed the tailoring of several stimulation schemes, which have improved treatment outcome.

There are two types of GnRH analogues: GnRH agonists incorporated into standard IVF procedure since the mid 1980s and GnRH antagonist which became available later.

The search for the "ideal" protocol to provide optimal care for our patients continues: a protocol intended to improve the patients' experience should not only provide advantages in terms of treatment burden, risk and distress, but also maintain IVF/intracytoplasmic sperm injection (ICSI) success.

Mechanism of action

For over 20 years, GnRH agonists have been used to prevent the mid-cycle LH surge that results from multiple follicular development. In the long protocol, GnRH agonist treatment is initiated in the mid-luteal phase (day 21) or on day 1 of the cycle. GnRH agonists bind to the pituitary receptors in the hypophysis and induce initially the release of high amounts of follicle stimulating hormone (FSH) and LH (flare-up effect) as well as an increase in the number of GnRH receptors (up-regulation). After prolonged use, however, internalization of the GnRH agonist/receptor complex occurs and it is accompanied by a decrease in the number of GnRH receptors (down-regulation). As a result, the pituitary becomes refractory to stimulation by GnRH, leading to a decrease of circulating gonadotropins. Pituitary desensitization is usually achieved after approximately two weeks of treatment, after which ovarian stimulation with exogenous gonadotropins can start.

GnRH antagonists were introduced in ART at the beginning of this decade using a completely different mechanism for inhibiting gonadotropin secretion. GnRH antagonists act by competitive blockade of the GnRH receptors preventing the action of endogenous GnRH pulses on the pituitary. The secretion of gonadotropins is decreased within hours of antagonist administration without an initial stimulatory response (no flare-up effect). Therefore, antagonists are only administered when there is a risk of a premature LH rise,

How to Improve Your ART Success Rates, ed. Gab Kovacs. Published by Cambridge University Press.

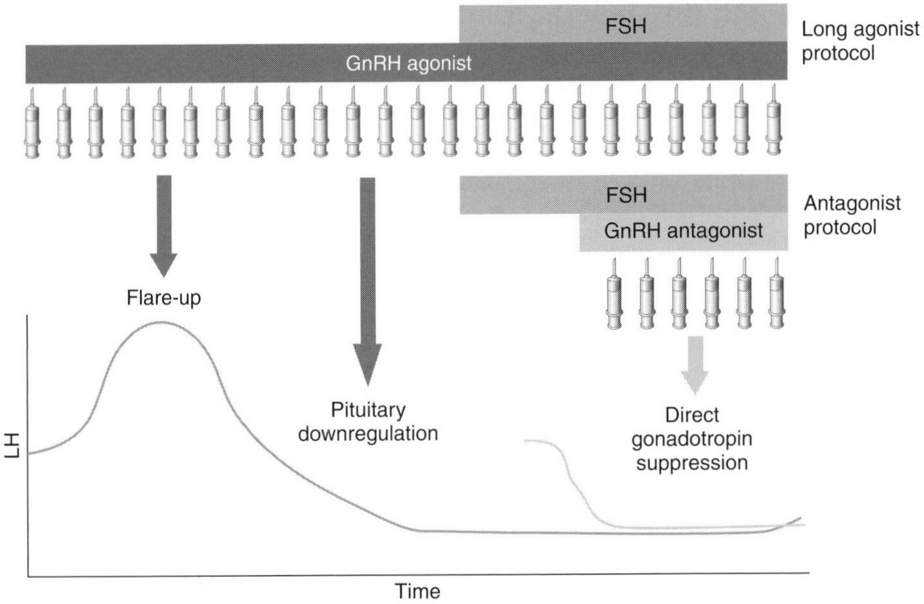

Figure 15.1 A comparison of treatment regimens using GnRH agonist (long protocol) and GnRH antagonist. Treatment duration is considerably longer with GnRH agonist than with GnRH antagonist use. (FSH = follicle stimulating hormone; LH = luteinizing hormone; GnRH = gonadotropin-releasing hormone.)

usually between days 5 and 7 of stimulation. Additionally, since there is no desensitization or down-regulation of the pituitary, cessation of GnRH antagonist treatment results in a rapid and predictable recovery of the pituitary-gonadal axis.

Ovarian stimulation protocols using GnRH agonists and GnRH antagonists are shown in Figure 15.1. The long GnRH agonist protocol is mostly used all over the world. Various modifications of the classic long agonist protocol have been developed in order to improve outcome and simplify the procedure; according to initiation and duration of the agonist use, a differentiation can be made between the so called "short" and " ultra-short" protocol, which are mainly used in low responders or older age groups because of the flare-up effect.

Advantages and disadvantages of GnRH agonists

It became clear that besides the elimination of premature LH surge, several advantages accompanied the use of GnRH agonists in ART, including the retrieval of more cumulus-oocyte complexes (COCs) and, in turn, the availability of more embryos for transfer and cryopreservation. Another important advantage of the GnRH agonist protocol is the possibility of an improved planning of IVF activities. At the other side there are a number of disadvantages with this technique, such as the flare-up effect (i.e., the initial unwelcome increase in the secretion of gonadotropins), which involves a long treatment period until desensitization and risk for causing cyst formation. The long period of desensitization implies an increased cost of treatment and is associated with oestrogen deprivation symptoms (weight gain, headache, hot flushes, night sweats, mood swings, breast tenderness, abdominal pain, diarrhea, and nausea).

Advantages and disadvantages of GnRH antagonists

Antagonists are associated with fewer side-effects in comparison with the GnRH agonists, because of their different mode of pharmalogical action on the pituitary. The antagonistic analogue has an immediate action and thus can be administered only when there is a need for suppressing LH surge, resulting in a shorter duration of stimulation and absence of side-effects caused by profound hypo-estrogenemia. Inadvertent administration of the GnRH analogue in early pregnancy can be avoided as the GnRH antagonist is administered in the mid-follicular phase [12]. Nevertheless, GnRH antagonists offer less flexibility regarding cycle programming compared with GnRH agonists [12].

The patients' experience may be improved through the use of GnRH antagonists rather than GnRH agonists. Patients undergoing IVF/IVSI frequently experience substantial treatment burden risk and psychological distress. Two factors constitute the bulk of treatment burden: length of treatment and side effects [3].

Efficacy of GnRH antagonists in IVF

The meaning of success in the context of IVF has been much debated in recent years, (as discussed in Chapter 46) although it is generally agreed that pregnancy rate and live birth rate are important factors as well as the welfare of mother and child [3].

There appears to be no clinically significant difference in terms of live birth rate between GnRH antagonists and agonists: two meta-analyses comparing the two classes of GnRH analogue calculated almost identical odds ratios (0.82, 0.86) for the probability of live birth, although the difference was statistically significant in one analysis [1] and not in another [11]. The difference is unlikely to be of clinical significance [3].

Regarding secondary outcomes, both meta-analyses [11] found shorter duration of GnRH analogue administration, decreased gonadotropin requirements and lower incidence of ovarian hyperstimulation syndrome (OHSS) in the antagonist group. On the contrary, significantly more COCs were retrieved in the agonist as compared with the antagonist group.

More than 20 different GnRH antagonist protocols have been reported [11, 12], this variety reflects an ongoing process of refinement and improvement [3]. A GnRH antagonist protocol, based on the knowledge of different studies optimizing the antagonist protocol, will lead to the optimal use of the GnRH antagonist in ovarian stimulation and enhance further the probability of pregnancy.

A GnRH antagonist protocol for normal responders, based on the current data and clinical experience, has been suggested and presented in Figure 15.2 [3].

Ovarian hyperstimulation syndrome

The most serious complication of ovarian stimulation for in vitro fertilization is the OHSS, a rare but potentially life-threatening condition, it is characterized by a cystic enlargement of the ovaries and an acute fluid shift from the intravascular to the third space, which may result in ascites, pleural effusions, pericardial effusion, and even generalized edema. This fluid shift is caused by an increase in vascular permeability and neoangiogenesis. Renal failure, thromboembolic complications and respiratory distress may occur.

Although many primary and secondary preventive measures have been taken to reduce the incidence of OHSS, complete prevention is still not possible without cycle cancellation in a GnRH agonist treatment protocol.

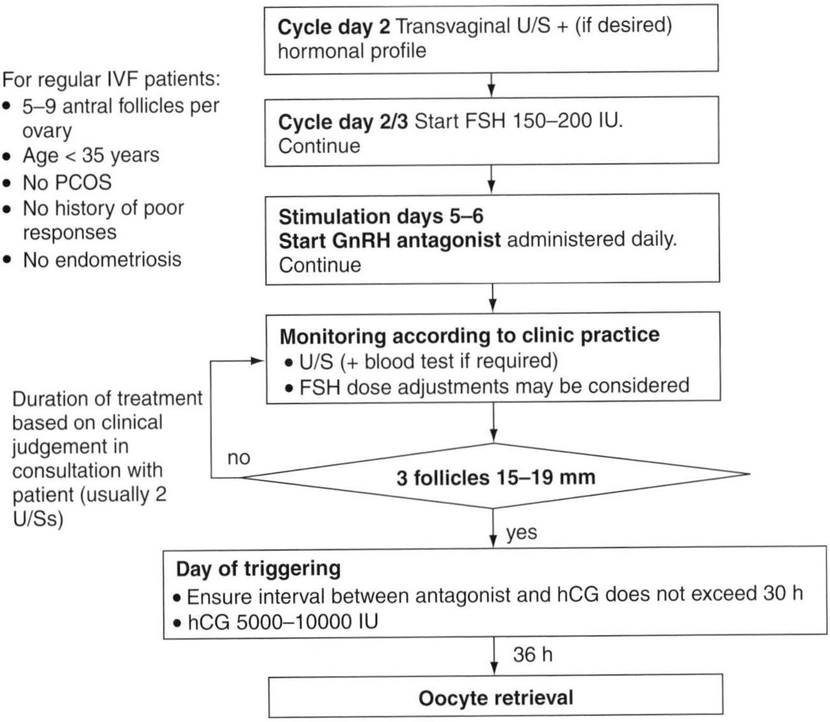

Cycle day 2 Transvaginal U/S + (if desired) hormonal profile
For regular IVF patients:
• 5–9 antral follicles per ovary
• Age < 35 years
• No PCOS
• No history of poor responses
• No endometriosis
Cycle day 2/3 Start FSH 150–200 IU. Continue
Stimulation days 5–6
Start GnRH antagonist administered daily. Continue
Monitoring according to clinic practice
• U/S (+ blood test if required)
• FSH dose adjustments may be considered
Duration of treatment based on clinical judgement in consultation with patient (usually 2 U/Ss)
no
3 follicles 15–19 mm
yes
Day of triggering
• Ensure interval between antagonist and hCG does not exceed 30 h
• hCG 5000–10000 IU
36 h
Oocyte retrieval

Figure 15.2 Suggested GnRH antagonist treatment protocol for normal responders. Reproduced with permission of Oxford University Press from Devroey P, Aboulghar M, Garcia-Velasco J, Griesinger G, Humaidan P, Kolibianakis E, Ledger W, Tomas C, Fauser BC. Improving the patient's experience of IVF/ICSI: a proposal for an ovarian stimulation protocol with GnRH antagonist co-treatment. *Hum Reprod* 2009; 24: 764–774. (U/S = ultrasound).

Evidence indicates that the use of GnRH antagonists instead of GnRH agonists reduces the relative risk of OHSS [1, 11]. Therefore GnRH antagonists are useful for primary prevention of OHSS and should be the first choice in high-risk patients.

Human chorionic gonadotropin (hCG), either exogenous or endogenous, is thought to play a crucial role in the development of the syndrome. The severe forms are almost always restricted to cycles where exogenous hCG has been given or with endogenous pregnancy derived hCG. In the natural cycle, ovulation is induced by the mid-cycle surge of LH (and FSH) from the pituitary, elicited by an increasing late follicular level of estradiol. As a substitute for the endogenous LH to induce final oocyte maturation, exogenous hCG (5000–10 000 IU) was successfully introduced more than 50 years ago. The significantly longer half-life of hCG as compared to LH, leads to a prolonged luteotrophic effect, development of multiple corpora lutea, and raised serum levels of estradiol and progesterone throughout the luteal phase, which increases the risk of OHSS [10].

By finding alternatives for hCG administration, it is theoretically possible to exclude the development of early OHSS.

Recombinant LH (rLH) has a shorter half-life than hCG and can induce oocyte maturation. It appears to be effective in reducing the incidence of OHSS, but is associated with lower pregnancy rates and high costs, and has never been produced commercially [10].

On top of the use of the GnRH antagonist protocol as a primary prevention, triggering of final oocyte maturation with a GnRH agonist has stirred a lot of interest. GnRH agonists had previously been shown to effectively stimulate ovulation and final oocyte maturation. However, with the introduction of the GnRH agonist for pituitary down-regulation prior to IVF/ICSI treatment in order to avoid a premature endogenous LH surge, this concept was clearly not applicable, as the simultaneous use of a GnRH agonist for down-regulation and triggering of final oocyte maturation is not possible. When GnRH antagonist protocols were introduced for the prevention of a premature LH surge, it became possible again to trigger ovulation with a bolus of a GnRH as an alternative to hCG. It has been shown that OHSS can be reliably prevented by replacing hCG with a single dose of GnRH agonist. The mechanism of action by which agonist prevents OHSS is rapid luteolysis. Nevertheless, due to a defective luteal phase post agonist triggering and therefore to a defective endometrial receptivity, the ongoing pregnancy rate is significantly lower [6]. Recently however, it has been advocated that a high-dosed luteal support until seven or even more weeks of gestation might overcome this luteal phase defect. Engmann *et al.* [4] showed an unaffected implantation rate with adequate luteal phase and early pregnancy estradiol and progestron supplementation. On the other hand, good clinical pregnancy rates could be obtained if a bolus of 1500 IU of hCG was administered 35 hours after triggering with the GnRH agonist [9]. However, OHSS was not excluded completely with this protocol.

Embryo quality seems not to be affected by GnRH agonist triggering; cryopreservation of all embryos followed by consecutive thaw cycles results in good pregnancy outcome [10].

Recent developments for ovarian stimulation in GnRH antagonist protocols

Low dose hCG in the late follicular phase

For many years, FSH was considered the only stimulatory factor needed for ovulation induction, acting through specific receptors present on granulosa cells of ovarian follicles. In a GnRH agonist protocol, it was demonstrated that the administration of low dosages of hCG (100–400 IU/day) can be successfully applied in patients undergoing ART to substitute for recombinant FSH in the final days of ovarian stimulation. Recently, a comparable protocol was succesfully used in a GnRH antagonist protocol. Low-dose hCG (200 IU/day) supplementation may improve pregnancy rates in antagonist protocols. Overall, these low-dose hCG-supplemented protocols are a cost-effective strategy [2].

Corifollitropin alfa

Due to the relatively short half-life of FSH preparations (32±12 hours) and rapid metabolic clearance, daily FSH injections are required to maintain the FSH concentration above the FSH threshold. The daily subcutaneous administration of the FSH preparations causes considerable discomfort to the patient.

Recombinant DNA technologies have been used to develop longer-acting therapeutic proteins. A new recombinant FSH was designated corifollitropin alfa. Recent trials demonstrated that one single sub-cutaneous injection of corifollitropin alfa is able to initiate and sustain multiple follicular growth for seven days in women undergoing ovarian stimulation for IVF/ICSI using GnRH antagonists or long GnRH agonist. This will simplify ovarian stimulation requiring daily injections [5].

Scheduling

In spite of the clear benefits associated with GnRH antagonists, GnRH agonists remain the GnRH analogue of choice in the majority of ART clinics. The flexibility of the long GnRH agonist protocol allows a more controlled organization of egg retrievals, in such a way that a significant decrease and even avoidance of oocyte retrievals during the weekend can be made possible, whereas the initiation of ovarian stimulation in GnRH antagonist cycles relies on the random occurrence of spontaneous menses. Since oral contraceptive pills pretreatment (discussed in Chapter 16) may reduce ongoing pregnancy rate.

In patients undergoing a GnRH antagonist protocol [7], other strategies of fine scheduling GnRH antagonist cycles to reduce weekend oocyte retrievals were studied. Adjusting the starting day of ovarian stimulation on cycle day 2 or 3 and advancing or delaying hCG administration by one day were found not to have an impact on live birth outcomes. A novel approach to further elaborate scheduling of GnRH antagonist cycles, namely the pretreatment with GnRH antagonists in the early follicular phase during three consecutive days prior to the onset of ovarian stimulation, was recently adopted (Blockeel *et al.*, unpublished data). Finally, programming with estradiol valerate during a variable number of days from the late luteal phase onwards, also allows organization of the center, without impairing pregnancy outcome [8].

Conclusion

Ovarian stimulation with GnRH antagonist co-treatment can provide live-birth rates (per embryo transfer) comparable to those achieved with the long GnRH agonist protocol, and has advantages in terms of tolerability and safety.

We should strive for an OHSS free clinic by using the GnRH antagonist co-treatment as standard protocol, triggering of final oocyte maturation with a GnRH agonist, freeze all embryos and transfer them in consecutive natural cycles, until luteal phase support in the fresh cycles has been optimized.

References

1. Al-Inany HG, Abou-Setta AM, Aboulghar M. Review: Gonadotrophin-releasing hormone antagonists for assisted conception: a Cochrane Review. *RBM Online* 2007;**14**:640–9.
2. Blockeel C, De Vos M, Verpoest W, *et al.* Can 200 IU of hCG replace recombinant FSH in the late follicular phase in GnRH antagonist cycle? A pilot study. *Hum Reprod* 2009;**24**:2910–16.
3. Devroey P, Aboulghar M, Garcia-Velasco J, *et al.* Improving the patient's experience of IVF/ICSI: a proposal for an ovarian stimulation protocol with GnRH antagonist co-treatment. *Hum Reprod* 2009;**24**:764–74.
4. Engmann L, Diluigi A, Schmidt D, *et al.* The effect of luteal phase vaginal estradiol supplementation on the success of in vitro fertilization treatment: a prospective randomized study. *Fertil Steril* 2008;**89**:554–61.
5. Fauser BC, Mannaerts BM, Devroey P, *et al.* Advances in recombinant DNA technology: corifollitropin alfa, a hybrid molecule with sustained follicle-stimulating activity and reduced injection frequency. *Hum Reprod* 2009;**15**:309–321.
6. Griesinger G. Ovarian hyperstimulation syndrome prevention strategies: use of gonadotrophin releasing hormone antagonists. *Semin Reprod Medicine* 2010a;**28**:493–99.
7. Griesinger G, Kolibianakis EM, Venetis C, Diedrich K, Tarlatzis B. Oral contraceptive

pretreatment significantly reduces ongoing pregnancy likelihood in gonadotropin-releasing hormone antagonist cycles: an updated meta-analysis. *Fertil Steril* 2010b;**94**:2382–4.

8. Guivarc'h-Levêque A, Arvis P, Bouchet JL, *et al.* Efficiency of antagonist IVF cycle programming by estrogens. *Gynecol Obstet Fertil* 2010;**38**:18–22.
9. Humaidan P, Bungum L, Bungum M, Yding Anderson C. Rescue of corpus luteum function with peri-ovulatory hCG supplementation in IVF/ICSI GnRH antagonist cycles in which ovulation was triggered with a GnRH agonist: a pilot study. *Reprod Biomed Online* 2006;**13**:173–8.
10. Humaidan MD, Quartarolo J, Evangelos G, Papanikolaou E. Preventing ovarian hyperstimulation syndrome: guidance for the clinician. *Fertil Steril* 2010;**94**:389–99.
11. Kolibianakis EM, Collins J, Tarlatzis BC, *et al.* Among patients treated for IVF with gonadotrophins and GnRH analogues, is the probability of live birth dependent on the type of analogue used? A systematic review and meta-analysis. *Hum Reprod Update* 2006;**12**:651–71.
12. Tarlatzis BC, Fauser BC, Kolibianakis EM, Diedrich K, Devroey P. GnRH antagonist in ovarian stimulation for IVF. *Hum Reprod Update* 2006;**12**:333–40.

Chapter 16

Should the oral contraceptive pill or progestogens be used to schedule controlled ovarian hyperstimulation?

Gab Kovacs

I believe that the first time oral contraceptives (OCPs) were incorporated into the controlled ovarian hyperstimulation (COH) protocol was in the early 1980s. The aim was to schedule oocyte collections for specific times, for example the availability of the microsurgeon to collect sperm samples for IVF [1]. Subsequently programming became an integral part of COH to batch the timing of oocyte collections which was essential for scheduling satellite programs, or to improve the efficiency of small IVF units which performed laboratory procedures at limited times, and sometimes for patient convenience.

The theory was that oral contraceptives would be administered to defer 'day 1' of the treatment cycle until a convenient day, so that cycles could be batched. In those days, gonadotropin-releasing hormone (GnRH) analogues were not available, so the cycle had to be monitored for luteinizing hormone (LH) rise. The use of the OCP was also reported from Clamart (France) by the Frydman/Testart Group in 1986 on a series of 35 patients, and across the Atlantic from Portland, Oregon in 1988 on 26 cycles. These initial studies were 'descriptive' and simply confirmed that the technique worked, and resulted in outcomes in the expected range. The first 'controlled study' came from Robert Casper's group in Toronto, where they compared the use of a 50 ug oestrogen monophasic pill as pre-treatment for 18 to 61 days to a clomiphene/hMG Boost/Flare cycle in 181 subjects, compared to 113 parallel, non randomized controls who did not receive pre-treatment. They found in the OCP group that there were no spontaneous LH surges, that the amount of hMG required was less, there were more follicles and oocytes collected, and in summary the protocol worked. Here was the first 'evidence' that using the OCP to programme cycles was 'OK'. When the GnRH agonists became available, the OCP was integrated into both the 'short' (Boost or Flare) protocol, and the long 'down-regulation protocol'. Supporting studies were published as small series from many countries.

At Monash IVF it became our practice to commence OCP on day 1 to 5 of a spontaneous cycle, and continue for at least 21 days, then overlap with the GnRH agonist (usually nafarelin acetate nasal spray [Pfizer Australia]) for four days, before ceasing the OCP, but continuing the GnRH agonist and measuring the estradiol level to confirm down-regulation seven days later, and then starting follicle stimulating hormone (FSH). This was called pill-down-regulation (PDR) and became widely used, and was the most commonly used COH protocol at Monash IVF, and it seemed to work.

How to Improve Your ART Success Rates, ed. Gab Kovacs. Published by Cambridge University Press.

When long down-regulation was introduced into the COH protocol and it was commenced in the luteal phase where it seemed most effective, inadvertent pregnancies sometimes occurred, causing anxiety about the effect of hormones on the early embryo. Integrating OCP into the down-regulation protocol also had the benefit that stimulation was always commenced at a time of menstruation and conceptions during treatment were avoided. Using the OCP and suppressing gonadotropin release from the early follicular phase also significantly decreased the formation of luteal cysts, one of the causes of unsuccessful down-regulation.

Adding the OCP not only had the advantages of programming, avoiding conception during treatment, and decreasing the incidence of cyst formation, but it also saved on the amount of GnRH agonist consumed, which was a cost saving.

Similar attempts at successfully programming cycles using progestogens were also reported. Both Ricardo Ash's (1989) and Polson/Lobo's (1990) group reported on using northindrone (norethisterone) successfully in pilot studies in Los Angeles.

Although there were several small series including observational studies, retrospective evaluations, comparisons with historical controls, reporting that both OCP and progestogen programming worked, some claiming benefits in birth rates, clinical pregnancy rates, or oocyte numbers, there was no high level 'evidence' whether the OCP programming improved or adversely affected outcomes. By 2008 GnRH antagonists were replacing the GnRH agonists in many protocols, as they were perceived to be more 'patient friendly' being shorter, with fewer side-effects and a lower incidence of ovarian hyperstimulation syndrome (OHSS). This prompted the first systematic review of controlled trials using OCP, but was confined to COH cycles using GnRH antagonists [2].

They concluded that the ongoing pregnancy rates were not significantly different whether OCP pretreatment was used (OR 0.74, 95% CI 0.53–1.03). However, the duration of gonadotropin stimulation expressed as weighted differences of means (WMD: +1.41 days, 95% CI +1.13 to +1.68) and gonadotropin consumption (WMD: +542 IU, 95% CI +127 to +956) were significantly increased after OCP pre-treatment. No significant differences were observed regarding the number of oocytes collected nor in fertilization rates. They suggested further studies were necessary for conclusions on pregnancy rates.

Further studies were published and are extensively reviewed in a recent Cochrane Review which published results for the use of hormonal pre-treatment (OCP and progestogens and estrogens) as part of COH protocols [3]. This review included a total of 1049 studies and after removing the duplicates there were approximately 900 studies left. Around 200 studies seemed eligible for inclusion, but after screening of titles and abstracts 23 studies on 2596 women were included in this review. It appears that all of the subjects reported in the 2008 meta-analysis [2] were included in this updated analysis.

All the details can be found in the Cochrane review and for the sake of simplicity no figures are quoted here except for significant findings, and readers are referred to the review [3].

Combined OCP versus no pre-treatment

This systematic review on the role of pre-treatment with the combined OCP prior to ART cycles, has pooled the results of studies for three of the six interventions. For the other interventions, the reviewers have not been able to pool any results, since only one study could be included in the subgroups of these interventions. The six interventions were:

OCP + Antagonist versus Antagonist
OCP + Antagonist versus Agonist

OCP + Agonist versus Agonist
OCP + Antagonist versus Agonist, low response
OCP + Antagonist versus Antagonist, low response
OCP + Agonist versus Antagonist, low response

The primary outcome studied was that of the number of live births achieved. No evidence of effect (no difference in results) was found with regard to the number of live births when using a pre-treatment, amongst any of the combinations studied above.

Secondary outcomes compared included:

- Number of ongoing pregnancies per woman randomized – *defined as evidence of a gestational sac with fetal heart motion at 12 weeks or later, confirmed with ultrasound.* Again there was no difference between OCP pretreatment groups
- Number of clinical/ongoing pregnancies per woman randomized – *defined as evidence of a gestational sac with fetal heart motion at six weeks or later, confirmed with ultrasound.*

It was only the comparison of the parameter of clinical/ongoing pregnancies between groups using the combined OCP with antagonist cycles, compared to no pre-treatment (antagonist alone), that was associated with significantly worse results for the OCP pre-treatment group. These results *OCP + Antagonist versus Antagonist* meta-analysis included five studies. Four randomized controlled trials were pooled in this subgroup, with a total of 847 women. In two of these studies, the number of ongoing pregnancies was used, since no data on clinical pregnancy rate were available. There was a statistically significant difference in the rates of clinical/ongoing pregnancies with fewer clinical/ongoing pregnancies occurring in the group pre-treated with a combined OCP (Peto OR 0.69; 95% CI 0.50–0.96, $p = 0.03$).

- The number of oocytes retrieved per woman randomized showed no difference in any of the subgroups.
- Days of gonadotropin treatment per woman randomized found a significant difference, with fewer days of gonadotropin treatment in the group that did not receive pre-treatment with a combined OCP (MD 1.44; 95% CI 1.15–1.72, $p < 0.00001$).
- The amount of gonadotropins administered per woman randomized again showed increased usage after OCP pre-treatment with antagonist when compared to both the antagonist (MD 231.14; 95% CI 161.50–300.78, $p < 0.00001$)and the agonist (MD 209.52; 95% CI 61.16–357.87, $p = 0.006$) group without OCP.
- Adverse events were also compared between the various groups using OCP pre-treatment. This included pregnancy loss, multiple pregnancy and OHSS, all of which found no difference with OCP pre-treatment. When it came to 'cyst formation' comparing *OCP + Agonist versus Agonist* only two studies reported on cyst formation, but results could not be pooled or analyzed because the number of women in each study or control group is unknown. The first study found that the number of women in which cyst formation occurred was none in the study group ($n = 51$ cycles) and 27 in the control group ($n = 51$ cycles). This result was statistically significant according to the authors ($p < 0.0001$). However, a cyst formation of 53% in the control group seems excessive, and throws doubt on this finding, although intuitively it seems correct.

The Cochrane Reviewers' conclusions were [3] that 'there were poorer pregnancy outcomes with a combined OCP pre-treatment'. However, they also concluded 'that major changes in ART protocols should not be made at this time, since the number of overall studies in the subgroups is small and reporting of the major outcomes is inadequate'. Whilst I agree with their recommendation against changes in protocols, I believe that their conclusion that 'there were poorer pregnancy outcomes with a combined OCP pre-treatment' are based on very limited data, only in clinical pregnancy rates/ongoing pregnancy rates not supported by live birth rates. Also, this 'poorer pregnancy outcome' was only observed for agonist cycles. There were two studies where agonists were used (*OCP + Agonist versus Antagonist*). Both studies reported the number of clinical pregnancies, but due to a lack of data the reviewers could not pool these results. Nevertheless, both studies found that their results showed no statistically significant differences. A more negative picture emerges from an updated meta-analysis by Griesinger and colleagues [4] after pooling data from six randomized controlled trials encompassing 1343 patients. Ongoing pregnancy rate (PR) per randomized woman was found to be just significantly lower in patients with OCP pre-treatment (RR 0.80, 95% CI 0.66–0.97; rate difference: −5%, 95% CI −10% to −1%; fixed effects model). Duration of stimulation (WMD: +1.33 days, 95% CI +0.61–2.05) and gonadotropin consumption (WMD: +360 IUs, 95% CI +158–563) were significantly increased after OCP pre-treatment, but there was no statistically significant gain in the number of cumulus–oocyte complexes (WMD: +0.6 cumulus–oocyte complexes, 95% CI −0.08–1.25).

My conclusion would be that one needs to compare all the benefits of OCP pre-treatment against the slightly decreased clinical/ongoing pregnancy rate before dispensing with OCP pre-treatment. The benefits and risks of OCP pre-treatment are summarized in Table 16.1. If there is a negative effect of OCP pre-treatment we have to postulate a mechanism. If it is an effect on the endometrium, then the duration of OCP pre-treatment is likely to have an influence, an aspect that has not been previously studied.

I have used an 'ultrashort pill-down regulation' regimen where the OCP is used for seven days only commencing on day 1 of cycle, it is overlapped with GnRH analogue for two days before discontinuing the OCP, and four days later an estradiol measurement is undertaken, and if downregulation is confirmed, FSH is commenced, whilst continuing the GnRH agonist. This protocol results in similar rates of downregulation, oocyte numbers and pregnancy rate as the conventional 21 day PDR (unpublished data). The protocol has also been adapted as 'flexi-short pill downregulation (F/SPDR)' where the duration of OCP taking can vary from a minimum of seven days to as many as required to programme the oocyte collection on the approximate appropriate days.

Table 16.1 Benefits and risks of oral contraceptive pill (OCP) pre-treatment for controlled ovarian hyperstimulation (COH) in IVF

Benefits • Prevents LH surge and suppresses FSH levels • Allows scheduling of treatment cycles • Facilitates synchronization of donor:recipient cycles for oocyte donation • Decreased risk of cyst formation • Decreased amount of GnRH analogoues used, cost saving • Avoidance of possible pregnancy in long down-regulation cycles
Risks • Decreased ongoing/clinical pregnancy rates in OCP anatagonist versus antagonist comparisons, not confirmed by live birth rates • May slightly lengthen the days of FSH and increase the quantity of FSH use (? clinically significant)

LH, luteinizing hormone; FSH, follice stimulating hormone; GnRH, gonadotropin – releasing hormone.

Although this chapter aimed to review the role of OCP, a short mention of the use of progestogens and estrogens is required for completeness, especially as these are both considered in the Cochrane Review 2010 [3]. Progestogens that have been used were either norethisterone 10 mg/day or medroxyprogesterone acetate 10 mg/day for durations of from 7 to 28 days. In the Review it was found that compared to placebo or no pre-treatment, a progestogen pre-treatment in GnRH agonist cycles was associated with more clinical pregnancies (Peto OR 1.95, $p = 0.007$) and fewer ovarian cysts (Peto OR 0.21, $p < 0.00001$).

Estrogens have also been used to delay day 1, either micronized 17-βE_2, or estradiol valerate, both 4 mg daily starting in the luteal phase as pre-treatment. The 2010 Cochrane Review [3] found that in estrogen pre-treated GnRH antagonist cycles, compared to no pre-treatment, more oocytes were retrieved (MD 2.01, $p < 0.00001$), but a higher amount of gonadotropin therapy was needed (MD 207.08, $p < 0.00001$). For the other outcomes no evidence of effect was found or there were not enough studies available in the subgroup for pooling [3].

Study or subgroup	Combined OCP Events	Combined OCP Total	No Rx Events	No Rx Total	Weight	Peto odds ratio Peto, fixed, 95% CI
1.2.1 COCP + Ant vs Ant						
Cédrin-Durnerin 2007 (1)	3	21	7	24	5.6%	0.43 [0.11, 1.74]
Huirne 2006b	4	32	8	32	7.0%	0.45 [0.13, 1.55]
Kolibianakis 2006	51	250	60	254	61.2%	0.83 [0.54, 1.26]
Rombauts 2006 (2)	20	117	26	117	26.2%	0.72 [0.38, 1.38]
Subtotal (95% CI)		**420**		**427**	**100.0%**	**0.74 [0.53, 1.03]**
Total events	78		101			
Heterogeneity: $Chi^2 = 1.50$, df = 3 ($P = 0.68$); $I^2 = 0\%$						
Test for overall effect: $Z = 1.80$ ($P = 0.07$)						
1.2.2 COCP + Ant vs Ag						
Huirne 2006a	17	91	20	91	44.4%	0.82 [0.40, 1.68]
Rombauts 2006 (3)	20	117	26	117	55.6%	0.72 [0.38, 1.38]
Subtotal (95% CI)		**208**		**208**	**100.0%**	**0.76 [0.47, 1.23]**
Total events	37		46			
Heterogeneity: $Chi^2 = 0.06$, df = 1 ($P = 0.81$); $I^2 = 0\%$						
Test for overall effect: $Z = 1.10$ ($P = 0.27$)						
1.2.3 COCP + Ant vs Ant, low response						
Kim 2005	8	27	5	27	100.0%	1.82 [0.53, 6.25]
Subtotal (95% CI)		**27**		**27**	**100.0%**	**1.82 [0.53, 6.25]**
Total events	8		5			
Heterogeneity: Not applicable						
Test for overall effect: $Z = 0.95$ ($P = 0.34$)						
1.2.4 COCP + Ant vs Ag, low response						
Kim 2005	8	27	6	28	100.0%	1.53 [0.46, 5.09]
Subtotal (95% CI)		**27**		**28**	**100.0%**	**1.53 [0.46, 5.09]**
Total events	8		6			
Heterogeneity: Not applicable						
Test for overall effect: $Z = 0.69$ ($P = 0.49$)						

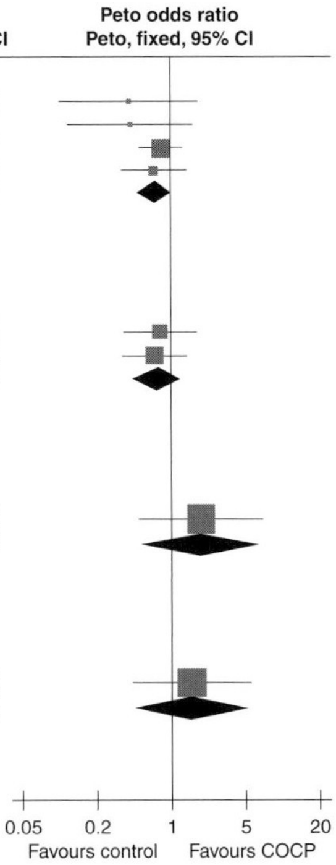

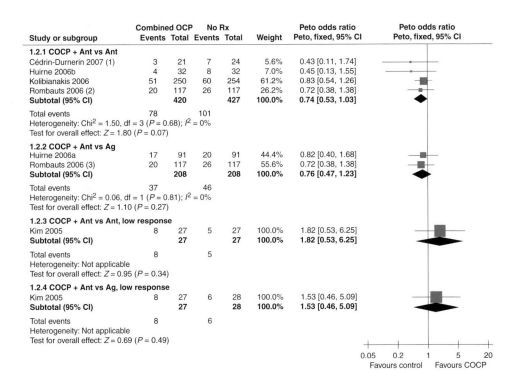

Test for subgroup differences: $Chi^2 = 3.06$, df = 3 ($p = 0.38$), $I^2 = 2.1\%$
(1) Data obtained from Dr. Cédrin-Durnerin.
(2) Includes 2 spontaneous pregnancies in the study group and 3 in the control group.
(3) Includes 2 spontaneous pregnancies in the study group.

Figure 16.1 Forest plot of comparison: Combined oral contraceptive pill (COCP) versus no treatment (Rx); outcome: ongoing pregnancies. *Cochrane Database of Systematic Reviews, reproduced with permission.*

References

1. Temple-Smith PD, Southwick GJ, Yates CA, Trounson AO, de Kretser DM. Human pregnancy by in vitro fertilization (IVF) using sperm aspirated from the epididymis. *J In Vitro Fert Embryo Transf* 1985;**2**: 119–22.
2. Griesinger G, Venetis CA, Marx T, *et al.* Oral contraceptive pill pretreatment in ovarian stimulation with GnRH antagonists for IVF: a systematic review and meta-analysis. *Fertil Steril* 2008;**90**: 1055–63.
3. Smulders B, van Oirschot SM, Farquhar C, Rombauts L, Kremer JA. Oral contraceptive pill, progestogen or estrogen pre-treatment for ovarian stimulation protocols for women undergoing assisted reproductive techniques. *Cochrane Database Syst Rev* 2010;**20**: CD006109.
4. Griesinger G, Kolibianakis EM, Venetis C, Diedrich K, Tarlatzis B. Oral contraceptive pretreatment significantly reduces ongoing pregnancy likelihood in gonadotropin-releasing hormone antagonist cycles: an updated meta-analysis. *Fertil Steril* 2010;**94**:2382–4.

Chapter 17

Dehydroepiandrosterone

Norbert Gleicher and David H. Barad

Introduction

Dehydroepiandrosterone (DHEA), a product of adrenal and ovarian steroidogenesis, is a mild androgen, which is primarily converted to testosterone but to a lesser degree also to estrogen. In 2000, Casson *et al.* were first to suggest that DHEA may beneficially affect ovarian function in women with diminished ovarian reserve (DOR), when reporting improving oocyte yields with IVF after relative short-term DHEA supplementation [1]. Their work, however, was not followed up until, approximately five years later, when our group became interested in DHEA, and in a series of studies determined that DHEA supplementation, indeed, significantly improves ovarian performance in women with DOR [2].

We demonstrated that DHEA not only improves oocyte yields but also embryo numbers, oocyte quality and, therefore, ultimately pregnancy chances with IVF, spontaneous pregnancy rates, cumulative pregnancy chances, and time to conception with infertility treatments [2]. The effectiveness of DHEA was recently also confirmed by a first small, prospectively randomized study [3].

While mode of action is not fully established, we demonstrated that DHEA reduces embryo aneuploidy [4] and diminishes spontaneous pregnancy loss by at least 50–80% [5]. A recent worldwide survey of IVF programs by www.IVF-worldwide.com suggested that approximately one quarter have started utilizing DHEA.

Indications for DHEA

We currently consider DHEA supplementation indicated in all women with DOR, and, especially after publication of a small prospectively randomized study [3] no longer consider such treatment experimental. Diminished ovarian reserve routinely affects aging women, and we, therefore, recommend DHEA supplementation to all women above age 40 years. However, DOR can also occur in younger females, and for such cases we have coined the acronym premature ovarian aging (POA), by others at times called occult primary ovarian insufficiency (OPOI).

We demonstrated that, assuming similar levels of DOR, DHEA was similarly effective at all ages, though younger women with POA demonstrate small advantages [2].

By itself, DHEA is neither panacea nor miracle drug, but used as part of a well-integrated diagnostic and therapeutic approach, it significantly improves pregnancy and delivery chances, even for women with very severe DOR. We so far have established close to 50 clinical

How to Improve Your ART Success Rates, ed. Gab Kovacs. Published by Cambridge University Press.

pregnancies in women with anti-mullerian hormone (AMH) below 0.4 ng/mL, many with undetectable levels of AMH (< 0.1 ng/mL).

Utilization of DHEA has remained controversial for lack of prospectively randomized studies. For lack of recruitable patients, we had to abandon two attempts to conduct such studies, one in New York City and the other in collaboration with colleagues in Europe [2]. However, in absence of Level I evidence, studies with Level II evidence can, and should, suffice to recommend treatment. We and others have reported on over a thousand DHEA supplemented patients, utilizing case control and other study formats. Moreover, Wiser *et al.* recently did report a first small, prospectively randomized clinical trial of DHEA supplementation, confirming its effectiveness in improving pregnancy chances with IVF [3].

Experimental use of DHEA

Some proposed applications, in our opinion, should still be considered experimental. Though they warrant further exploration, this should be done under study protocols and with appropriate informed consent. Mamas and Mamas, for example, reported a small case series of patients with alleged premature ovarian failure (POF), also called primary ovarian insufficiency (POI) [6]. Some of these patients, however, were actually not POF but POA patients.

Their claim of spontaneous pregnancies in POF/POI patients after DHEA supplementation, therefore, requires confirmation. Our center currently is conducting a prospectively randomized study of POF/POI patients (registration number NCT00948857). Enrollment is slow, and only one spontaneous pregnancy has so far been recorded.

Our center is also currently conducting a prospectively randomized study of women with so-called unexplained infertility (registration number NCT00650754), investigating whether DHEA-induced improvements in ovarian function may result in spontaneous pregnancies in such patients.

Finally building on the observations that DHEA reduces embryo aneuploidy [4] and miscarriage rates [5] in DOR patients, a similar effect can, possibly, be also anticipated in normally fertile females at older ages. The investigation of DHEA as a supplement to decrease aneuploidy among normal older patients, akin to folic acid for prevention of neural tube defects, therefore, would seem useful.

Diagnosis of DOR

Everything, of course, begins with timely and correct diagnosis. Even in competent fertility centers, and especially in younger women, a diagnosis of POA is frequently overlooked. This can be avoided if, in addition to follicle stimulating hormone (FSH), other ovarian reserve (OR) parameters are utilized. At our center, this is AMH, which especially in younger women demonstrates better specificity than FSH (see also Chapter 1).

Even more importantly, however, we utilize age-specific normal ranges for FSH and AMH to define DOR. This is a crucial distinction to the practice still widely followed in most IVF centers, which uses standard cut-offs for all ages. Figure 17.1 demonstrates our center's age-specific normal ranges for FSH and AMH, based on age-specific 95% CIs. As the figure demonstrates, women with normal age-specific OR should, until age 45, never reach a cut off of 10.0 mIU/mL, a level still widely utilized to define DOR at all ages. Indeed, up to age 35, ca. 8.0 mIU/mL should not be exceeded.

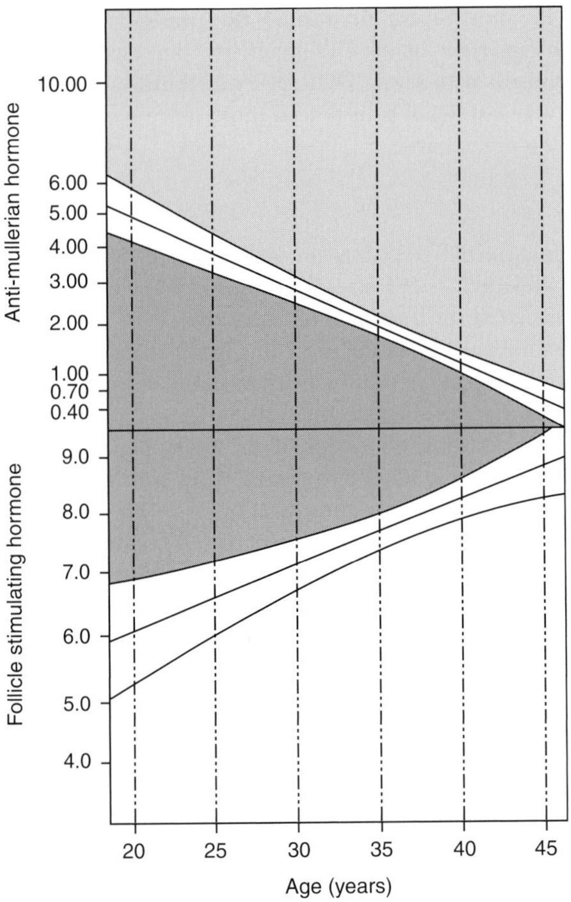

Figure 17.1 Age-specific anti-mullerian hormone (AMH) and follice stimulating hormone (FSH) levels.

Age-specific AMH and FSH levels are based on 95% CIs of levels in each age group. Patients used to establish these cut offs were infertile women with considerable prevalence of diminished ovarian reserve (DOR). Presented values are, therefore, only applicable to our center's patient population. Centers with lower prevalence of DOR, likely, have to consider slightly higher AMH and lower FSH cut offs than shown here. Ideally, age-specific values should be established in fertile populations.

As the figure also demonstrates, normal ranges for AMH are narrower than those of FSH. While the literature does not agree on specific cut-offs, below which women are defined as DOR patients, normal age-specific ranges decline in parallel to rising normal age-specific FSH ranges, as women age. So, for example, an AMH 1.0 ng/mL reflects normal between 40 and 43 years, an age range where most women are already considered to suffer from DOR. Our center defines DOR as any AMH level below the 95th CI for age.

We also reported that, independent of female age, AMH of 1.05 ng/mL denotes a rather well-defined borderline between mild and more severe DOR. Anti-mullerian hormone above this level, following DHEA supplementation, offers significantly higher pregnancy and live birth chances at all ages.

Accurate and timely diagnosis, of course, allows for timely treatments (we below outline our approach to ovarian stimulation). Timely treatment means DHEA supplementation of at least six weeks prior to IVF cycle start and appropriately selected ovarian stimulation, resulting in timely adjustments of stimulation protocols, fewer poor quality ovarian stimulations, and cycle cancellations. As always explained to patients, our center treats *ovarian*, not *chronological*, ages of patients.

This kind of full integration of diagnosis, DHEA pretreatment, ovarian stimulation, and other treatment options (see below) then leads to improved pregnancy chances and better live birth rates in patients with even the most severe forms of DOR. Considering the low pregnancy chances and high miscarriage risks of all DOR patients, but especially the extremely poor outcome chances of patients with severe DOR, every established pregnancy is especially 'valuable.' Attention to every last detail is of crucial importance if every additional oocyte and/or embryo can make a difference.

Treatment protocols

We prescribe pharmaceutical grade micronized DHEA at an oral dosage of 25 mg TID. Patients initiate treatment at least six weeks before IVF start, and continue supplementation until a second, normally rising pregnancy test (or treatment termination).

Most patients are primed with estradiol patches, in the preceding luteal phase, ca. 10–12 days prior to ovarian stimulation start. Our center's routine ovarian stimulation involves a microdose agonist protocol (Lupron, 50 ug SQ bid), starting on day 2, and followed by ovarian stimulation with gonadotropins, starting on day 4 of the cycle. Gonadotropin dosages in DOR patients vary from a minimum of 450 IU to 600 IU daily, with all given as FSH, except for 150 IU of human menopausal gonadotropins (hMG).

The rest of IVF cycle management follows routine criteria, except that our center does not require minimum follicle numbers to reach retrieval. Especially in women with DOR, already on maximal stimulation, we consider cancellation ineffective since better outcomes in subsequent cycles are unlikely.

Since findings of abnormal autoimmunity are frequent amongst IVF patients, especially in association with POA, all DOR patients receive a daily baby aspirin and 10 mg of prednisone. In the presence of established autoimmunity, a prophylactic dose of heparin or lovenox (exoxaparin) is added, starting the day after egg retrieval.

All patients receive intravaginal and intra-muscular progesterone support in the luteal phase, based on our understanding that the functionally 'older' ovary requires more progesterone support.

Treatment outcomes

We previously noted that in matched studies at our center, DHEA-supplemented patients with DOR repeatedly outperformed controls in practically all IVF outcome parameters [2]. This has now also been confirmed by other investigators, including in a first prospectively randomized clinical trial in Israel [3].

It, therefore, should not surprise that DHEA objectively improves OR, as assessed by AMH [7]. Indeed, amongst patients who achieve pregnancy after DHEA supplementation, a large majority can be found amongst those who demonstrate improvements in AMH values with DHEA treatment. Improving AMH values, therefore, represent a positive prognostic sign during DHEA supplementation [7].

We also already noted that close to 50 pregnancies in DHEA-supplemented women with very low AMH levels (undetectable levels, defined as < 0.1 ng/mL, up to maximally 0.4 ng/mL) have so far been established. This, by itself, represents a remarkable achievement, as women with such minimal OR, currently, at most centers, are not entered into treatment with use of autologous oocytes. Even more remarkable, however, was the observation that these pregnancies were only rarely miscarried, corresponding to the previously noted observation that miscarriages in DOR patients on DHEA supplementation, in general, are surprisingly rare [5].

Revising the concept of ovarian aging

That DHEA apparently reduces embryo aneuploidy and miscarriage rates in women with DOR is not only clinically important. This observation also mandates reconsideration of the current understandings of ovarian aging. Under current dogma, oocytes women are born with 'age' as women age. Such aged oocytes are then at increased risk for non-dysjunctional events, leading to more aneuploidy and, consequently, more spontaneous pregnancy loss. Current understanding, therefore, places oocytes at the center of ovarian aging.

It would, however, appear unreasonable to assume that any therapeutic intervention can still nurse back to health already damaged oocytes. The fact that DHEA achieves lower embryo aneuploidy and miscarriage rates is, therefore, not comprehendible under the current ovarian aging concepts.

Searching for a hypothesis of ovarian aging that would explain such DHEA abilities, only one possible explanation appears reasonable: ovarian aging cannot be oocytes-based, since, considering these DHEA effects, one has to assume availability of practically undamaged oocytes. Only healthy, 'young' oocytes can lead to approximately 15% miscarriage rates, reported after DHEA supplementation, and representing average spontaneous pregnancy loss in normal, fertile, average populations [5].

Considering options further, a model of ovarian aging arises, which no longer assumes aging oocytes as women age. To the contrary, this new model assumes that, while still unrecruited, primordial follicles remain 'ageless.' Follicles entering maturation after recruitment, therefore, do so with, in principle, ageless oocytes. The reason why older women produce oocytes of poorer quality, characterized by more non-dysjunctional events, is, instead, their aging ovarian environment in which follicle maturation takes place.

Ovarian aging is, thus, not characterized by, a-priori, aging oocytes but by aging ovarian environments, which in secondary fashion adversely affect maturing oocytes.

While the possibility of rescue of already damaged oocytes by DHEA appears highly unlikely, improvements of aging ovarian environments by supplementation with DHEA appear as a perfectly reasonable scenario, which, in secondary fashion, of course, will also impact oocyte quality, aneuploidy risk, and, ultimately, miscarriage rates.

There is a significant decline in DHEA in all people with advancing age, and the overwhelming importance of androgens for normal follicle maturation has only recently been well demonstrated in a mouse model.

Under such a modified concept of ovarian aging, DHEA should be seen as only a forerunner for a whole new class of fertility medications, which, finally, after 50 years of concentration on only the last two weeks of follicle maturation (the gonadotropin-sensitive stage), hopefully, will focus on the preceding months. Significant additional progress in treating women with DOR can then be expected.

Conclusion

The utilization of DHEA not only improves treatment results in women with DOR but also leads to a modified understanding of the ovarian aging process. Considering already published outcome data and the modified model of ovarian aging presented here, DHEA, likely, is only a forerunner of a completely new class of medications with potential to reconstitute aging ovarian environments. Should this concept be proven correct, a revolution in the treatment of DOR will significantly prolong reproductive lives of older women.

References

1. Casson PR, Lindsay MS, Pisarska MD, Carson SA, Buster JE. Dehydroepiandrosterone supplementation augments ovarian stimulation in poor responders: a case series. *Hum Reprod* 2000;**15**;2129–32.

2. Barad DH, Brill H, Gleicher N. Update on the use of dehydroepiandrosterone supplementation among women with diminished ovarian function. *J Assist Reprod Genet* 2007;**24**:629–34.

3. Wiser A, Gonen O, Ghetler Y, *et al.* Addition of dehydroepiandrosterone (DHEA) for poor-responder patients before and during IVF treatment improves the pregnancy rate: A randomized prospective study. *Hum Reprod* 2010;**25**:2496–2500.

4. Gleicher N, Weghofer A, Barad D. Increased euploid embryos after supplementation with dehydroepiandrosterone (DHEA) in women with premature ovarian aging. *Fertil Steril* 2007;**88**(Suppl1):S232

5. Gleicher N, Ryan E, Weghofer A, Blanco-Mejia S, Barad DH. Miscarriage rates after dehydroepiandrosterone (DHEA) supplementation in women with diminished ovarian reserve: a case control study. *Reprod Biol Endocrinol* 2009;**7**:108.

6. Mamas L, Mamas E. Premature ovarian failure and dehydroepiandrosterone. *Fertil Steril* 2009;**91**:644–6.

7. Gleicher N, Weghofer A, Barad DH. Improvement in diminished ovarian reserve after dehydroepiandrosterone supplementation. *Reprod Biomed Online* 2010;**21**:360–5.

Chapter 18

Luteinizing hormone supplementation in ART

Colin M. Howles

Introduction

Exogenous gonadotropins can be applied to treat anovulation or to stimulate multiple follicular development in women who are candidates for ART. Although both follicle-stimulating hormone (FSH) and luteinizing hormone (LH) are involved in the natural menstrual cycle, the use and benefit of exogenous LH in protocols for ovarian stimulation in ART has long been subject to discussion [1]. In part, this is due to the widespread use of gonadotropin-releasing hormone (GnRH) long agonist protocols for pituitary downregulation. Such protocols can result in levels of LH similar to those seen in hypogonadotrophic hypogonadism (HH), defined by LH levels ≤ 1.2 IU/L, for which exogenous LH supplementation is recommended [2].

More recently, GnRH antagonist protocols have become more widely used in ART. As both LH and oestradiol levels may fall substantially during GnRH antagonist protocols, it has been suggested that LH supplementation may have benefit, but the evidence to date is limited.

In this chapter, the author will provide a concise overview with the aim of demonstrating that in unselected patient populations there is no benefit, whilst in women classified as poor or hyporesponders to FSH and those of advanced reproductive age (i.e., those aged ≥ 35 years), LH supplementation can improve ART outcomes.

Folliculogenesis and hormonal regulation of ovulation in the menstrual cycle

The classic 'two cell – two gonadotropin' model proposed that both FSH and LH are required for oestradiol synthesis; LH binds to theca cells to induce synthesis of androgens, which diffuse out into the circulation and into the granulosa cells where, through the FSH-stimulated action of aromatase, they are converted to oestrogen. This theory was subsequently revised to take into account the induction of granulosa cell LH receptor expression by FSH during advanced stages of antral follicular development. Thus, LH regulates and integrates both granulosa and theca cell function during late preovulatory development. At this stage, FSH and LH work together to induce local production of growth factors needed for the paracrine regulation of follicular maturation and a lack of either gonadotropin may be compensated for by higher levels of the other. Luteinizing hormone may exert a beneficial effect on oocytes via its effects on cumulus cells, which play a vital role in the maturation of oocytes during folliculogenesis, and has been shown to reduce the apoptosis rate of cumulus

How to Improve Your ART Success Rates, ed. Gab Kovacs. Published by Cambridge University Press.

cells, thereby prolonging their duration of support for the developing oocyte, increasing its chances of fertilization and subsequent implantation. During natural menstrual cycles, FSH levels initially rise and then, primarily under the influence of oestradiol, decline, whereas LH is secreted in pulses, rising during the mid-follicular phase of the cycle. In 1987, to explain the monthly production of one oocyte by most women of reproductive age, Baird proposed that, during the intercycle rise in FSH levels, a threshold is reached and the 'window of recruitment' is opened to allow projection of the largest, healthiest follicle for ovulation, whilst the remaining follicles become atretic.

The LH ceiling and threshold

The concept of an LH ceiling was proposed by Hillier in 1994 [3] and has been confirmed by others [4]. High LH doses have been associated with poor oocyte quality, reduced fertilization rates, reduced rate of embryo implantation, and a high rate of miscarriage. Evidence for an LH threshold comes from a multicenter study of women with HH by the European Recombinant Human LH Study Group, published in 1998 [2], which showed that an LH dose of ≥ 75 IU was needed for optimal follicular maturation in most cases.

The role of LH in HH

Luteinizing hormone supplementation is mandatory for normal, healthy follicular development and oocyte maturation in patients with HH, as demonstrated by significantly lower efficacy of stimulation with FSH alone compared with FSH plus LH in a study by the European Recombinant Human LH Study Group [2]. Based on these results, a product containing a fixed combination of recombinant human FSH (r-hFSH) and r-hLH in a 2:1 ratio (Pergoveris®, Merck Serono S. A. – Geneva, Switzerland [an affiliate of Merck KGaA, Darmstadt, Germany]) has been developed for follicular maturation in women with severe gonadotropin deficiency [5].

The role of exogenous LH in ART

Supplementation with LH can be provided through treatment with recombinant human LH (r-hLH) or urinary derived human menopausal gonadotropin (hMG). Even in so-called 'purified' hMG, in addition to FSH and LH, there are non-specific proteins extracted from the urine of postmenopausal women. Human chorionic gonadotropin (hCG), which has LH-like activity but a longer half-life, is added to the preparation to standardize the two gonadotropins in a 1:1 ratio. The advantages of r-hLH are its purity and precision and flexibility of dosing [5].

There have been two meta-analyses published comparing the utilization of r-hLH plus FSH vs FSH alone in women co-treated with GnRH agonists and antagonists in ART protocols and these will now be reviewed. In addition, the first systematic review and the most recent meta-analysis published on hMG vs r-hFSH will also be considered.

Women treated with GnRH agonist and antagonist protocols

In women undergoing pituitary down-regulation with GnRH agonist long protocols, LH levels can fall to below those that characterize HH. As an alternative to GnRH agonists, GnRH antagonists may be administered at any time during the early or mid-follicular phase of a treatment cycle to prevent a premature LH rise. Protocols that use GnRH antagonists in the late follicular phase induce a sharp decrease in serum LH levels. The need for LH supplementation in these women has been debated and results from different studies have been conflicting and inconclusive.

An early Cochrane systematic review of four randomized controlled trials comparing r-hFSH and hMG protocols in young normogonadotrophic women undergoing a GnRH agonist long protocol performed in 2003 (1214 women) found no differences between treatments in pregnancy and live birth rates or secondary outcomes [6]. In the most comprehensive meta-analysis performed to date (16 studies involving 4040 women), treatment with hMG resulted in fewer oocytes (−1.54; 95% CI −2.53 to −0.56; $p < 0.0001$) compared to r-hFSH and a higher total dose of hMG was necessary (mean difference, 235.46 IU/L [95% CI 16.62–454.30; $p = 0.03$]; standardized mean difference, 0.33 [95% CI 0.08–0.58; $p = 0.01$]). Finally, the pregnancy relative risk and absolute risk differences for *fresh transfers* were not significantly different [7]. These authors also explore in some detail the results from previous meta-analyses and conclude that there is clear heterogeneity.

In 2007, a systematic review and meta-analysis of seven studies (701 women representing a normal in vitro fertilization/intracytoplasmic sperm injection [IVF/ICSI] population) was performed in which supplemental LH was given to women treated with FSH and GnRH analogues (five studies with agonists and two with antagonists); it concluded that the addition of LH did not improve the live birth rate or other secondary endpoints [8].

In the same year (2007), a Cochrane systematic review of 14 trials compared r-hLH plus r-hFSH vs r-hFSH in IVF/ICSI in 2612 women; 11 trials involving 2396 women used a GnRH agonist and three trials used a GnRH antagonist. There was no evidence of a statistical difference in pregnancy outcomes when r-hLH was used [9]. However, the authors stated that pooled pregnancy estimates may not have been significant due to the small numbers and that results suggested a beneficial effect of co-treatment with r-hLH with respect to pregnancy loss and poor responders (see Figure 18.1).

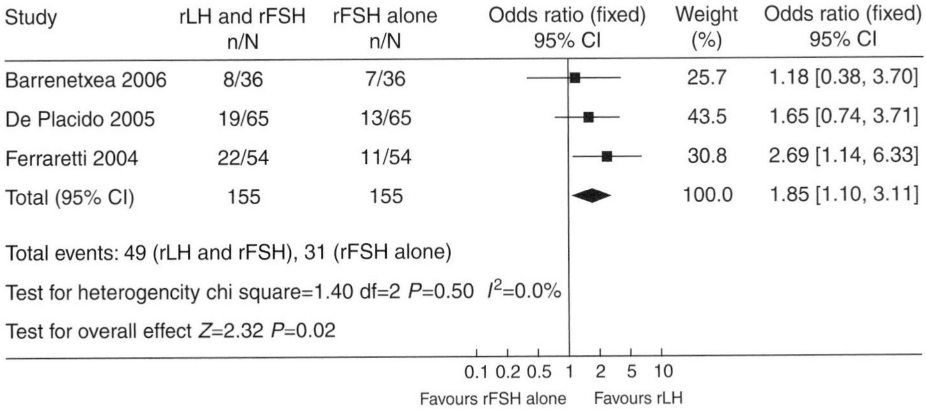
Study
rLH and rFSH n/N
rFSH alone n/N
Odds ratio (fixed) 95% CI
Weight (%)
Odds ratio (fixed) 95% CI
Barrenetxea 2006
8/36
7/36
25.7
1.18 [0.38, 3.70]
De Placido 2005
19/65
13/65
43.5
1.65 [0.74, 3.71]
Ferraretti 2004
22/54
11/54
30.8
2.69 [1.14, 6.33]
Total (95% CI)
155
155
100.0
1.85 [1.10, 3.11]
Total events: 49 (rLH and rFSH), 31 (rFSH alone)
Test for heterogencity chi square=1.40 df=2 P=0.50 I²=0.0%
Test for overall effect Z=2.32 P=0.02
0.1 0.2 0.5 1 2 5 10
Favours rFSH alone
Favours rLH

Figure 18.1 Analysis of ongoing pregnancy rates in randomized trials comparing recombinant FSH alone versus recombinant FSH plus recombinant LH for controlled ovarian stimulation in GnRH agonist downregulated IVF or ICSI treatment cycles in poor responders. Reproduced with permission from Mochtar *et al.* The Cochrane Collaboration [9]. Copyright © Cochrane Collaboration.

CI, confidence interval; FSH, follicle-stimulating hormone; GnRH, gonadotropin-releasing hormone; ICSI, intracytoplasmic sperm injection; IVF, in vitro fertilization; LH, luteinizing hormone.

Women with a suboptimal response to FSH

It has been reported that in about 10–15% of young women, ovarian response to r-hFSH stimulation in the GnRH agonist protocol is suboptimal, despite the presence of normal FSH and/or LH circulating levels (for review see Alviggi [10]). Poor responders to FSH are those in whom an insufficient follicular growth results in cycle cancellation or retrieval of less than four oocytes. Additionally, a higher incidence of an LH-beta variant polymorphism has been reported in women who demonstrate a hyporesponse to FSH [10]. Unlike poor responders, hyporesponders to FSH have normal follicular development up to days 5–7, but this response plateaus on days 8–10 [10]. A significant improvement of a suboptimal response to r-hFSH by r-hLH supplementation was first reported in a study of 12 women (17 cycles) who had required high doses of r-hFSH during previous cycles for follicles to mature sufficiently. In this study, supplementation with r-hLH significantly increased fertilization and clinical pregnancy rates.

Other studies of women hyporesponsive to FSH have also shown that the clinical response to FSH treatment can be improved by LH supplementation [10]. In such women, LH supplementation has been shown to be more effective in terms of ovarian stimulation outcomes (number of oocytes retrieved and mature oocytes) than increasing the FSH dose. In these women, an LH dose of 150 IU was better than a 75 IU dose. Supplementation with LH was also shown to be better than hMG supplementation in terms of clinical outcomes, as well as being associated with a lower total FSH dose requirement [10].

Women of advanced reproductive age (≥ 35 years)

It is well documented that the likelihood of successful outcomes decreases progressively in women over the age of 35 years and poor ovarian response to stimulation becomes more common in this age group as the ovaries become less sensitive to FSH and LH with increasing age [11]. Supplementation with LH in this subgroup has been tested in a series of studies; however, not all supported improved outcomes [12].

In a prospective randomized study, involving 231 normogonadotrophic women undergoing ART with GnRH agonist co-treatment, a subgroup aged ≥ 35 years who received exogenous LH supplementation had significantly increased implantation rates [13]. Similarly, results from another randomized study have shown improved clinical pregnancy rates with LH supplementation compared with FSH alone in women aged ≥ 35 years and undergoing their first assisted reproduction cycle [14]. A recent randomized study in women undergoing co-treatment with a GnRH agonist for ICSI and aged 35–39 years reported significantly higher rates of implantation and live birth per started cycle in those given r-hLH supplementation from the mid-stimulation phase [15].

In a further large, single-center, randomized controlled trial, 333 women aged < 36 years and 292 women aged 36–39 years undergoing a first or second IVF cycle received pre-treatment with an oral contraceptive pill and a GnRH antagonist following FSH or FSH plus LH administration. In this study, supplementation with 75 IU/day LH was shown to significantly increase implantation rates in the older but not the younger women OR 1.56, 95% CI 1.04–2.33, $p = 0.03$) [16]. A trend towards a better pregnancy rate was also observed (OR 1.37, 95% CI 0.86–2.18, $p = 0.18$).

Conclusion

In women with HH, it is generally accepted that LH supplementation is needed for normal, healthy follicular development, and oocyte maturation. In a general population of normogonadotrophic women undergoing ART, irrespective of whether a GnRH agonist or GnRH antagonist is co-administered, the addition of r-hLH to treatment protocols does not appear to provide any additional benefits. Subgroups of normogonadotrophic women who may receive benefit from r-hLH supplementation for IVF and ICSI include the following: women aged ≥ 35 years and women who are hyporesponsive to FSH. The latter group of women may be further identified by specific genetic biomarkers that are currently being investigated.

References

1. Chappel SC, Howles C. Reevaluation of the roles of luteinizing hormone and follicle-stimulating hormone in the ovulatory process. *Hum Reprod* 1991;**6**:1206–12.
2. European Recombinant Human LH Study Group. Recombinant human luteinizing hormone (LH) to support recombinant human follicle-stimulating hormone (FSH)-induced follicular development in LH- and FSH-deficient anovulatory women: a dose-finding study. *J Clin Endocrinol Metab* 1998;**83**:1507–14.
3. Hillier SG. Current concepts of the roles of follicle stimulating hormone and luteinizing hormone in folliculogenesis. *Hum Reprod* 1994;**9**:188–91.
4. Balasch J, Fabregues F. LH in the follicular phase: neither too high nor too low. *Reprod Biomed Online* 2006;**12**:406–15.
5. Bosch E. Recombinant human FSH and recombinant human LH in a 2:1 ratio combination: a new tool for ovulation induction. *Exp Rev Obstet Gynecol* 2009;**4**:491–8.
6. van Wely M, Westergaard LG, Bossuyt PM, van der Veen F. Human menopausal gonadotropin versus recombinant follicle stimulation hormone for ovarian stimulation in assisted reproductive cycles. *Cochrane Database Syst Rev* 2003: CD003973.
7. Lehert P, Schertz JC, Ezcurra D. Recombinant human follicle-stimulating hormone produces more oocytes with a lower total dose per cycle in assisted reproductive technologies compared with highly purified human menopausal gonadotrophin: a meta-analysis. *Reprod Biol Endocrinol* 2010;**8**:112.
8. Kolibianakis EM, Kalogeropoulou L, Griesinger G, *et al.* Among patients treated with FSH and GnRH analogues for in vitro fertilization, is the addition of recombinant LH associated with the probability of live birth? A systematic review and meta-analysis. *Hum Reprod Update* 2007;**13**:445–52.
9. Mochtar MH, van der Veen F, Ziech M, van Wely M. Recombinant luteinizing hormone (rLH) for controlled ovarian hyperstimulation in assisted reproductive cycles. *Cochrane Database Syst Rev* 2007: CD005070.
10. Alviggi C, Mollo A, Clarizia R, De Placido G. Exploiting LH in ovarian stimulation. *Reprod Biomed Online* 2006;**12**:221–33.
11. Weissman A, Howles CM. Treatment strategies in assisted reproduction for the low responder patient. In: Gardener E, Weissman A, Howles CM, Shoham Z, editors. *Textbook of Assisted Reproductive Techniques*. 3rd ed. London: Informa Healthcare, 2008.
12. Fabregues F, Creus M, Penarrubia J, *et al.* Effects of recombinant human luteinizing hormone supplementation on ovarian stimulation and the implantation rate in down-regulated women of advanced reproductive age. *Fertil Steril* 2006;**85**:925–31.
13. Humaidan P, Bungum M, Bungum L, Yding Andersen C. Effects of recombinant LH supplementation in women undergoing assisted reproduction with GnRH agonist down-regulation and stimulation with recombinant FSH: an opening study. *Reprod Biomed Online* 2004;**8**:635–43.
14. Marrs R, Meldrum D, Muasher S, *et al.* Randomized trial to compare the effect of recombinant human FSH (follitropin alfa)

with or without recombinant human LH in women undergoing assisted reproduction treatment. *Reprod Biomed Online* 2004;**8**:175–82.

15. Matorras R, Prieto B, Exposito A, *et al.* Mid-follicular LH supplementation in women aged 35–39 years undergoing ICSI cycles: a randomized controlled study. *Reprod Biomed Online* 2009;**19**:879–87.

16. Bosch E, Labarta E, Simón C, Remohi J, Pellicer A. Impact of luteinizing hormone supplementation on gonadotropin releasing hormone antagonist cycles: an age-adjusted analysis. *Fertil Steril* 2011;**95**(3):1031–6.

Chapter 19

The use of growth hormone in IVF

Luk Rombauts

Introduction

Since the introduction of IVF three decades ago, outcomes have steadily improved to the point where IVF units can now reliably offer most of their patients high implantation rates. Unfortunately, poor responders have not benefited to the same degree. This group of patients is still very difficult to manage and many strategies have been explored to improve their pregnancy rates. One such strategy is the use of growth hormone (GH) as an adjuvant for controlled ovarian stimulation (COH) during IVF treatment.

Mode of action

Growth hormone is a 191-amino acid, single-chain polypeptide. It is produced, stored, and secreted by the somatotroph cells in the anterior pituitary gland.

The secretion of GH is principally under the control of two hypothalamic hormones. Growth hormone releasing hormone (GHRH) up-regulates the GH gene transcription and somatostatin has an inhibitory effect on the secretion of GH by the pituitary gland. Ghrelin, a gut-derived hormone, potentiates the release of GH by simultaneously facilitating the release of hypothalamic GHRH and inhibiting the action of somatostatin at the level of the pituitary [3].

Growth hormone secretion is pulsatile with prolonged periods of low serum GH concentrations between peaks. Testing for GH deficiency has therefore relied heavily on standardized stimulation tests, which allows for a better discrimination between normal and GH-deficient subjects. Studies have shown that intra-abdominal fat mass is the most important negative predictor of peak GH levels, while lean body mass was not significantly associated with GH status. Age, gender, and physical fitness also influence the peak levels, but to a lesser extent. A slow decline in serum GH concentrations is seen with aging [3].

Pituitary GH release stimulates the secretion of insulin-like growth factor 1 (IGF-1, formerly known as somatomedin C), primarily by the liver after which it enters the circulation to reach its target tissues. Growth hormone can also stimulate the production of IGF-1 within the target organs itself, so IGF-1 can thus be considered both an endocrine and a paracrine/autocrine mediator [3].

In addition to stimulating the growth of the long bones in children and adolescents, growth hormone has many other physiological effects, some of which include increased calcium retention, increasing muscle mass, gluconeogenesis, and lipolysis.

How to Improve Your ART Success Rates, ed. Gab Kovacs. Published by Cambridge University Press.

Rationale for IVF

The ovary is another peripheral target organ for IGF-I. Granulosa cells secrete IGF-1 following stimulation by GH, FSH, and estradiol. The role of intrafollicular IGF-1 is to regulate granulosa cell function by augmenting the actions of FSH, such as granulosa cell proliferation, the secretion of estradiol and inhibin, and the synthesis of LH receptors. IGF-1 also exerts a paracrine role by up-regulating basal and LH-stimulated theca cell production of androgens and progesterone [2].

There is also clinical evidence that GH may play a role in folliculogenesis and oocyte development. The concentration of different follicular fluid hormones correlates with the ability of human oocytes to form morphologically normal and implantation-competent embryos. Higher follicular fluid concentrations of GH are associated with rapid cleavage, good embryo morphology, and a high embryo implantation potential. Mendoza *et al.* also reported lower follicular fluid GH concentrations in older women [5].

The rationale of GH administration during COH in IVF is therefore based on the assumption that increased serum concentrations of GH will increase the secretion of IGF-1 by the ovary, leading to a cascade of intrafollicular events which all converge to promote oocyte development and maturation.

Approved medical use

Recombinant human GH (hGH) is believed to be safe when it is used in the paediatric management of growth insufficiency and adult growth hormone deficiency. Adult GH-deficient patients treated with hGH experience decreased body fat, increased muscle mass, energy levels, bone density and sexual function, and improved immune system function.

Medical treatment with hGH may result in negative side-effects such as joint swelling, joint pain, and carpal tunnel syndrome and sleep loss, which are reversible and not usually associated with short-term use. Long-term use is also associated with an increased risk of diabetes.

Pharmaceutical recombinant hGH is a powder and must be stored in a refrigerator. It is reconstituted with bacteriostatic water just prior to injection. In the initial GH studies doses of 16.5 IU were divided into three doses per week. Smaller and more frequent doses are now advocated as equally effective whilst causing less side effects. Generally, lower doses such as 4–8 IU per week are prescribed and are divided into two doses per day for six days a week. The dose should be individualized and it is often recommended to start with a dose of 0.5 IU s.c. per day and to slowly increase the dosage in 0.5 IU monthly increments as required.

Use of GH in IVF

There have been a number of small randomized controlled trials (RCTs) performed to date and two systematic reviews have critically analyzed and summarized our current knowledge on the topic. The two systematic reviews are broadly in agreement with each other.

The first systematic review is by Kyrou *et al.* [4]. They performed a review of the literature to evaluate any interventions aimed at improving pregnancy rates in poor responders undergoing IVF. Many different strategies were analyzed, but the one that appeared to be the most beneficial was the addition of GH during the COH phase of IVF treatment. They included five studies with a total of 182 women. A subset of four studies including 82 couples allowed them to analyze the summary point estimate for the birth rate which they calculated to be more than five-fold increased following GH treatment (OR 5.22, 95% CI 1.09–24.99).

Table 19.1 Growth hormone (GH) versus placebo

	OR	95%CI
Routine use		
Live birth rate per woman	1.32	0.40–4.43
Pregnancy rate per woman	1.78	0.49–6.50
Poor responders		
Live birth rate per woman	5.39	1.89–15.35
Pregnancy rate per woman	3.28	1.74–6.20

Adapted from Duffy *et al.* [1]. Odds ratios > 1 favour GH treatment.

The most recent meta-analysis is an update by Duffy *et al.* [1] of a previously published Cochrane review. A total of 440 subfertile couples were included from 10 studies they retained after critical review. Their results showed no difference in outcome measures and adverse events for the use of adjuvant GH in IVF protocols in unselected patients. Restricting the meta-analysis to poor responders, however, indicated a statistically significant difference in both live birth rates and pregnancy rates favouring the use of adjuvant growth hormone (OR 5.39, 95% CI 1.89–15.35 and OR 3.28, 95% CI 1.74–6.20 respectively). Importantly, no increase was seen in adverse events.

Both systematic reviews provide evidence that adjuvant GH treatment during IVF may increase the live birth rate in poor responders. It is important, however, to clarify a number of points.

All of the randomized trials that have been carried out to date are small. The number of patients recruited in each study ranged from only 14 to 61. In addition, women over the age of 40 years were excluded from all but one study.

There is also the question of administration and drug dosing. Some RCTs administered hGH on a daily basis whereas others administered the drug on alternate days. There was also significant variability in the dose when the different studies were compared: the dose of hGH ranged from 8 IU to 24 IU s.c. per day. Although the administration of hGH during COH only lasts approximately two weeks, the doses used in the studies are high compared with hGH regimens for approved clinical use. This raises the question of possible risks and side-effects, neither of which have been documented adequately in the RCTs to date.

Significant heterogeneity between studies was also due to differing definitions of a poor responder, making it hard to determine which subset of patients would benefit most. The reasons for poor ovarian response are indeed poorly understood, and it is likely that they vary significantly from patient to patient. Despite these difficulties Duffy *et al.* [1] attempted a sub-group analysis that showed that women who are considered poor responders because of previous sub-optimal response had a statistically significantly higher pregnancy rate, but it failed to provide evidence for an improved live birth rate with GH. This was more likely due to the fact that only 2 studies with a total of 38 patients were available for this subanalysis.

Future challenges

At best, the available evidence so far on adjuvant GH treatment during IVF is suggestive of a positive impact on ART outcomes in poor responders, but not for the routine patient.

However, the confidence intervals around the odds ratios derived from the latest meta-analysis indicate that there is still a large amount of uncertainty. More studies of better quality and larger size are required to increase our overall confidence that the addition of hGH to COH really improves the healthy take-home baby rate, the outcome that matters most to IVF patients.

Such a study is now under way, spearheaded by Professor Rob Norman from the Robinson Institute in Adelaide. The LIGHT (Live birth, In vitro fertilization and Growth Hormone Treatment) study is an Australian and New Zealand multicenter randomized, double blind placebo-controlled study assessing the effect of recombinant human growth hormone on live birth rates in women who are poor responders undergoing an IVF/ICSI cycle (ANZCTR Number: ACTRN12609001060235).

Patients will be eligible if they are between 18 and 40 years old with a body mass index of < 32 kg/m^2, require IVF/ICSI treatment, have never recorded an FSH level of > 15 IU/L and currently have regular spontaneous menstrual cycles between 21 and 35 days in length. They still should have both ovaries and have had a previous IVF/ICSI cycle resulting in the collection of less than five oocytes.

The study aims to overcome several of the shortcomings of previous studies. Most importantly the study is adequately sized to assess whether the live birth rates are indeed higher in poor responders when they add hGH to their stimulation protocol. A total of 389 women will be recruited (177 in each arm and allowing for a 10% dropout/cancellation rate). When completed this will almost double the number of assessable patients for a new Cochrane review update. The sample size of the study provides the power to detect an increase in live births from 10% to 20% (one-sided Fisher exact test at 5% significance level).

Great care went into the randomization design. The process will be performed by block randomization for each infertility center. Randomized patients will be sequentially allocated pre-numbered drug boxes. Growth hormone or placebo will be administered subcutaneously from day 1 of ovarian stimulation, until the day of the ovulation-triggering injection with recombinant human chorionic gonadotropin (hCG). All medical professionals will remain blinded to the drug allocation.

The study will randomize patients to a placebo or a daily GH dose of 12 IU for each day of FSH treatment. As mentioned before this dose is relatively high compared to the dose used in approved indications and it will thus be important to actively monitor and report adverse effects, serious adverse effects and congenital birth defects. In addition, an independent Safety and Monitoring Committee has been set up to ensure the safe conduct of the trial.

Conclusion

There is currently enough evidence to be moderately confident that adjuvant GH treatment for poor responders undergoing IVF/ICSI treatment results in higher delivery rates in this difficult patient group. Some caution is required, however, when interpreting the point estimates of this treatment effect. In the latest Cochrane review [1], the summary odds ratio suggests a more than five-fold increase in delivery rates in the hGH-treated patients. However, the very wide 95% confidence intervals indicate that there is great uncertainty about the real magnitude of the effect size. In the absence of adequate safety data this evidence should therefore be considered carefully with the patient before commencing hGH treatment. Fortunately, fertility specialists can look forward to the results of a large randomized, double blind placebo-controlled study which may bring more clarity in the not too distant future.

References

1. Duffy JMN, Ahmad G, Mohiyiddeen L, Nardo LG, Watson A. Growth hormone for in vitro fertilization (Review). *Cochrane Database Syst Rev* 2010:CD000099.
2. Hiller SG. Cellular basis of follicular endocrine function. In: Hillier SG, ed. *Ovarian Endocrinology*. Oxford: Blackwell Scientific Publications, 1991; 73–106.
3. Jørgensen JOL, Hansen TK, Møller N, Christiansen JS. Normal physiology of growth hormone in adults. In www.endotext.org website, updated February 27, 2007, Section Editor Ashley Grossman; published by MDText.com, Inc, S. Dartmouth, MA.
4. Kyrou D, Kolibianakis E, Venetis C, *et al.* How to improve the probability of pregnancy in poor responders undergoing in vitro fertilization: a systematic review and meta analysis. *Fertil Steril* 2009;**91**:749–66.
5. Mendoza C, Cremades N, Ruiz-Requena E, *et al.* Relationship between fertilization results after intracytoplasmic sperm injection, and intrafollicular steroid, pituitary hormone and cytokine concentrations. *Hum Reprod* 1999;**14**:628–35.

Chapter 20

Prevention of ovarian hyperstimulation syndrome

Mohamed Aboulghar

Introduction

Ovarian hyperstimulation syndrome (OHSS) is the most serious complication of ovulation induction. As OHSS has no definitive treatment, prevention has become the most important aspect of the management.

Identification of patients at risk of OHSS

The first step in prevention of OHSS is to identify patients at high risk of developing the syndrome. These include patients with a history of severe OHSS in a previous IVF cycle and patients diagnosed as having polycystic ovarian syndrome (PCOS). In a future IVF cycle for those patients, the lowest possible dose of follice stimulating hormone (FSH) should be given as a starting point. Patients should be closely monitored using ultrasound and serial serum estradiol (E2) measurements.

Type of GnRH analogue used for controlled ovarian stimulation

In two recent meta-analyses comparing the outcome of GnRH agonist versus antagonist, both showed that the incidence of OHSS was significantly reduced in the antagonist protocol. It seems logical that patients with a history of OHSS and patients who are considered at high risk of developing OHSS could be treated by a GnRH-antagonist protocol.

Prevention of OHSS in high-risk patients during stimulation

During ovarian stimulation, patients are considered at risk if a large number of follicles are visualized in both ovaries as well as increasing E2 levels, above 3000 pg/ml while the follicles are not ready for triggering ovulation. Preventive measures include several options.

Withholding human chorionic gonadotropin

Withholding human chorionic gonadotropin (hCG) and continuation of GnRHa will abolish the development of OHSS, but at the expense of cancelling the cycle, which creates a frustrating situation for both the physician and the patient. It is now uncommonly used, and is resorted to in rare circumstances when the risk is very high.

Coasting

Coasting is a technique which involves withdrawing exogenous gonadotropins and withholding hCG until the patient's serum E2 level decreases to a safer level. The technique of

How to Improve Your ART Success Rates, ed. Gab Kovacs. Published by Cambridge

coasting appeals to both physicians and patients, and it also allows for the timely transfer of fresh embryos. The timing of stopping of FSH and starting coasting is controversial. Mansour *et al.* reported in the largest study in the literature [1] coasting started according to the size of the leading follicles rather than the level of E2. When the leading follicles reached 15–16 mm in mean diameter and the E2 level was above 3000 pg/ml, FSH was stopped. The follicles continued to grow while the E2 first increased and then started falling down. We should wait until E2 falls to less than 3000 pg/ml before giving hCG. During coasting, the small immature follicles, being less receptive to FSH will undergo apoptosis.

The number of days without FSH that is needed before giving hCG varied from 2 to 9 days. It is believed that coasting should not be limited to an arbitrary number of days, instead, it should continue until E2 reaches a safe level. Prolonged coasting for four or more days significantly reduced the IVF pregnancy rate.

Coasting probably works by inducing apoptosis in the granulosa cells and reducing vascular endothelial growth factor (VEGF) protein secretion and gene expression.

Coasting has helped to reduce the incidence of OHSS markedly, however, complete prevention with coasting was not possible.

Intravenous albumin

Several randomized studies used 50 g albumin which was infused at the time of oocyte retrieval to prevent OHSS. There was a marked discrepancy in the results of different studies. Some studies showed that it is very effective, others showed it has no value in prevention of OHSS.

The effectiveness of human albumin administration in prevention of severe OHSS was published in a Cochrane review [2]. Seven randomized controlled trials were identified, five of which met the inclusion criteria and enrolled 378 women (93 in the albumin-treated group; 185 in the control group). There was significant reduction in severe OHSS on administration of human albumin (OR 0.28; 95% CI 0.11–0.73). Relative risk was 0.35 (95% CI 0.14–0.87) and absolute risk reduction was 5.5. For every 18 women at risk of severe OHSS, albumin infusion will save one more case.

A new update of the Cochrane review by the same group on the effectiveness and safety of administration of intravenous fluids as albumin, hydroxyethyl starch, Haemaccel and dextran in prevention of severe OHSS in IVF/intracytoplasmic sperm injection (ICSI) treatment cycles is currently in press in the Cochrane library.

Ten RCTs involving 2048 randomized women have been included in this review. There was no evidence of statistically significant difference in severe OHSS incidence after administration of human albumin (OR 0.72, 95% CI 0.49–1.06).There was a statistically significant decrease in severe OHSS incidence with administration of hydroxyethyl starch (three RCTs, OR 0.12, 95% CI 0.04–0.40).

It seems that the early enthusiasm on the value of IV albumin was based on small numbers of studies, on the other hand the value of hydroxyethyl starch in prevention of OHSS awaits further trials to confirm the preliminary positive results.

Triggering ovulation and OHSS

In a prospective randomized study which compared 2000 IU, 5000 IU, and 10 000 IU of hCG to trigger ovulation, there was no significant difference in number of retrieved oocytes between 5000 IU and 10 000 IU; however, 2000 IU yielded a significantly lower number of oocytes. It seems logical that the dose of hCG in patients at risk for OHSS should be only 5000 IU. On the other hand, in a recent pilot study, infertile patients at high risk of developing OHSS were given half the current minimum dose of hCG (i.e., 2500 IU). No women developed moderate or severe OHSS.

A low dose of hCG appears to reduce the incidence of OHSS without compromising success rates.

GnRH agonist for triggering ovulation

The longer half-life of hCG is associated with a sustained luteotrophic effect, and supra-physiological serum concentrations of oestradiol and progesterone throughout the luteal phase. A single GnRH-agonist injection (500 mg leuprolide acetate s.c.) resulted in a combined LH and FSH surge lasting 34 h. Therefore, the shorter duration of LH-like activity after GnRH agonist compared with hCG administration may indeed reduce stimulation of the ovary in the luteal phase. Most of the studies reported the protective effect of GnRH agonist administration for triggering ovulation hence reducing the incidence of OHSS.

A recent meta-analysis [3] showed that the use of GnRH agonist to trigger final oocyte maturation in IVF, in GnRH antagonist cycles, yields a number of oocytes capable of undergoing fertilization and subsequent embryonic cleavage, which is comparable to that achieved with hCG. However, the likelihood of an ongoing clinical pregnancy after GnRH-agonist triggering was significantly lower as compared with standard hCG treatment (OR 0.21; 95% CI 0.05–0.84; $p = 0.03$).

Dopamine agonists for prevention of OHSS

The administration of hCG leads to vascular permeability enhancement resulting in loss of fluid to the third space and the full blown syndrome as a consequence. Vascular endothelial growth factor has emerged as the main angiogenic factor responsible for increased vascular permeability.

The hCG action on vascular permeability can be reversed by SU5416, a VEGFR-2 inhibitor, providing new insights into the development of strategies to prevent and treat the syndrome. The dopamine agonist cabergoline can reverse VEGFR-2 and the increased vascular permeability.

The concept has been tested in humans and it was observed that cabergoline can significantly reduce the incidence of moderate OHSS as well as pelvic fluid accumulation and hemoconcentration when compared with placebo in oocyte donors at risk of OHSS. Implantation and ongoing pregnancy/live birth rates of IVF patients at risk of OHSS appear to not be affected by cabergoline administration. Cabergoline, however, has been associated with valvular heart disease when administered chronically in patients with Parkinson's disease.

Quinagolide is a non-ergot-derived dopamine D2 receptor agonist, with lack of effect on the serotonin (5-hydroxytryptamine [5-HT]) receptor subtype 5-HT2b at relevant concentrations. It is also differentiated by pharmacokinetic profile, with a much shorter half-life, thus minimizing exposure during organogenesis when used in an IVF setting. These two features make quinagolide an interesting dopamine agonist for use in prevention of OHSS. In the first randomized, double-blind study to evaluate the efficacy of three weeks of treatment with three different doses of quinagolide versus placebo in preventing the development of OHSS in patients undergoing COH for ART [4].

The incidence of moderate/severe early OHSS was 23% (12/53) in the placebo group and 12% (6/51), 13% (7/52) and 4% (1/26) in the quinagolide 50, 100 and 200 mg/day groups, respectively. The moderate/severe early OHSS rate was significantly lower with all quinagolide groups combined compared with placebo [$p = 0.019$; OR 0.28, CI 0.09–0.81)]. The incidence of ultrasound evidence of ascites among patients with no clinical pregnancy was significantly reduced from 31% (8/26) with placebo to 11% (8/70) with all quinagolide groups combined, although there was no difference for those with clinical pregnancy.

The use of GnRH antagonist

Recently it was shown in a retrospective uncontrolled study that GnRH antagonist administration resulted in a rapid reduction of oestradiol concentrations in women pretreated with long GnRH-agonist protocol, and suggested that this may reduce the incidence of OHSS. In a prospective randomized study comparing coasting ($n = 96$) and GnRH-antagonist administration ($n = 94$) plus one 75 IU ampoule of human menopausal gonadotropin (hMG) daily until the day of hCG administration in patients at risk of OHSS. The primary outcome measure was high-quality embryos. The secondary outcome measures were days of intervention, number of oocytes, pregnancy rate, number of cryopreserved embryos, and incidence of severe OHSS.

There were significantly more high-quality embryos (2.87 ±1.2 versus 2.21 ±1.1; $p < 0.0001$) and more oocytes (16.5 ±7.6 versus 14.06 ±5.2; $p = 0.02$) in the GnRH-antagonist arm as compared with the coasting arm. There were more days of coasting as compared with days of antagonist administration (2.82 ±0.97 versus 1.74 ±0.91; $p < 0.0001$). In conclusion, GnRH antagonist was superior to coasting in producing significantly more high-quality embryos and more oocytes as well as reducing the time until hCG administration. There was no significant difference in pregnancy rate between the two groups. No OHSS developed in either group. The shorter intervention period in the antagonist arm and the administration of a small dose of hMG continuously may maintain the granulosa cells and support the production of good-quality oocytes and embryos.

Metformin

The use of insulin-sensitizing agents, such as metformin, in women with PCOS who are undergoing ovulation induction of IVF cycles has been widely studied. Metformin was used by women undergoing IVF/ICSI for more than five weeks before and during treatment and during luteal phase. There was no significant difference in clinical pregnancy rate between both groups but there was significant reduction in the incidence of OHSS in the group taking metformin. In a randomized, placebo-controlled, double-blinded study. Patients with PCOS undergoing IVF/ICSI treatment using a long GnRH-agonist protocol were randomized to receive 850 mg metformin or placebo tablets twice daily from the start of the down regulation process until the day of oocyte collection. A significant decrease in the incidence of severe OHSS was observed (metformin 3.8%, placebo 20.4%; $p = 0.023$), and this was still significant after adjustment for body mass index, total recombinant FSH done and age (OR 0.15; 95% CI 0.03–0.76; $p = 0.022$).

A systematic review compared whether metformin co-administration with gonadotropins for IVF improves outcome in women with PCOS. Metformin co-administration to IVF treatment does not improve pregnancy rate (OR 1.29; 95% CI 0.84–1.98) or live birth (OR 2.02, 95% CI 0.98–4.14) rates but reduces the risk of OHSS (OR 0.21; 95% CI 0.11–0.41, $p < 0.00001$).

In conclusion, there is evidence that metformin reduces the incidence of OHSS in PCOS patients undergoing ovarian stimulation for IVF [5].

Conclusion

Prevention of OHSS during ovarian stimulation is the most important step in the management of this serious complication, which is associated with serious morbidity and possible mortality in a young healthy woman. Currently, there is no curative treatment of OHSS and the available treatment is symptomatic, hence prevention becomes an essential step in the management.

References

1. Mansour R, Aboulghar M, Serour G, Amin Y, Abou-Setta AM. Criteria of a successful coasting protocol for the prevention of severe ovarian hyperstimulation syndrome. *Hum Reprod* 2005;**20**:3167–2.
2. Aboulghar M, Evers JH, Al-Inany H. Intravenous albumin for preventing severe ovarian hyperstimulation syndrome: a Cochrane review. *Hum Reprod* 2002;**17**:3027–32.
3. Griesinger G, Diedrich K, Tarlatzis BC, Kolibianakis EM. GnRH-antagonists in ovarian stimulation for IVF in patients with poor response to gonadotrophins, polycystic ovary syndrome, and risk of ovarian hyperstimulation: a meta-analysis. *Reprod Biomed Online* 2006;**13**:628–38.
4. Busso C, Fernandez-Sanchez M, Garcia-Velasco JA, *et al.* The non-ergot derived dopamine agonist quinagolide in prevention of early ovarian hyperstimulation syndrome in IVF patients: a randomized, double-blind, placebo-controlled trial. *Hum Reprod* 2010;**25**:995–1004.
5. Tso LO, Costello MF, Albuquerque LE, Andriola RB, Freitas V. Metformin treatment before and during IVF or ICSI in women with polycystic ovary syndrome. *Cochrane Database Syst Rev* 2009;**15**: CD006105.

Chapter 21

Is in vitro maturation the best approach?

Baris Ata, Hai Ying Chen, Ayse Seyhan and Seang Lin Tan

Introduction

In vitro fertilization is regarded the most effective treatment of subfertility, with results achieved by most treatment centers exceeding spontaneous conception rates in healthy fertile couples. However, this has been achieved with the simultaneous transfer of multiple embryos. In order to generate multiple embryos controlled ovarian hyperstimulation (COH) with exogenous gonadotropins has become an integral part of IVF treatment. Unfortunately, COH is not without limitations. Firstly, the cost of drugs poses a substantial financial burden and at times prevents a couple's access to treatment. Secondly, COH requires frequent monitoring scans and creates further direct and indirect costs, loss of working time and inconvenience. Furthermore, the most important medical problem associated with COH is the risk of ovarian hyperstimulation syndrome (OHSS) which is a potentially lethal condition, most commonly occurring as an iatrogenic complication of COH. More recently, COH has been suggested to have detrimental effects on developing oocytes, embryos derived from these oocytes, and/or endometrial receptivity.

In vitro maturation (IVM), a technique which has the potential to provide the pregnancy rates of conventional IVF in selected cases while avoiding the risks and costs associated with COH, could be considered a better option. The small antral follicles present in the human ovary at every stage of the menstrual cycle harbor immature oocytes which can resume meiosis upon removal from the follicle. Collection and IVM of these already existing immature oocytes provides multiple mature oocytes that can be fertilized in vitro.

In vitro maturation techniques have improved since 1991, when the first live birth following transfer of embryos derived from immature oocytes collected from unstimulated ovaries was reported. Essentially, all assisted reproduction technology (ART) laboratory procedures can be performed with in vitro matured oocytes if the need arises. The first successful IVM cycles combined with preimplantation genetic screening and percutaneous testicular sperm aspiration have been reported by our team. The technique has enabled successful treatment of patients with empty follicle syndrome in previous stimulated IVF cycles. Patients can undergo several IVM cycles and we previously reported a series of patients who achieved repeated live births with IVM treatment. In vitro matured oocytes and embryos derived from them can be successfully cryopreserved. Currently, IVM pregnancy rates exceed 35% per cycle in appropriately selected patient groups.

At the McGill Reproductive Center monitoring of an IVM cycle starts with a baseline scan performed in the early follicular phase of the menstrual cycle, preferably between days

How to Improve Your ART Success Rates, ed. Gab Kovacs. Published by Cambridge

2 and 5 of a natural menstrual cycle or a withdrawal bleed, induced with progestogen administration in amenorrheic women. This is done to rule out the presence of an ovarian cyst or uterine pathology. A second scan is performed when it is anticipated that the largest follicle has reached 10–12 mm in diameter and the endometrial thickness is at least 6 mm. We have reported that the implantation and clinical pregnancy rates were the highest in cycles where human chorionic gonadotropin (hCG) was given when the leading follicle was 12 mm. We routinely administer hCG at a dose of 10 000 IU 38 hours before immature oocyte collection. We administer 150 IU/day of human menopausal gonadotropin (hMG) to women whose endometrial thickness was less than 6 mm on the day of the second scan and whose follicles were still small. The aim is to boost endogenous estrogen levels while supporting the growth of the follicles in the cohort. Given the shorter duration of proliferative phase in IVM cycles, we initiate estrogen on the day of oocyte collection and postpone progesterone supplementation to day of fertilization for luteal phase support.

We recently demonstrated similar aneuploidy rates in IVM embryos and IVF embryos. Once pregnancy is achieved, pregnancy outcome of IVM treatment is equivalent to IVF treatment outcome. In a retrospective analysis of 1581 women who had a positive pregnancy test following ART with IVM, IVF or intracytoplasmic sperm injection (ICSI) in our unit during a five-year period, pregnancy loss rates seem similar following IVM and conventional IVF (17.5% for IVM pregnancies, 17% for IVF, and 18% for ICSI pregnancies, $p = 0.08$). Although the clinical miscarriage rate was significantly higher in IVM pregnancies (25.3%) than in IVF (15.7%) and ICSI (12.6%) pregnancies ($p < 0.01$), the difference can be attributed to the higher incidence of polycystic ovarian syndrome (PCOS) among IVM patients. While only 8% and < 1% of women in the IVF and ICSI groups had PCOS, respectively, the incidence of PCOS in the IVM group was 80%. The clinical miscarriage rates in women with PCOS were statistically similar after IVM and after IVF (24.5% versus 22.2%, $p = 0.72$).

Obstetric outcomes including cesarean delivery rate, birth weight, incidence of low birth weight, and very low birth weight infants, APGAR scores were not found to be different between infants conceived with IVM or IVF. Currently available data suggest the incidence of congenital abnormalities is not increased with IVM. Compared with spontaneous conceptions, the observed odds ratios for any congenital abnormality were 1.42 (95% CI 0.52–3.91) for IVM, 1.21 (95% CI 0.63–2.32) for IVF and 1.69 (95% CI 0.88–3.26) for ICSI, respectively. The physical growth and neuromotor development of IVM children also appears to be similar to that of spontaneously conceived children.

Currently, IVM is not only a recognized treatment alternative for couples who need ARTs, but also is considered as an innovative fertility preservation method which extends the options for patients with various diseases that preclude treatment with conventional methods.

Potential advantages of IVM in different patient groups

High responders to ovarian stimulation

Young women with high antral-follicle counts achieve the highest pregnancy rates with IVM. Such women also have a high risk of OHSS following COH. Therefore IVM may be considered perhaps a better treatment option for women with polycystic ovaries (PCO) or PCOS who need treatment with ART. In 2009, we achieved an embryo implantation rate of 19.5% and a clinical pregnancy rate per embryo transfer of 55.2% in women with PCO or PCOS with an average age of 32.6 ± 3.6 years. Successful results have been reported by other centers around the world. Pregnancy rates seem to be significantly higher when an in vivo matured oocyte has been collected.

Normal responders to ovarian stimulation

The high pregnancy rates with IVF have been achieved with simultaneous transfer of multiple embryos, which has resulted in a tremendous increase in multiple pregnancies. In fact in the year 2006 approximately one third of all live births following ART in the USA were the result of a multiple infant delivery. Recognition of the disappointing obstetric and perinatal outcomes of these iatrogenic multiple pregnancies have led to both voluntary and in some countries legal restrictions in the number of transferred embryos per treatment cycle. The uptake of single embryo transfers is increasing, and advances in embryology, laboratory and cryopreservation technologies further encourage this 'transfer less' approach around the world. This fact renders the additional benefit of COH in ART cycles questionable. In vitro maturation has the potential to provide similar pregnancy rates following fresh embryo transfer with IVF if single embryo transfer is to become the norm. At least one in vivo matured oocyte is retrieved in a substantial proportion of IVM cycles. The possibility of repeating treatment in consecutive menstrual cycles in case of treatment failure can be considered another advantage of IVM.

Poor responders to gonadotropin stimulation

Some women develop very few mature follicles despite aggressive COS in repeated cycles with different protocols. For women in whom poor ovarian response does not seem to be due to a rectifiable cause inherent to the particular treatment cycle; i.e., inappropriate choice of stimulation protocol, skipped medication, etc., justification of trying other stimulated cycles is questionable and IVM may provide a better option in such cases.

When gonadotropin stimulation fails to provide the desired number of in vivo matured oocytes in women with genuinely decreased ovarian reserve, IVM in an unstimulated cycle or combined with natural-cycle IVF may provide a reasonable option. In fact, in eight women with a poor response, defined as ≤ four follicles growing or oocytes collected in a previous stimulated IVF cycle, we achieved a similar number of embryos available for transfer in the subsequent IVM cycle. Six women reached embryo transfer (75%), and one achieved a live birth, yielding a 16.7% live birth rate per transfer in this small group of genuine poor responders.

Oocyte donation

Oocyte donors routinely undergo COH in order to maximize the number of mature oocytes available for donation. However, COH puts young donors with high ovarian reserve under a high risk of OHSS. The inconvenience of the numerous injections required and concern by some women about risk of cancer associated with repeated use of ovulation induction drugs cause reluctance on the part of some potential oocyte donors. In vitro maturation provides a good option for oocyte donation cycles as young women with high antral follicle counts comprise the best candidates for IVM and yield good pregnancy rates. Avoiding ovarian stimulation decreases the risks and inconvenience for oocyte donors. We collected on average 12.8 immature oocytes from 12 oocyte donors with a mean age of 29 years. Sixty-eight per cent of the oocytes matured in vitro and 62 embryos were available for transfer to 12 recipients with a mean age of 37.7 years. On average, four embryos were transferred (range 2–6) and a clinical pregnancy rate of 50% was achieved. Two women had first-trimester miscarriages while four had healthy live births, yielding a live birth rate of 33%.

Fertility preservation

In vitro fertilization and embryo cryopreservation (EC) is the only method of female fertility preservation that is endorsed by the American Society of Clinical Oncology and American Society of Reproductive Medicine. However, conventional IVF and embryo cryopreservation most importantly requires a male partner, takes 2–5 weeks to complete, and produces relatively high estradiol levels, which may be deleterious in certain hormone sensitive malignancies. In vitro maturation expands the fertility preservation options for women who are not candidates for IVF – EC for various reasons. Women with hormone-sensitive tumors may undergo immature oocyte collection and cryopreserve resultant embryos. In addition to eliminating the need for expensive drugs and the inconvenience of injections, IVM enables oocyte retrieval at any phase of the menstrual cycle and completion of the fertility preservation procedure in 2–10 days, preventing a delay in treatment of the primary disease.

We reported three women without male partners seeking fertility preservation prior to chemotherapy, who presented for the first time in the luteal phase of their menstrual cycle and were to undergo gonadotoxic treatment immediately. Five to seven immature oocytes were recovered with luteal-phase oocyte retrieval from these patients. Three to five MII oocytes were vitrified following IVM. Two of these three women later underwent one and two more collections, respectively, in the follicular phase of the next cycle(s) and additional immature oocytes were vitrified following IVM. Recently, similar maturation and fertilization rates have been reported for immature oocytes collected in follicular phase or luteal phase of the menstrual cycle.

Immature oocytes can also be collected from ovarian biopsy specimens and can be vitrified following IVM. This combination of ovarian-tissue cryobanking and IVM represents a new strategy for fertility preservation. We retrieved 11 immature oocytes from a wedge resection specimen in a 16-year-old patient with mosaic Turner syndrome (20% 45XO and 80% 46XX karyotype). Eight of these oocytes were vitrified following IVM. In 4 women with cancer, we harvested 11 immature and 8 mature oocytes from wedge biopsy specimens. Eight of the 11 immature oocytes reached MII stage following IVM and were vitrified.

In vitro maturation combined with embryo or oocyte vitrification provides previously unavailable options for some patients and improves the services provided by a fertility preservation program.

Conclusion

Although IVM is a relatively new technology, clinical experience with this technique is rapidly increasing. Patients who are at high risk of OHSS, those with unexpectedly hyper- or poor responses during COH, those with recurrent unexplained IVF failures, as well as those who are facing imminent gonadotoxic chemotherapy can benefit from advantages of IVM. In the era of mild approaches and single embryo transfers the additional benefit of stimulated IVF is being questioned. At least one in vivo matured oocyte is collected in a substantial proportion of IVM cycles. This number is significantly increased in women who have been given low dose gonadotropins for 1 to 3 days. These facts suggest that IVM can be a viable option for the regular normo-responder women as well. Currently, IVM represents the least invasive and the simplest option for ART patients, and with further improvement in success rates, it can become the 'ultimate' patient-friendly protocol.

References

1. Son WY, Chung JT, Herrero B, *et al.* Selection of the optimal day for oocyte retrieval based on the diameter of the dominant follicle in hCG-primed in vitro maturation cycles. *Hum Reprod* 2008;**23**:2680–5.
2. Zhang XY, Ata B, Son WY, Buckett WM, Tan SL, Ao A. Chromosome abnormality rates in human embryos obtained from in-vitro maturation and IVF treatment cycles. *Reproductive BioMedicine Online* 2010;**21**:552–9.
3. Buckett WM, Chian RC, Holzer H, Dean N, Usher R, Tan SL. Obstetric outcomes and congenital abnormalities after in vitro maturation, in vitro fertilization, and intracytoplasmic sperm injection. *Obstet Gynecol* 2007;**110**:885–91.
4. Buckett WM, Chian RC, Dean NL, *et al.* Pregnancy loss in pregnancies conceived after in vitro oocyte maturation, conventional in vitro fertilization, and intracytoplasmic sperm injection. *Fertil Steril* 2008;**90**:546–50.
5. Demirtas E, Elizur SE, Holzer H, *et al.* Immature oocyte retrieval in the luteal phase to preserve fertility in cancer patients. *Reprod Biomed Online* 2008;**17**:520–3.
6. Maman E, Meirow D, Brengauz M, *et al.* Luteal phase oocyte retrieval and in vitro maturation is an optional procedure for urgent fertility preservation. *Fertil Steril* 2011;**95**:64–7.
7. Huang JY, Tulandi T, Holzer H, Tan SL, Chian RC. Combining ovarian tissue cryobanking with retrieval of immature oocytes followed by in vitro maturation and vitrification: an additional strategy of fertility preservation. *Fertil Steril* 2008;**89**:567–72.

Chapter 22

How to monitor for best results

Jack Yu Jen Huang, Hey-Joo Kang and Zev Rosenwaks

Over the past decade, we have witnessed remarkable improvements in pregnancy success rates following IVF. While many attribute this progress to innovations in the IVF laboratory, one cannot over-emphasize the fact that refinements in our approach to and optimization of ovarian stimulation protocols have also played critical roles. Experience has shown that a philosophy which encompasses individualized, moderate stimulation protocols yields the best outcomes. This approach involves the selection of an appropriate (individualized) controlled hyperstimulation (COH) protocol, careful monitoring of follicle growth and serum estradiol (E_2) levels, adjustment of gonadotropin dosage to avoid hyper-response, and individualized timing of human chorionic gonadotropin (hCG) administration. We believe that such an intensive monitoring approach during ovarian stimulation results in improved oocyte and embryo quality and higher implantation and pregnancy rates. Most importantly, this approach reduces the incidence of complications, especially ovarian hyperstimulation syndrome (OHSS).

In this chapter, we will describe our approach to and strategies of monitoring and selecting ovarian stimulation protocols, all aiming at optimizing IVF outcomes.

Individual patient characteristics guide the initial stimulation protocol

The central question when designing an initial IVF protocol builds upon whether the patient will likely be a good or poor responder to exogenous gonadotropin therapy. Since there is no single predictive marker of ovarian reserve, a constellation of factors is used to reach this decision.

The history and physical exam provide the first building blocks in protocol design. Patient age, reproductive history, parity, and cycle regularity all contribute to an assessment of response to gonadotropin therapy. For example, parous women have an improved prognosis and may require less aggressive stimulation. In the setting of oligo or amenorrhea, systemic evaluation should be undertaken to sort out hypothalamic from ovarian etiologies. The physical exam should focus on body mass index (BMI), evidence of hirsutism, and coexistent thyroid disorders. A BMI in either extreme can portend an exaggerated response to gonadotropins, whether in the setting of a low BMI and hypogonadotropic hypogonadism or obesity with evidence of hirsutism suggesting polycystic ovarian syndrome.

Transvaginal ultrasounds can provide objective evidence of ovarian reserve through an assessment of ovarian volume as well as antral follicle count (AFC). If the patient is

How to Improve Your ART Success Rates, ed. Gab Kovacs. Published by Cambridge
 University Press.

mid-follicular or in the luteal phase, a proper assessment of AFC can be challenging. Hence, an assessment in the succeeding follicular phase may be necessary before determining total gonadotropin dose.

Information from hormonal assays is the final step in building an initial stimulation protocol. Day 3 testing with normative values of follicle stimulating hormone (FSH) < 12 mIU/ml and E_2 levels < 70 pg/ml can assist in predicting response to gonadotropin therapy. Although E_2 is not an independent ovarian reserve marker, a high level may suppress FSH values as well as signal early recruitment of a dominant follicle. More recently, anti-Müllerian hormone (AMH) has been found to be a convenient and effective predictor of ovarian reserve. AMH is produced by preantral and small antral follicles and correlates with size of the residual follicular pool (see Chapter 1). Levels are independent of FSH and E_2 concentrations and vary minimally within and between menstrual cycles. There is currently no universal agreement on the threshold value for AMH as a predictor of ovarian response or pregnancy outcome, therefore normative values should be established within each endocrine laboratory.

The aggregate of the history, physical exam, AFC and hormonal assays predicts a good or poor responder and should be the basis of designing an initial IVF protocol. Ovarian reserve testing should not be used to deny treatment, but rather to help predict prognosis and guide choice of treatment.

Designing a stimulation protocol for the good responder

Once an individual is deemed a good responder, the focus of stimulation is judicious administration of an initial gonadotropin dose to mitigate the risk of OHSS. When determining the correct starting dose, one should remember that there are minimal consequences to erring on the conservative side. When necessary, one can increase the gonadotropin dosage on day 3 of stimulation in the setting of low E_2 levels without compromising oocyte yield or pregnancy outcomes. Conversely, the consequences of administering extremely high gonadotropin doses at the start of stimulation cannot always be reversed even with dose reduction later on in the follicular phase.

Dual suppression with oral contraceptive pills (OCPs) for three weeks in the preceding cycle while overlapping the third week with a gonadotropin-releasing hormone (GnRH) agonist assists in diminishing recruitment of a large cohort of antral follicles (see Figure 22.1). In addition, close monitoring of potential hyper-responders is necessary to titrate and adjust the gonadotropin dosage. Despite these efforts, if an exaggerated response is seen, "coasting" – withholding gonadotropins while continuing a GnRH agonist – is used to starve the smaller follicles while allowing larger, more mature follicles to develop. We have found that coasting for more than five days is associated with reduced oocyte yields and lower pregnancy rates.

For hyper-responders at risk of developing OHSS, who are being stimulated with GnRH agonist/gonadotropin protocols, reducing the ovulatory hCG trigger dose should be considered. Individualization of hCG dose has been based on the E_2 levels on the day of hCG as follows: 5000 IU for E_2 levels of 1500 to 2000 pg/ml; 4000 IU in patients with levels between 2000 to 2500 pg/ml and 3300 IU for E_2 levels greater than 2500 but less than 3000 pg/ml. When E_2 levels exceed 3000 pg/ml, the decision to administer hCG or cancel the cycle should be made with consideration given to coexistent risk factors. hCG should generally be withheld when E_2 levels exceed 3500 pg/ml as patient safety is paramount.

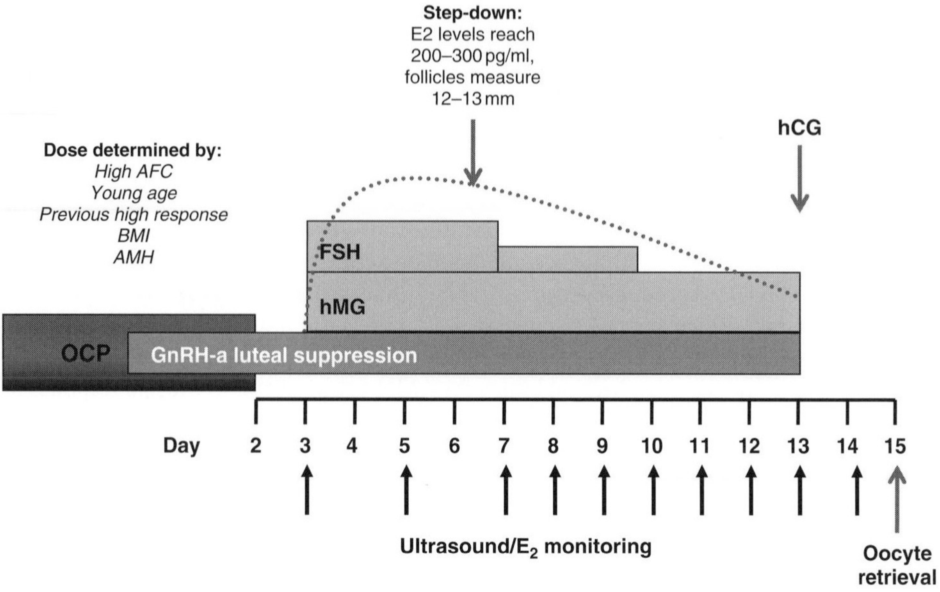

Figure 22.1 A typical oral contraceptive pill (OCP)/gonadotropin – releasing hormone (GnRH) agonist dual suppression gonadotropin stimulation protocol. Starting and step-down dosages are individualized according to patient characteristics and response. (Dotted line represents theoretical follicle stimulating hormone (FSH) levels).

In lieu of the dual suppression protocol, some patients who are predicted to be high responders are candidates for a low-dose 75–150 IU gonadotropin/GnRH antagonist protocol (see Figure 22.2). Although this protocol has traditionally been reserved for poor responders, there are several advantages to utilizing them in good responders. Antagonist protocols reduce the duration of stimulation and cumulative number of injections. This in turn reduces the physical and psychological treatment burden and has been shown to result in fewer patient dropouts without compromising pregnancy rates.

Indeed, antagonist protocols have been increasingly applied to good responders due to their added advantage of diminishing the risk of OHSS. More importantly, gonadotropin ovarian stimulation with GnRH antagonist luteinizing hormone (LH) suppression allows the option of triggering ovulation with either hCG or a GnRH agonist. It has been demonstrated that OHSS can be prevented by replacing hCG with a bolus injection of a GnRH agonist in GnRH antagonist protocols. The mechanism of action by which this approach prevents OHSS is rapid luteolysis. Whereas hCG levels (and LH activity) following a single 10 000 unit hCG bolus remain in the circulation for 7–10 days, endogenous LH levels after GnRH agonist trigger return to pre-injection baselines within 24–48 hours. However, there are drawbacks to using the GnRH agonist as the sole ovulatory trigger. GnRH agonists may not be effective in patients with overly suppressed LH secretion or those with hypothalamic amenorrhea. These subjects often fail to elicit an adequate LH response resulting in cycle cancellations or the retrieval of mostly immature oocytes. Moreover, when applied to autologous oocyte cycles, the use of GnRH agonist alone for ovulation trigger appears to be associated with lower

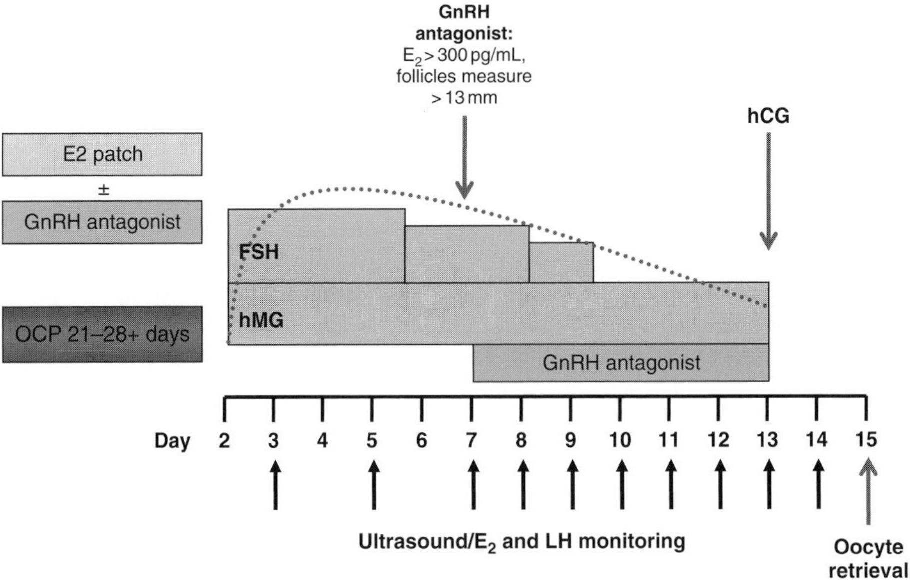

Figure 22.2 Step-down gonadotropin ovarian stimulation protocol with gonadotropin – releasing hormone (GnRH) antagonists. Pre-treatment with estradiol, GnRH antagonist or oral contraceptive pill (OCP) is dependent on patient characteristics. [Dotted line represents theoretical follicle stimulating hormone (FSH) levels].

clinical and ongoing pregnancy rates as well as an increase in pregnancy losses. Presumably, the poor results are related to impaired steroid secretion and luteal phase defects.

In an effort to reduce the potential drawbacks of the GnRH agonist ovulatory trigger, we have explored the use of concomitant hCG at doses between 1000–2500 units to supplement the post trigger LH activity. We have found that oocyte yields, pregnancy, and live birth rates are comparable to those seen following traditional hCG trigger. Thus, the "dual GnRH agonist/1500 IU hCG trigger" appears to be effective in promoting final oocyte maturation and providing adequate luteal support while reducing the risk of OHSS.

Designing a stimulation protocol for the poor responder

Controlled ovarian hyperstimulation protocols for poor responders are designed to improve the overall hormonal milieu, optimize concordant follicle growth, and prevent early follicle selection. Poor responders often exhibit an earlier rise in FSH levels in the late luteal phase, which can result in recruitment of fewer follicles and discordant follicle growth. Luteal E_2 administration can be utilized to suppress FSH secretion in order to minimize early selection of a single follicle and promote homogeneity of follicular growth during gonadotropin stimulation. This approach appears to improve synchronous follicle development in women with elevated baseline FSH levels. When FSH suppression with E_2 is found to be inadequate or when follicular heterogeneity persists, concomitant administration of GnRH antagonists in the late luteal phase may be more effective (see Figure 22.2).

The OCP-microdose flare protocol is another commonly applied COH strategy for poor responders. The oral contraceptive pill is administered for 14–21 days. Twice daily microdose Lupron (MDL) (40 ug) is started on the third day following the last dose of OCP. High dose gonadotropin (300 to 450 IU) stimulation is started on the third day of MDL. The proposed advantage of MDL is its usefulness in stimulating endogenous FSH release without increasing ovarian androgen production or rescuing the corpus luteum of the antecedent cycle.

In the standard "co-flare" protocol, 1 mg of leuprolide acetate is administered on cycle day 2 to cycle day 4. This protocol takes advantage of the initial activation of pituitary GnRH receptors and the consequent rise of endogenous gonadotropins, which augments the stimulatory impact of administered gonadotropins. High dose gonadotropin (300–450 IU) stimulation is usually started on cycle day 3. Theoretical concerns about the co-flare protocol are related to the enhanced ovarian androgen production and corpus luteum rescue, all of which can potentially affect oocyte quality and pregnancy rates.

In general, total gonadotropin dose should not exceed 450 IU in women with BMI of less than 25. For obese women without evidence of polycystic ovarian disease, it may be prudent to raise the total gonadotropin dose to 600 IU/day in efforts to reduce the risk of cycle cancellation.

Hormonal assessment and cycle monitoring

Pre-cycle assessment

Baseline blood work and pelvic ultrasound are performed on menstrual cycle day 2 for patients treated with GnRH antagonist protocols and on menstrual cycle day 3 for patients treated with the long GnRH agonist protocols. Normal baseline parameters include FSH less than 13 mIU/ml, radioimmunoassay (RIA) E_2 less than 75 pg/ml, and progesterone less than 1 ng/ml. Pelvic ultrasound is performed to evaluate endometrial thickness, assess the AFC and the presence of ovarian cysts. Based on this collective data, the final protocol and starting gonadotropin dose should be reassessed to optimize IF outcomes.

Management techniques for patients with elevated FSH or E_2 levels include cycle cancellation or delay of treatment start with administration of OCP for a period of two weeks. In these instances, luteal priming with estrogen patches and GnRH antagonist should be considered for subsequent IVF cycles.

The management of an ovarian cyst is based on its size stability, any prior known pathologic tissue diagnosis, and production of estrogen. While the presence of a small, simple appearing cyst with an E_2 level less than 70 pg/ml may not warrant cycle cancellation, the presence of functional ovarian cysts with elevated E_2 levels has been shown to adversely affect IVF outcomes. Management options include cancellation of cycle, administration of GnRH antagonist for 3–5 days until resolution of the cyst or treatment with OCP for 2–4 weeks.

We have recently shown that a thickened baseline endometrial stripe, defined as greater than 5 mm, on day 3 in long GnRH-agonist protocol is associated with reduced implantation, clinical pregnancy, and live birth rates. Compared to cycles where stimulation began on day 3, cycles where starts were delayed for 3–4 days to allow for endometrial sloughing had significantly higher clinical pregnancy (49% versus 37%) and live birth (39% versus 22%) rates.

Monitoring of follicle growth and hormonal levels

In an initial IVF cycle, patient response to COH is verified after 2–3 days of gonadotropin stimulation. Occasionally an early exaggerated E_2 response requires immediate reduction in gonadotropin dosage. Most commonly, the gonadotropin dose remains unchanged for the first 4–5 days in order to allow the gonadotropin threshold to reach a steady state. Once a steady state is established and E_2 levels reach 200–300 pg/ml – concomitant with lead follicle (s) size of 12–13 mm – we begin to reduce the gonadotropin dose in a step-down manner (see Figure 22.1). Initially, we reduce the dose by 25%, although in some instances it can be dropped by 50% from the initial starting doses. The step-down protocol appears to pharmacologically mirror FSH dynamics of the natural cycle. It endeavors to promote larger follicles to grow in a relatively low FSH milieu while starving the smaller follicles, thus improving synchronization of follicular development. An additional but equally important advantage of the step-down protocol is its potential for reducing the incidence of OHSS. In this context, assessing steady rising E_2 levels confirms progressive follicular growth. In women undergoing GnRH antagonist ovarian stimulation protocols, we routinely monitor serum LH levels to ensure that premature luteinization has not occurred.

Timing of hCG injection

The timing of hCG injection should be individualized based on several factors, including follicle diameter, E_2 level, prior cycle response, and embryo quality within the context of the particular COH protocol. For good responders in an initial IVF cycle, hCG is administered when two lead follicles reach 17 mm in average diameter. For patients on a combined clomiphene citrate/gonadotropin protocol, hCG is administered when the lead follicular diameter is 19–20 mm in average diameter.

If the initial IVF cycle has failed, a careful review of the response to stimulation, oocyte yield, maturity rating, and embryo quality should be undertaken. In patients exhibiting poor oocyte/embryo quality especially in the presence of a high proportion of polyspermic fertilization, one should be suspicious of oocyte post maturity. This is particularly true when all or almost all the retrieved oocytes are mature (metaphase II oocytes). In such circumstances, the patient may benefit from triggering ovulation at smaller lead follicle diameters in subsequent cycles. This approach has been highly successful in improving oocyte/embryo quality and achieving pregnancy. Patients should be informed of the plan and given an explanation for earlier hCG administration, but should also be cautioned that such an approach may yield fewer mature oocytes. On the other hand, in patients where mostly immature oocytes are retrieved, consideration should be given to delay hCG administration in the subsequent cycle. In these cases, the protocol should be adjusted in anticipation of additional stimulation days and aiming at higher E_2 levels. Another important parameter for administrating hCG is a plateau or doubling of E_2 levels on consecutive days after the lead follicle(s) has reached ≥ 16 mm in diameter. Moreover, should this be observed in an unsuccessful cycle, consideration should be given to administering hCG at smaller follicle diameters in the succeeding cycle.

Monitoring following hCG injection

We measure serum E_2 and hCG levels, follicular diameter and endometrial thickness on the day following hCG injection. In patients who were triggered with GnRH agonist alone or with a dual hCG/GnRH agonist trigger, serum LH is also measured. Serum hCG and LH levels serve as quality assurance measure to ensure hCG and GnRH agonist have been administered properly. In the event that appropriate levels of hCG or LH are not observed, a repeat dose is given and serum E_2 and hCG levels are assessed the following day. If the E_2

level decreases by greater than 30%, consideration should be given to cycle cancellation, as this could be a harbinger of poor IVF outcome.

Patients with E_2 levels greater than 3000 pg/ml on hCG day or E_2 levels greater than 4000 pg/ml on the day after hCG are monitored closely for signs and symptoms of OHSS. Evaluation on the third, and when appropriate, the fifth day following oocyte retrieval is performed. This evaluation includes a complete physical examination, measurement of waist circumference, weight, pelvic ultrasound for ovarian size, and presence of ascites. In addition, evaluation of hematocrit, liver enzymes, and kidney function tests are assessed. If the patient exhibits signs of early OHSS, it is prudent to cryopreserve all viable embryos and avoid pregnancy.

Conclusion

The success of IVF treatment can be optimized by adopting an individualized, patient-centered approach to COH. Key components involve selection of appropriate COH protocol, close monitoring of follicle growth and serum E_2 levels, adjustment of gonadotropin dose to avoid hyper-response, and individualized timing of hCG injection. This approach to IVF can improve oocyte and embryo quality, pregnancy and implantation rates, and most importantly, minimizes the risk of OHSS. The cost-effectiveness of such intensive monitoring during COH has been questioned. However, we believe close monitoring during COH is paramount to ensuring patient safety and should be adopted as the standard of care.

References

1. Davis OK, Rosenwaks Z. Superovulation strategies for assisted reproductive technologies. *Semin Reprod Med* 2001;**19**:207–12.
2. Kligman I, Rosenwaks Z. Differentiating clinical profiles: predicting good responders, poor responders, and hyperresponders. *Fertil Steril* 2001;**76**:1185–90.
3. Chen D, Burmeister L, Goldschlag D, Rosenwaks Z. Ovarian hyperstimulation syndrome: strategies for prevention. *Reprod Biomed Online* 2003; 7:43–9.
4. Macklon NS, Stouffer RL, Giudice LC, Fauser BC. The science behind 25 years of ovarian stimulation for in vitro fertilization. *Endocr Rev* 2006;**27**:170–207.
5. Fauser BC, Diedrich K, Devroey P. Predictors of ovarian response: progress towards individualized treatment in ovulation induction and ovarian stimulation. *Hum Reprod Update* 2008;**14**:1–14.
6. Huang JYJ, Rosenwaks Z. Preventive strategies of ovarian hyperstimulation Syndrome. *J Exp Clin Med* 2010;**2**:53–62.

Chapter 23

Sperm selection for assisted conception

R. J. Aitken

Introduction

The development of safe, effective, efficient methods for the isolation of human spermatozoa is a major feature of current research into the optimization of assisted conception therapy. The objective of such research is to deliver methods that will efficiently generate populations of motile, functional spermatozoa that are competent to fertilize the oocyte in vitro and initiate normal embryo development. If sperm quality is so seriously impaired that conventional fertilization is impossible, then the sperm isolation procedure should be competent to recover spermatozoa that are, at least, capable of supporting normal embryonic development following intracytoplasmic sperm injection (ICSI).

The methods that have been used to isolate sperm populations for assisted conception purposes include: (1) repeated cycles of centrifugation (typically 600 *g* for five minutes) and resuspension with a simple culture medium; (2) swim-up from a washed pellet; (3) swim-up (or swim down) from semen followed by a centrifugation and resuspension step to remove any traces of seminal plasma; (4) centrifugation through discontinuous density gradients composed of media such as Percoll® (colloidal silica coated with polyvinyl pyrrolidone), Puresperm® or ISolate® (colloidal silica with covalently bound silane), and (5) a recently introduced electrophoretic method [1, 2]. In addition, a variety of procedures, including filtration through columns containing glass wool, glass beads, or Sephadex, are available for further purifying the sperm suspensions once they have been isolated using the above techniques. In addition, treatment with magnetic Dynabeads® or ferrofluids coated with anti-CD45 monoclonal antibodies has been used to rid sperm suspensions of contaminating leukocytes [3]. Assessment of which of these techniques is the most appropriate for clinical application depends upon an understanding of the fundamental principles underpinning their effectiveness as sperm isolation strategies.

Basic principles of sperm isolation

Fundamental to the process of sperm isolation is an awareness of the vulnerability of human spermatozoa to oxidative stress. These cells are vulnerable to such damage because they are well endowed with targets for oxidative attack, particularly polyunsaturated fatty acids (50% of the fatty acid in a human sperm cell is docosahexaenoic acid with six double bonds per molecule) and DNA. The vulnerability of these highly specialized cells is further compounded by the limited volume and restricted distribution of cytoplasmic space which, in

How to Improve Your ART Success Rates, ed. Gab Kovacs. Published by Cambridge University Press.

somatic cells, would house critical antioxidant defence enzymes such as catalase, superoxide dismutase, or glutathione peroxidase [1, 4]. Because of this inherent vulnerability, spermatozoa are highly reliant on the antioxidant properties of the extracellular fluids in which they are bathed to provide antioxidant protection. It is for this reason that seminal plasma has evolved into one of the most powerful antioxidant fluids known to man.

Such antioxidant protection is necessary because, at the moment of ejaculation, spermatozoa come into contact with leukocytes for the very first time. Although the source of these leukocytes is still the subject of debate, it is highly likely that they enter the seminal plasma via the urethra and secondary sexual glands. Every human semen sample is contaminated with leukocytes, a majority of which are neutrophils and macrophages that are actively generating reactive oxygen species (ROS) [5]. Thus, whatever sperm isolation protocols we use we should try to ensure that spermatozoa and leukocytes do not come into contact with each other without the protection afforded by seminal plasma. It is for this reason that sperm preparation techniques that involve the isolation of spermatozoa directly from seminal plasma, whether this is discontinuous gradient centrifugation, swim-up from unfractionated semen, or electrophoretic separation, usually generate sperm populations that are more motile and functional than those prepared by repeated centrifugation or swim-up from a washed pellet [1, 6]. With the latter techniques, the spermatozoa are suddenly exposed to a free radical attack originating from the seminal leukocyte population in the absence of antioxidant protection. Furthermore, some culture media, such as Hams F10, are supplemented with transition metals, such as iron, that only exacerbate the oxidative stress experienced by the spermatozoa by promoting the lipid peroxidation reactions that have such a devastating effect on sperm function [7].

Even when sperm populations have been isolated direct from seminal plasma on Percoll gradients, or to a lesser extent by swim-up, they may still be contaminated with leukocytes. A detailed assessment of leukocyte contamination in sperm preparations submitted for ART demonstrated that around 30% of such preparations were still contaminated with leukocytes. Moreover the level of leukocyte contamination detected in such samples was negatively associated with fertilization rates following IVF [8].

If, even after preparing sperm samples directly from semen in the recommended manner, leukocyte contamination is still a problem, there are three major courses of action that might be pursued:

1) detect the leukocytes using a simple, sensitive chemiluminescent assay employing formyl peptides or opsonized zymosan as a stimulant and then, if these cellular contaminants are present, use magnetic beads coated in anti-CD45 (the common leukocyte antigen) to effect their removal [3].
2) Incorporate antioxidants into the medium to counteract the negative impact of leukocyte contamination. In this context, glutathione, N-acetylcysteine, hypotaurine, and catalase have all been shown to exert a protective effect in vitro [9].
3) Supplement the medium with reagents such as EDTA, DETAPAC or apotransferrin in order to chelate cytotoxic transition metals and neutralize the stimulatory impact of ROS on lipid peroxidation.

DNA damage

In times past, it was envisaged that the only attribute of sperm quality that had to be preserved during sperm isolation was the capacity of these cells for fertilization. We now know that another important property that spermatozoa must confer upon the zygote is the capacity for normal embryonic development. In this context a variety of factors may be important including: (1) a functional centrosome to regulate cell division in the embryo, (2) remodelled chromatin characterized by the presence of protamines 1 and 2 in a ratio of 1:1, as well as appropriately modified histones, (3) a population of mRNA and miRNA species that are carried into the zygote by the fertilizing spermatozoon and may contribute to the regulation of early embryonic development, (4) an appropriate pattern of DNA methylation, and (5) intact nuclear DNA.

The latter is thought to be a particularly important aspect of sperm quality. DNA damage in spermatozoa has been linked with a wide variety of adverse clinical outcomes including impaired fertilization, disrupted pre-implantation development, an increased risk of miscarriage, and a wide variety of defects in the offspring ranging from complex neurological conditions such as autism or spontaneous schizophrenia to childhood cancer [4].

Although definitive evidence is lacking, it is possible that DNA damage in the male germ line makes a significant contribution to the elevated incidence of birth defects observed following ART, when compared with the naturally conceived population. Furthermore, there is good evidence for an increase in imprinting disorders, notably the Beckwith–Wiedemann and Angelman syndromes, in children produced by assisted conception, which may be associated with defects in the methylation status of spermatozoa. It is also known that singleton infants produced by ART are significantly more likely to be admitted to a neonatal intensive care unit, to be hospitalized, and to stay in hospital longer than their naturally conceived counterparts. In addition, recent independent studies have revealed an eight-fold increase in the incidence of undescended testicles in boys conceived by ICSI, while another analysis demonstrated abnormal retinal vascularization in such children [4]. In order to negate the male contribution to such abnormalities, the spermatozoa we isolate for assisted conception purposes should not only be capable of fertilization but also possess as little DNA damage as possible.

In considering the impact of sperm preparation techniques on sperm DNA integrity, it is important to stress that a majority of the DNA damage we see in the spermatozoa of male patients is, like defective sperm function, oxidatively induced. DNA damage is also tightly correlated with defects in the remodelling of sperm chromatin during spermiogenesis [10]. On the basis of these results, we have proposed a two-step hypothesis for the induction of DNA damage in the male germ line [4]. In the first step, spermiogenesis becomes disrupted leading to the generation of spermatozoa possessing poorly remodelled chromatin and lacking a full complement of protamines. In the second step, these vulnerable cells become oxidatively attacked leading to the rapid formation of base adducts, particularly 8-hydroxy-2′-deoxyguanosine. The formation of such adducts then destabilizes the DNA backbone leading to the formation of abasic sites and, ultimately, the appearance of DNA strand breaks.

Thus whatever approach we adopt in the preparation of spermatozoa for ART, it should avoid the formation of oxidative DNA damage. A number of studies have demonstrated that the preparation of spermatozoa by, for example, discontinuous gradient centrifugation produces populations possessing low levels of DNA damage [11]. Although this is a positive finding, it should be noted that such assessments of sperm DNA integrity with TUNEL or Comet assays do not take account of cell viability. A recent technical development in this area has, for the first time, permitted the simultaneous assessment of DNA damage and cell vitality by flow cytometry [12]. Application of this methodology clearly demonstrated that a majority of the DNA damaged spermatozoa found in the ejaculate are, in fact, dead. This study also confirmed previous reports indicating that discontinuous gradient centrifugation leads to the production of sperm suspensions exhibiting significantly more vitality and (as a result) significantly less DNA damage than unfractionated sperm suspensions. However when only the viable cells were considered, discontinuous gradient centrifugation was shown to actually induce a significant increase in oxidative DNA damage that, in the patient population, translated into an increase in the levels of DNA fragmentation [12]. Thus, even when care is taken to isolate spermatozoa using state-of-the–art preparation techniques, DNA damage may still be induced in these cells. New technologies are clearly needed.

Electrophoretic sperm isolation

Ainsworth *et al.* described an alternative method of isolating spermatozoa for assisted conception purposes in 2005 [6]. This procedure relied upon two fundamental principles: (1) that normal functional spermatozoa are negatively charged and thus move towards the anode in an electric field and (2) that spermatozoa are amongst the smallest cells in the body and will pass through a 5 μm filter. The electrophoretic device described in the above publication uses electric current to pull negatively charged spermatozoa through a polycarbonate filter and into a collection chamber. The separation system is depicted in Figure 23.1 and consists of a cassette comprising two 400 μl chambers separated by a polycarbonate filter containing 5 μm pores and bounded by a 15 kDa polyacrylamide membrane to allow the free circulation of buffer. Semen is introduced into one chamber, current applied (75 mA at variable voltage) and within seconds a purified suspension of spermatozoa can be collected from the adjacent chamber in an appropriate buffer.

The method is extremely rapid, and isolates sperm populations possessing good motility, excellent morphology, and low rates of DNA damage. Furthermore these cell populations are essentially free of contamination by leukocytes and precursor germ cells. The method is also effective with a wide range of starting materials including testicular biopsies and cryostorage media [6].

Given the initial promise of this system, it was employed in a case study of a couple experiencing prolonged infertility associated with high rates of DNA damage in the male partner's spermatozoa [13]. In this example, the patient produced an oligozoospermic ejaculate on the day of oocyte retrieval containing 3.2 million spermatozoa/ml and an equivalent number (2.1 million/ml) of contaminating round cells. Of the spermatozoa that were present, 30% were vital, 18% were motile and 26% were TUNEL positive. Following electrophoretic separation, a purified sperm population was generated that was 62% vital, 24% motile and 14% TUNEL positive. Assessment of these samples by SCSA revealed a DNA fragmentation index that fell from 41% in the ejaculated sample to 15% in the electrophoretically separated population. The isolated spermatozoa were then used in ICSI; five out of seven oocytes were fertilized, and two of the embryos were transferred on day 3. Embryo transfer was followed by pregnancy and, later, the birth of a healthy girl with no complications.

This case report was then followed up by a more extensive clinical trial in order to compare the electrophoretic method with conventional density gradient centrifugation in a clinical setting [14]. Each semen sample was randomly split between preparation using the electrophoretic system and preparation by standard density gradient centrifugation. Furthermore, each cohort of oocytes was split for insemination using either electrophoretically- or density-gradient prepared spermatozoa. In the event, both methods of sperm preparation yielded comparable rates of sperm recovery, motility, and DNA fragmentation. Furthermore there

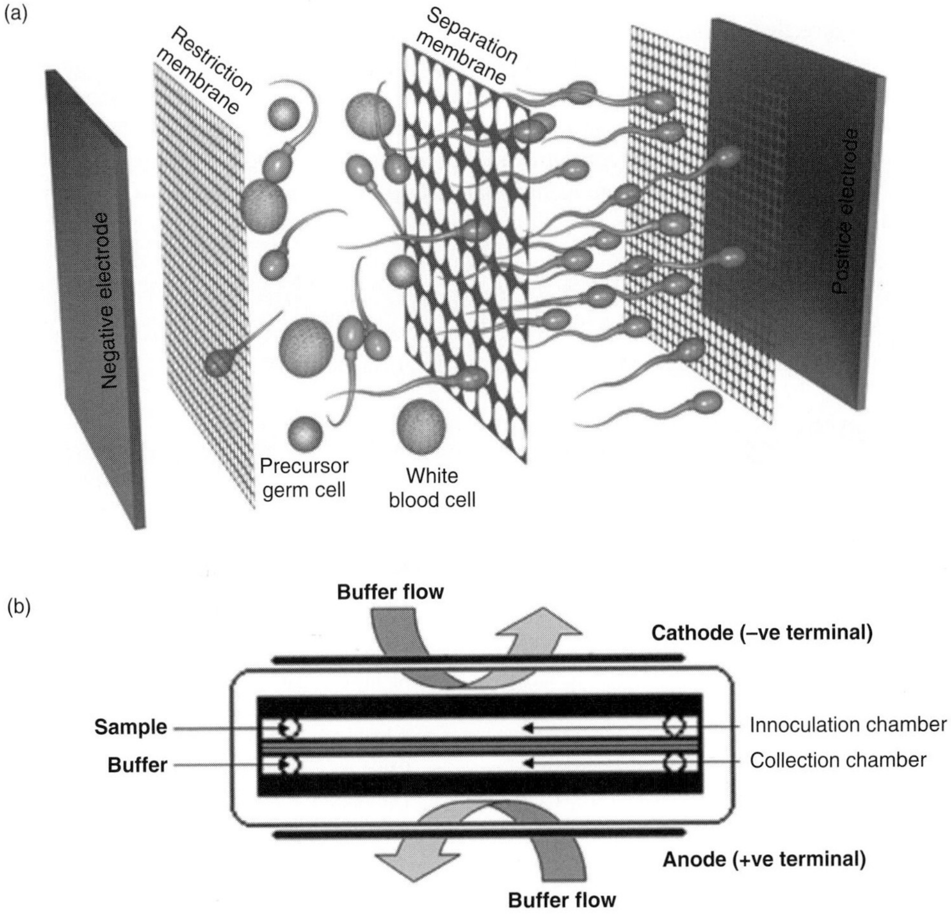

Figure 23.1 Schematic representation of the cartridge-based electrophoretic separation technology. (a) Directional movement of competent spermatozoa in the applied electric field and resultant passage through polycarbonate 5 µm separation membranes results in the rapid production of highly purified sperm populations. (b) Topography of the cartridge configuration including restriction and separation membranes, indicating buffer flows and sample inoculation and collection locations. Figure based on reference 15, with permission from Oxford University Press.

were no significant differences between these methods in the ability of the spermatozoa to achieve fertilization (62.4% versus 63.6%), cleavage (99.0% versus 88.5%), and high-quality embryos (27.4% versus 26.1%). Thus, this novel approach to sperm isolation appears to be as effective a sperm preparation regime as density gradient centrifugation, while taking a fraction of the time.

Conclusion

In order to ensure high rates of fertilization and normal embryonic development to term, it is essential that oocytes are inseminated with carefully prepared sperm suspensions. The latter should be free of cellular contamination and comprise only the most viable, motile, functional spermatozoa in the ejaculate. It is also extremely important that the selection technique isolates cells that are, as far as possible, free of DNA damage. In order to avoid the iatrogenic induction of damage to spermatozoa during their preparation, it is also important to isolate these cells directly from seminal plasma. This can be easily achieved by allowing the cells to swim out of seminal plasma, providing the intrinsic motility of the spermatozoa is adequate to the task. Alternatively, the spermatozoa can be isolated from semen using discontinuous gradient centrifugation or a new electrophoretic approach. Preliminary results suggest that the latter represents an extremely rapid, effective means of isolating high quality cells for insemination. Additional clinical trials are now needed to substantiate this early promise.

Acknowledgments

Grateful thanks are due to the ARC, Newcastle Innovation, the ARC Centre of Excellence in Biotechnology and Development and NuSep for financial support.

References

1. Aitken RJ, Clarkson JS. Significance of reactive oxygen species and antioxidants in defining the efficacy of sperm preparation techniques. *J Androl* 1988;**9**:367–76.
2. Mortimer D. Sperm preparation methods. *J Androl* 2000;**21**:357–66.
3. Aitken RJ, Buckingham DW, West K, Brindle J. On the use of paramagnetic beads and ferrofluids to assess and eliminate the leukocytic contribution to oxygen radical generation by human sperm suspensions. *Am J Reprod Immunol* 1996;**35**:541–51.
4. Aitken RJ, De Iuliis GN, McLachlan RI. Biological and clinical significance of DNA damage in the male germ line. *Int J Androl* 2009;**32**:46–56.
5. Aitken RJ, Baker HW. Seminal leukocytes: passengers, terrorists or good samaritans? *Hum Reprod* 1995;**10**:1736–9.
6. Ainsworth C, Nixon B, Aitken RJ. Development of a novel electrophoretic system for the isolation of human spermatozoa. *Hum Reprod* 2005;**20**:2261–70.
7. Gomez E, Aitken J. Impact of in vitro fertilization culture media on peroxidative damage to human spermatozoa. *Fertil Steril* 1996;**65**:880–2.
8. Krausz C, Mills C, Rogers S, Tan SL, Aitken RJ. Stimulation of oxidant generation by human sperm suspensions using phorbol esters and formyl peptides: relationships with motility and fertilization in vitro. *Fertil Steril* 1994;**62**: 599–605.
9. Baker HW, Brindle J, Irvine DS, Aitken RJ. Protective effect of antioxidants on the impairment of sperm motility by activated polymorphonuclear leukocytes. *Fertil Steril* 1996;**65**:411–9.
10. De Iuliis GN, Thomson LK, Mitchell LA, *et al.* DNA damage in human spermatozoa is highly correlated with the efficiency of chromatin remodeling and the formation of 8-hydroxy-2′-deoxyguanosine, a marker of oxidative stress. *Biol Reprod* 2009;**81**:517–24.
11. Donnelly ET, O'Connell M, McClure N, Lewis SE. Differences in nuclear DNA fragmentation and mitochondrial integrity of semen and prepared human spermatozoa. *Hum Reprod* 2000;**15**:1552–61.
12. Mitchell LA, De Iuliis GN, Aitken RJ. The TUNEL assay consistently underestimates DNA damage in human spermatozoa and is influenced by DNA compaction and cell vitality: development of an improved methodology. *Int J Androl* 2011;**34**:2–13.
13. Ainsworth C, Nixon B, Jansen RP, Aitken RJ. First recorded pregnancy and normal birth after ICSI using electrophoretically isolated spermatozoa. *Hum Reprod* 2007;**22**:197–20.
14. Fleming SD, Ilad RS, Griffin AM, *et al.* Prospective controlled trial of an electrophoretic method of sperm preparation for assisted reproduction: comparison with density gradient centrifugation. *Hum Reprod* 2008;**23**:2646–51.

Chapter 24

ICSI for all?

David Mortimer and Sharon T. Mortimer

Introduction

Intracytoplasmic sperm injection (ICSI) is the most significant advance in ART for the alleviation of male factor subfertility of the past three decades. However, its use has become increasingly widespread and indiscriminate in ART clinics, extending well beyond the real reasons for its application, which are as follows.

- Cases of severe male factor subfertility where there is actual evidence for a serious risk of impaired sperm function that would lead to reduced or failed fertilization in vitro, such as autoimmune infertility caused by antibodies directed against the sperm head, and many (but certainly not all) cases of retrograde ejaculation.
- Couples in whom conventional IVF has failed due solely to sperm dysfunction, such as failure to acrosome react.
- Use of spermatozoa recovered surgically from the male reproductive tract.
- Cases where pre-implantation genetic testing is to be performed for monogenic conditions, so as to avoid possible contamination with DNA from spermatozoa still attached to the zona pellucida.
- Use of spermatozoa that were cryopreserved in finite limited quantities, e.g., prior to chemo- or radiotherapy or prior to vasectomy, or with known poor cryosurvival.

The proposition for the widespread, even "universal", use of ICSI is based on the perception of a higher fertilization rate than by conventional IVF, and the desire to avoid unexpected IVF fertilization failure. Although wishing to avoid having to explain to a man why his sperm "didn't work" is quite understandable, the indiscriminate, even total, use of ICSI is increasingly being seen as unacceptable, and some jurisdictions have regulated against this approach. For example, an expert Panel Report for the Ontario (Canada) Ministry of Children and Youth Services states that ICSI should be provided only for individuals where either severe male factor infertility is present, or there is demonstrated fertilization failure in a previous IVF cycle. Clearly, a "poor" semen analysis, even one with several characteristics below the World Health Organization reference values for recently fertile men, is not adequate justification for using ICSI.

This chapter will analyze the basis for this reasoning, and identify the risks to which couples are exposed by the unjustified use of ICSI; a debate that has been raging for the past decade [1–4].

How to Improve Your ART Success Rates, ed. Gab Kovacs. Published by Cambridge University Press.

How much ICSI is necessary?

Based on our experience, and that of many centers with which we have been associated over the past 15 years, even though 90% or more of couples might be defined as having a male factor according to current WHO semen analysis reference values, ICSI is necessary in no more than about 40% of cases [1]. The only exception to this is for centers that specialize in treating men with spinal cord injuries or have a very specific focus on severe male factor subfertility.

Fertilization rates are not higher using ICSI

While various studies have reported higher fertilization rates with ICSI than with IVF, this is unproven [5], and clearly untrue in centers with good IVF systems [6]. While ICSI fertilization rates of up to 85% of MII oocytes injected have been published, most centers report values around 65–80%, with oocyte damage rates of about 5%. Many laboratories also report standard IVF fertilization rates of 65–80% of oocytes inseminated. However, with a typical prevalence of 85% MII oocytes this actually equates to a fertilization rate of 76–94% of MII oocytes inseminated, i.e., equivalent to the best ICSI fertilization rates, with no oocytes destroyed inadvertently. For a typical stimulated cycle, this represents, on average, one or two fewer zygotes when ICSI is used in a case where IVF would have worked [e.g., 6], or a decrease in overall outcome potential of 10–20% after including thawed embryo transfers.

What is the real risk of total IVF fertilization failure?

Many centers have published a prevalence of total IVF fertilization failure (TIFF) of 5–10%, or even higher, yet others report values of 2% [2]. This discrepancy, and the finding of high rates of TIFF, are the result of two main issues: (1) poor andrological (more correctly, spermatological) evaluation of the male partners and (2) poor sperm handling/preparation/capacitation systems that result in impaired sperm function in vitro. Centers with these issues create a self-fulfilling prophecy: sperm will show poor function, thereby reducing IVF fertilization rates and causing a high prevalence of TIFF. Although ICSI would eliminate this iatrogenic problem of TIFF due to poor sperm function, what is really needed is just better IVF.

With optimized IVF lab systems TIFF rarely exceeds 2–3%, against a generally established background ICSI fertilization failure rate of about 1%. Certainly patients could choose to use ICSI if they found a 1–2% incremental risk of TIFF to be unacceptable, but it would be irresponsible to allow them to believe that the prevalence of TIFF is 10% or higher.

Does ICSI have any real benefit in non-male factor cases?

Although numerous studies have considered whether ICSI might improve outcomes compared to IVF in couples with non-male factor infertility, including a Cochrane Review (www.CochraneLibrary.net), no clear benefit has been defined beyond avoiding some cases of TIFF, even when only a few oocytes are available for insemination [5].

Does using IVF/ICSI "splits" have any real value?

A number of centers employ IVF/ICSI "splits", where the available oocytes are assigned to two groups, one for conventional insemination and the other for ICSI. The rationale is that because these centers' sperm assessments cannot identify those men whose spermatozoa have impaired fertilizing potential, this approach is "easier" than upgrading the diagnostic andrology testing to include sperm functional assessments. However, with "splits" it is not uncommon for the "better looking" cumulus-corona-oocyte complexes to be assigned to ICSI. As a result, another self-fulfilling prophecy is created: that ICSI achieves a higher fertilization rate.

Is a "poor" semen analysis justification for using ICSI?

No. The limited prognostic value of descriptive semen analysis characteristics has long been known, rendering simple assessments of sperm concentration, motility, and even normal sperm morphology (even by properly trained, expert semen analysis technologists) of limited value in defining sperm fertilizing ability. For example, many morphologically abnormal spermatozoa fertilize oocytes, and we have routinely employed IVF in men with <4% normal forms and achieved normal IVF fertilization rates – so long as the teratozoospermia index (TZI) is below the threshold value of 1.60.

Sperm preparation and selection issues

There are well-documented processes of sperm selection in vivo during their passage through the female reproductive tract and the oocyte vestments, with the acquisition of fertilizing ability being closely regulated in those spermatozoa that ultimately fertilize oocytes [7, 8].

Sperm preparation using a technique that selects properly mature spermatozoa with better functional potential and low levels of DNA damage, and protects them from oxidative damage by reactive oxygen species (ROS) during handling, is essential for both IVF and ICSI. Even though sperm fertilizing ability is unimportant for ICSI, the quality of the male genetic contribution to the embryo is still critical – and perhaps even more so since male factor cases have inherently higher levels of sperm DNA damage.

Sperm selection for ICSI is important to exclude dead spermatozoa that will be undergoing autolysis, and hence at much greater risk of having damaged DNA. Various techniques for selecting "better" spermatozoa, such as using hyaluronan-binding, have been reported but are not yet in routine clinical use [8].

Although there is no specific relationship between sperm phenotype and genotype (beyond diploid spermatozoa having larger heads), men with oligoasthenoteratozoospermia have increased levels of ROS, DNA fragmentation and chromosomal aberrations in their spermatozoa. Because these are the men who will more likely require ICSI to achieve a conception, sperm selection is critical in these cases.

The use of high optical magnification to select spermatozoa without vacuoles for ICSI (IMSI: intracytoplasmic morphologically-selected sperm injection) seems to increase the success rate of ICSI [9], but comes at a high cost, both in terms of the microscopes required and the greatly increased time taken to perform a case (often 1.5–2 hours). Moreover, from the "standard ICSI" fertilization and pregnancy rates reported in these studies, it does seem that IMSI is only of value in extreme cases; which is fortunate as its routine use for all ICSI cases would be enormously expensive in equipment and human resources.

What are the biological risks associated with ICSI?

While the increased prevalence of sex chromosome aneuploidy and imprinting disorders in ICSI-derived offspring have been shown to be more related to the higher prevalence of such disorders in couples receiving ICSI treatment, scientific evidence for adverse effects upon the oocyte, fertilization, and subsequent embryonic development, is accumulating [reviews: 2, 3].

- During normal fertilization in Eutheria the acrosome is lost prior to sperm-oocyte fusion, and the remaining sperm plasma membrane is incorporated as a patch into the oolemma as part of the fusion process. However, during ICSI, both the intact acrosome and the sperm plasma membrane are inserted directly into the ooplasm. Experiments in mice have shown that the cholesterol content of the plasma membrane of uncapacitated spermatozoa (more specifically, its oxidation by ROS within the ooplasm), and/or the protease(s) contained within the acrosome, can affect sperm chromatin remodelling, leading to DNA damage. Removal of these structures prior to ICSI in this species reduced aberration rates in the resultant embryos to those of IVF-derived embryos.
- Since the sperm plasma membrane is inserted into the ooplasm at ICSI, whatever is bound to its outer surface (including bacteria, viruses, and DNA) is also transferred into the ooplasm. Indeed, ICSI-based sperm-mediated gene transfer is now a well-established and highly efficient technique for generating transgenic animals [10]. The risk of inadvertent ICSI-mediated transgenesis is a serious risk that must be avoided whenever possible.
- The pattern of sperm-induced Ca^{2+} oscillations during rabbit oocyte activation is different following ICSI compared to normal sperm-oocyte fusion, and this has been associated with impaired blastocyst formation, perhaps due to difficulties in going through cell cycle checkpoints [11]. A study on sibling human oocytes has also shown that the ICSI procedure itself can be detrimental to embryonic development in vitro [6].
- Fertilization failure of human oocytes following ICSI is largely due to incomplete oocyte activation, defects in pronuclear apposition, and abnormal sperm head decondensation [11]. Abnormal sperm head decondensation can be due to abnormalities in either the spermatozoon or the oocyte (perhaps as a result of incomplete cytoplasmic maturity, which is frequently asynchronous with nuclear maturation in oocytes following controlled ovarian hyperstimulation). Sperm-based issues include "super-stabilized" chromatin resulting from zinc deficiency in the seminal plasma, and abnormal chromatin condensation and/or incomplete replacement of histones by protamines during defective spermiogenesis – which is reflected in impaired sperm morphology, a common reason for performing ICSI.
- Finally, in the absence of any serious IVF treatment option, laboratory staff could lose the necessary skills related to the handling and processing of spermatozoa. This could then lead to sub-optimal practices and culture conditions, as well as elevated risks of iatrogenic sperm DNA damage and an overall detrimental impact on treatment outcomes, all of which must be avoided when striving for best practice.

Increased financial burden to patients from ICSI

Financial modelling has shown that in the UK it would cost £60 000 for every extra pregnancy achieved if ICSI is used instead of IVF [2].

In Canada, where pregnancy rates by IVF and ICSI are equivalent, ICSI typically costs about $1500 ($1000 to $1500) extra per treatment cycle, and is currently used in just over 70% of the 10 400 treatment cycles started annually. Therefore, if only 40% of cycles need ICSI the extra financial burden (primarily to patients since ART is still mostly in the private sector in Canada) is approximately $4.5M annually.

An IVF lab's "standard" semen analysis frequently fails to meet the expected minimum standards for accuracy and precision. However, the typical *incremental* cost of proper sperm testing in Canada to include assessments that allow the assignment to conventional IVF with only a 1% or so increased risk of TIFF, is approximately \$200. Compared with the standard ICSI supplement, this would represent an average saving of about \$1200 for up to 50% of patient cycles.

The best practice way forward

Based on this analysis, the following general conclusions can be drawn:

1) ICSI will remain, for the foreseeable future, an essential part of our armamentarium for helping infertile couples with a severe male factor achieve their goals of a healthy baby.
2) ICSI is not "better" than IVF using any established outcome metric. Indeed, it yields fewer embryos per treatment cycle, which may have impaired developmental potential compared to IVF-derived embryos.
3) ICSI costs more than IVF because of the capital cost of ICSI workstations, extra consumables, and embryologist time (and IMSI even more so). Most centers identify this cost up-front, but even if a center charges the same for both treatment modalities, the cost is still higher.
4) The argument of universal use of ICSI to avoid low or no fertilization at IVF is a simplistic approach to the issue of managing occult male factor subfertility that cannot be considered best practice. Proper sperm assessments would allow the great majority of patients to undertake IVF with an increased TIFF risk of about 1%; naturally, those who are not prepared to accept this small risk can always choose ICSI, with its associated other risks.

Recommended minimum sperm assessment ("sperm screen") package

a) Comprehensive semen analysis according to WHO/ESHRE methods, but including assessment of *rapid progressive* (WHO "grade *a*") motility and the TZI. Assessments should have an uncertainty of measurement of ≤10%.
b) Direct Immunobead test for sperm surface antibodies, including isotyping in cases of >50% bead binding.
c) Computer-aided sperm analysis (CASA) assessment of sperm kinematics on progressively motile seminal spermatozoa.
d) A "trial wash" preparation, ideally using a two-step density gradient centrifugation technique (lower layer specific gravity = 1.1 g/ml).
e) CASA-based longitudinal assay of sperm hyperactivation after incubation under capacitating conditions, ideally including an agonist treatment as positive control.

References

1. Mortimer D. Structured management as a basis for cost-effective infertility care. In: Gagnon C, ed. *The Male Gamete: From Basic Science to Clinical Applications.* Vienna (IL, USA): Cache River Press 1999;363–70.
2. Ola B, Afnan M, Sharif K, *et al.* Should ICSI be the treatment of choice for all cases of in-vitro conception? Considerations of fertilization and embryo development, cost-effectiveness and safety. *Hum Reprod* 2001;**16**:2485–90.

3. Varghese AC, Goldberg E, Agarwal A. Current and future perspectives on intracytoplasmic sperm injection: a critical commentary. *Reprod Biomed Online* 2007;**15**:719–27.

4. Kim HH, Bundorf MK, Behr B, *et al.* Use and outcomes of intracytoplasmic sperm injection for non-male factor infertility. *Fertil Steril* 2007;**88**:622–8.

5. Borini A, Gambardella A, Bonu MA, *et al.* Comparison of IVF and ICSI when only few oocytes are available for insemination. *Reprod Biomed Online* 2009;**19**:270–5.

6. Griffiths TA, Murdoch AP, Herbert M. Embryonic development *in vitro* is compromised by the ICSI procedure. *Hum Reprod* 2000;**15**:1592–6.

7. Mortimer D. Sperm transport in the female genital tract. In: Grudzinskas JG, Yovich JL, eds. *Gametes – The Spermatozoon.* Cambridge: Cambridge University Press, 1995;157–74.

8. Franken DR, Bastiaan HS. Can a cumulus cell complex be used to select spermatozoa for assisted reproduction? *Andrologia* 2009;**41**:369–76.

9. Berkovitz A, Eltes F, Lederman H, *et al.* How to improve IVF-ICSI outcome by sperm selection. *Reprod Biomed Online* 2006;**12**:634–8.

10. Moisyadi S, Kaminski JM, Yanagimachi R. Use of intracytoplasmic sperm injection (ICSI) to generate transgenic animals. *Comp Immunol Microbiol Infect Dis* 2009;**32**:47–60.

11. Rawe VY, Olmedo SB, Nodar FN, *et al.* Cytoskeletal organization defects and abortive activation in human oocytes after IVF and ICSI failure. *Mol Hum Reprod* 2000;**6**:510–6.

Chapter

25

Day of embryo transfer

David K. Gardner and Denny Sakkas

Introduction

With the development and the subsequent clinical validation of physiological culture systems over the past decade, it has become possible to culture, as a matter of routine, the human embryo to the blastocyst stage. Prior to these advances it was simply not feasible to grow the human embryo routinely past the eight-cell stage in the laboratory. Consequently, during the first 20 years of clinical IVF embryo transfers have been performed on days 1 to 3, the former being the choice primarily when laboratory conditions were unfavorable [1]. Given that sufficient investment in the embryology laboratory has been undertaken [2] and that sufficient quality control and quality assurance procedures are in place [3], then it is possible to culture highly viable human blastocysts. Therefore, for the first time in human IVF there is now the possibility of transferring the human embryo at any stage of development during the preimplantation period. This raises the question of which day is optimal for embryo transfer? Here we provide data to identify which day(s) of development the human embryo should be replaced in the uterus.

The oviduct and uterine environments

Analysis of the composition of the female reproductive tract has revealed that the embryo is exposed to gradients of nutrients as it progresses from the oviduct to its site of implantation within the uterus [4]. These gradients mirror the changing requirements of the embryo as it develops, with the embryo entering the uterus after compaction. So if a human embryo is transferred asynchronously, then it will be required to adapt to its environment. Of note, the embryo is most sensitive to its environment prior to compaction, while it resides in the oviduct, and therefore, any stress will be greatest at the cleavage stages [5]. Significantly, asynchronous transfer of embryos to the uterus in all mammalian species studied to date leads to compromised embryo development and significant loss of viability [6]. Delaying embryo transfer to the uterus until after compaction greatly reduces embryonic stress. Interestingly, the human stands alone against all other eutherian species in that one can place the preimplantation embryo into the uterus prior to compaction, and the formation of a morula, and still get live young. Interestingly, or conveniently, this species difference is hardly ever referred to.

Potential advantages of blastocyst transfer

What are the perceived advantages to the culture and transfer of the human blastocyst? A list of identified advantages is shown in Table 25.1. By transferring the embryo post-compaction

How to Improve Your ART Success Rates, ed. Gab Kovacs. Published by Cambridge University Press.

Table 25.1 Potential benefits of blastocyst transfer

• Synchronization of embryonic stage with the female tract; reduces cellular stress on the embryo
• Minimize exposure of embryo to hyperstimulated uterine environment
• Reduction in uterine contractions; reduces chance of embryo being expelled
• Embryo selection; ability to identify those embryos with limited, as well as those with the highest developmental potential, also assessing the embryo post genome activation
• Ability to undertake cleavage stage embryo biopsy without the need for cryopreservation when the biopsied blastomere has to be sent to a different locale for analysis
• High implantation rates means reducing the need to transfer multiple embryos

at the blastocyst stage, one not only synchronizes embryo development with the female reproductive tract, but also places the embryo in the uterus at a time when there are greatly reduced uterine contractions, thereby negating the possibility of the embryo being expelled [7]. Another key advantage of delayed embryo transfer at the blastocyst stage is that the embryonic genome is activated and the embryo has begun differentiation. i.e., one is able to assess the embryo proper. Prior to compaction one is primarily considering a cleaving oocyte, and subsequently one may not have all the necessary information upon which to perform embryo selection. With such proposed advantages, what are the clinical data?

Clinical application of blastocyst transfer

The first prospective randomized trial comparing human embryo transfer on either day 3 or day 5 in good prognosis patients, i.e., good ovarian reserve, revealed a significantly higher implantation and pregnancy rate when transfer occurred at the blastocyst stage [8]. Subsequent studies have revealed that not only are pregnancy rates higher with day 5 embryo transfer, but that transfer on day 3 is associated with higher pregnancy losses [9]. Since the first prospective randomized trial in 1998 there have been at least a further 50 trials, 18 of which have been randomized. In the most recent Cochrane review it was determined that live birth rate following day 5 transfer was significantly higher compared to transfer on day 3 [10]. This difference was especially evident in good prognosis patients. However, in the trials analyzed, rates of embryo freezing were higher when embryo transfer was performed on day 2 or 3, and the failure to have any embryos for transfer was higher on day 5. As culture systems continue to be improved, together with the introduction of vitrification as the primary cryopreservation protocol, it will be interesting to re-evaluate cryopreservation rates and the incidence of cancelled transfers for the different days of transfer. However, when there are good numbers of eight-cell embryos, i.e., three or more, then data indicate that day 5 transfer will give higher pregnancy rates. Whether transfer of embryos on day 4 at the morula stage will become a clinical treatment has yet to be established, but good pregnancy rates have already been established with this approach [11].

Single embryo transfer

Given that a major goal of human IVF is the birth of a healthy singleton child born through the transfer of a single embryo, elective single embryo transfer (SET) is becoming more

Table 25.2 Viability of human embryos conceived in vitro using an oocyte donor model ($n = 950$ patients)

Mean blastocyst development (%)	65.1
Mean no. blastocysts transferred	2.05
Mean age of recipient (years)	40.3
Fetal heart (per blastocyst transferred; %)	68
Clinical pregnancy rate (per retrieval; %)	85.2
Twins (%)	59.9

Pronucleate oocytes were cultured for 48 h in medium G1 at 5% $O2$, 6% $CO2$ and 89% $N2$. On day 3 of development embryos were washed and transferred into medium G2 under the same gaseous environment. Embryos were cultured in groups of four in 50-µL drops of medium under Ovoil (Vitrolife AB, Gothenburg, Sweden) in 60-mm Falcon Primaria (BD Bio sciences, Franklin Lakes, NJ, USA) dishes. All embryos were transferred on day 5 of development in a medium with a high concentration of hyaluronan [2].

widespread in the IVF community. The main hindrance to its introduction has been suboptimal laboratory conditions, combined with inappropriate stimulation regimens. Consequently, it was considered acceptable to transfer multiple embryos in an attempt to maintain IVF success rates [12]. With the recent improvements in the IVF laboratory, combined with patient stimulation regimens designed to generate fewer, healthier oocytes, SET is now a feasible patient treatment. The move to SET is especially relevant to good prognosis patients and oocyte donation programs. In the case of the latter, blastocysts can have implantation rates close to 70% [Table 25.2], and hence the transfer of just two blastocysts gives a greater than 50% chance of twins [2]. Analysis of day of transfer in SET through prospective randomized trials has confirmed the improved outcome associate with day 5 compared to day 3 transfers [13, 14]. Furthermore, initial concerns regarding an increased incidence of monozygotic twinning associated with blastocyst transfer do not appear to have been realized [15].

Conclusion

With the relatively recent introduction of better laboratory conditions it has become possible to culture the human embryo throughout the preimplantation period [2]. For the successful implementation of improved culture systems, one cannot overstate the significance of adequate quality control/quality assurance in the IVF laboratory. Without an appropriate means of pre-testing all contact supplies etc., and the ability to implement some form of quality management system, then all the improvements in the world cannot be translated into high and reproducible pregnancy rates. It has been demonstrated that when laboratory conditions are not ideal, then it would be more appropriate to place the embryos into the uterus sooner than later [1]. Clearly, with the investment in appropriate laboratory personnel and resources, such situations should be few and far between. The available literature indicate that embryo transfer on day 5 is associated with better outcomes and that with the increasing move to SET, single blastocyst transfer will become the preferred treatment option for several groups of patients, especially good prognosis and oocyte donor cases.

References

1. Quinn P, Stone BA, Marrs RP. Suboptimal laboratory conditions can affect pregnancy outcome after embryo transfer on day 1 or 2 after insemination in vitro. *Fertil Steril* 1990;**53**:168–70.
2. Gardner DK. Dissection of culture media for embryos: the most important and less important components and characteristics. *Reprod Fertil Dev* 2008;**20**:9–18.
3. Mortimer DM, S. *Quality and risk management in the IVF laboratory.* Cambridge: Cambridge University Press 2005.
4. Gardner DK, Lane M, Calderon I, Leeton J. Environment of the preimplantation human embryo in vivo: metabolite analysis of oviduct and uterine fluids and metabolism of cumulus cells. *Fertil Steril* 1996;**65**:349–53.
5. Gardner DK, Lane M. Ex vivo early embryo development and effects on gene expression and imprinting. *Reprod Fertil Dev* 2005;**17**:361–70.
6. Barnes FL. The effects of the early uterine environment on the subsequent development of embryo and fetus. *Theriogenology* 2000 15;**53**:649–58.
7. Fanchin R, Ayoubi JM, Righini C, *et al.* Uterine contractility decreases at the time of blastocyst transfers *Hum Reprod* 2001;**16**:1115–9.
8. Gardner DK, Schoolcraft WB, Wagley L, *et al.* A prospective randomized trial of blastocyst culture and transfer in in-vitro fertilization. *Hum Reprod* 1998;**13**:3434–40.
9. Papanikolaou EG, Camus M, Fatemi HM, *et al.* Early pregnancy loss is significantly higher after day 3 single embryo transfer than after day 5 single blastocyst transfer in GnRH antagonist stimulated IVF cycles. *Reprod Biomed Online* 2006;**12**:60–5.
10. Blake DA, Farquhar CM, Johnson N, Proctor M. Cleavage stage versus blastocyst stage embryo transfer in assisted conception. *Cochrane Database Syst Rev* 2007:CD002118.
11. Feil D, Henshaw RC, Lane M. Day 4 embryo selection is equal to Day 5 using a new embryo scoring system validated in single embryo transfers. *Hum Reprod* 2008;**23**:1505–10.
12. Gerris J. Single-embryo transfer versus multiple-embryo transfer. *Reprod Biomed Online* 2009;**18** Suppl 2: 63–70.
13. Gardner DK, Surrey E, Minjarez D, *et al.* Single blastocyst transfer: a prospective randomized trial. *Fertil Steril* 2004;**81**:551–5.
14. Papanikolaou EG, Camus M, Kolibianakis EM, *et al.* In vitro fertilization with single blastocyst-stage versus single cleavage-stage embryos. *New Engl J Med* 2006;**354**:1139–46.
15. Papanikolaou EG, Fatemi H, Venetis C, *et al.* Monozygotic twinning is not increased after single blastocyst transfer compared with single cleavage-stage embryo transfer. *Fertil Steril* 2010;**93**:592–7.

Chapter 26

The beneficial effects of culture medium supplementation with growth factors in the development of human embryos in vitro

Klaus E. Wiemer

Introduction

The determination of proper overall culture conditions as well as clarification of metabolic requirements for human embryos has been an ongoing endeavor. Early attempts to provide developing human embryos with proper substrate(s), macromolecules, and cytokines was attempted through the use of somatic cell co-culture [see 1 for review]. The use of this culture methodology most likely improved embryo development by at least two modes of action: (1) by secreting various molecular weight growth factors and (2) by extracting factors/impurities or reducing nutrient levels in the culture medium. Eventually, the use culture media based upon simple balanced salt solutions gave way to complex formulations containing carbohydrates, amino acids (essential and non-essential), chelating agents, and other energy substrates. The advent of these complex media systems were of paramount importance for the routine development of human zygotes into competent blastocysts without the use of somatic cell support. Nonetheless, these culture media have been supplemented in part with proteins and other macromolecules in the form of human serum albumin (HSA) or more complex albumin products containing alpha- and beta-globulins (CHSA).

The beneficial effects of HSA supplementation in conjunction with the new generation of culture media have provided countless IVF laboratories with high quality blastocysts for transfer and/or cryopreservation. However, the addition of complex proteins found in CHSA and other protein supplements may better mimic in some manner the conditions found in vivo due in part to the growth factors that are present in many of the more complex albumin preparations commercially available today. These albumin products might also act as carriers for lipid soluble vitamins and other bioactive lipids for embryos during in vitro development. In other words, the addition of albumin and its fractions might improve the solvent nature of the culture media that is more similar to that found in the microenvironment within the oviduct. The use of these more complex albumin products is also a means for clinical embryologists to introduce globulins into their culture media since these products are not normally found in culture media formulations.

How to Improve Your ART Success Rates, ed. Gab Kovacs. Published by Cambridge University Press.

The ability to fully elucidate the autocrine/paracrine relationship between the oviduct/uterus and developing human embryo has been extremely difficult to establish given the scarcity of available material. Most would agree that the majority of early human embryonic development occurs within the hormonally regulated environment of the oviduct. The resulting embryo is bathed in a solution of fluids containing a multitude of micro and macromolecules which most likely play a specific as well as passive role in supporting proper embryonic development.

Considerable evidence now exists that expression of several growth factor ligands and receptors are present in embryos of several species including humans as well as within the lumen of the oviductal cells themselves [2, 3, 4]. These factors include members of the insulin-like growth factors (IGF), interleukin (IL-1, IL-6), granulocyte macrophage colony-stimulating-factor (GM-CSF), leukemia inhibitory factor (LIF), platelet activating factor (PAF), platelet-derived growth fact (PDGF), and other factors. These factors most likely exert their effects by modulating gene expression in the developing embryo. The temporal nature of gene expression is based upon the stage of the embryos as well.

Discussion

During in vivo development, maternally and embryonic-derived growth factors play a role in preimplantation development. As an example, the presence of apoptotic cells is generally higher in in vitro produced mouse embryos. This would suggest that the secretory cells within the reproductive tract provide important factors for the developing embryo. The fact that the supplementation of culture media with transforming growth factor alpha (TGF-a) or insulin-like growth factor-1 (IGF-1) decreases apoptosis in mouse embryos indicates that this growth factor improves cell survival. In addition, some of these growth factors are also produced by the embryos themselves. For example, mouse embryos possess ligands for TGF-a on the inner cell mass (ICM) and trophectoderm cells. When mouse embryos are cultured in small volumes of media, the result is improved development and reduced levels of apoptosis. It is possible that the ICM is producing TGF-a and binds the receptor sites on its own trophectoderm cells. Subsequently, these factors which are produced by the embryos themselves have a mutually beneficial effect on the cohort of embryos within the small volume of media. Members of the epidermal growth factor (EGF) family are also produced by the embryo itself and have been shown to decrease apoptosis as well. These are examples of how the use of group culture might be applicable to human IVF in order to take advantage of the factors produced by the embryos themselves. However, the number of embryos, the quality of embryos from secretory standpoint and volume of media might have an impact on any potential benefit.

Not all factors are expressed throughout preimplantation embryonic development. The expression of several growth factor ligands and receptors are present only after activation of the embryonic genome. This temporal expression is a common characteristic of many of the important growth factors in mammalian embryos. For example, the growth factor LIF is not produced by the embryo until it reaches the blastocyst stage; however, it is obligatory for implantation. In addition, not all growth factor expressions are common between species. For example, EGF is expressed by human but not cow embryos.

Like most other species, the addition of growth factors to culture medium for human preimplantation development has had beneficial effects on embryo development and quality. Examples of some of the growth factors that have proven to have beneficial effects are: GM-CSF, EGF, IGF, LIF, PAF, and PDGF. Insulin has also proven to have embryotrophic qualities for human embryos. Although the embryo cannot make insulin, it has receptor sites on the blastomeres and can respond to its presence. Insulin appears to have metabolic and cell growth promoting properties. Specifically, insulin increases protein synthesis and lactate production. One can only assume that this would transpire into higher quality embryos with improved implantation potential. The addition of IGF-1 and GM-CSF has improved the percentage of embryos that develop to the blastocyst stage. The use of these factors has specifically been shown to improve the total number of cells with the ICM of the blastocyst. In addition, IGF-1 has proven to decrease the rate of apoptosis in human blastocysts as well. It appears that IGF-1 has a function in cell survival [5].

GM-CSF is a growth factor that is produced by the oviduct and uterus in the human following estrogen priming. During in vivo development, this factor promotes development of preimplantation embryos and is involved in regulating blastocyst development and reduces the incidence of apoptosis. Similar findings have been reported with the addition of this growth factor as well to culture media used to support human preimplantation development in vitro. Culture of human embryos in the presence of GM-CSF has shown increased rates of blastocyst formation as well as total number of cells allocated to the ICM and trophectoderm. In addition, the incidence of cell death was lower in embryos cultured in the presence of this factor. In particular, the incidence of cell death was higher within the ICM of embryos that were cultured in the absence of GM-CSF [5].

An additional factor that is unique in terms of clinical application in assisted reproduction is hyaluronan. Hyaluronan (HN) is a non-sulfated glycosaminoglycan that is associated with extracellular matrix tissue that exhibit rapid rates of growth and is found in large quantities in the reproductive tract including follicular fluid. It is thought to play an important role in cell migration and proliferation, and is unique for human IVF because it is often added prior to fresh embryo transfer as well as replacement of cryopreserved embryos. The exact mechanism whereby this factor can improve outcomes is not clear. It is possible that HN might improve cell adhesion or cell matrix adhesion during blastocyst implantation.

The culture media formulations in use today contain the necessary substrates in order to support the development of competent blastocysts. For this reason, most IVF laboratories with high standards of quality control and assurance can replace blastocysts on a routine basis. In addition, the use of triple gas incubators has improved the efficiency at which embryos develop to the blastocyst stage. This author has performed routine blastocyst culture for many years using HSA as the protein source with success. The overall rates of blastocyst development varied from 55 to 60% using a HSA (unpublished results). There was no impact of ICSI on rate of development. The rate of high quality blastocyst formation using HSA varied from 30 to 40% of all embryos placed into culture (unpublished results). High quality blastocysts are defined as developmentally expanded blastocysts or greater with a well-defined robust ICM as well as possessing a trophectoderm made up of many epithelial-shaped cells in conjunction with a well-organized cavity. However, our center began to supplement the culture media with commercially available more complex albumin products that contain alpha- and beta globulins. We noted an immediate change in overall embryo development. Namely, the cleavage intervals increased for embryos on days 2 and 3 of development (day 0 equals day of retrieval). The proportion of four cells on day 2 increased from 48% to 62% and the proportion of 6–10 cells on day 3 increased from 58% to 73% by using albumin products that contain globulins (unpublished data). These results, noted on day 3, afforded us the possibility to select more patients for extended culture. In addition, the proportion of embryos that developed to blastocysts as well as high quality blastocysts increased to approximately 66% and 48%, respectively. We are fairly certain that this enhancement in overall embryo performance is based upon using a more complex albumin product. However, we are not convinced that improved developmental rates were solely due to the globulins since there are a multitude of factors that might be present in these more complex yet less defined solutions. The beneficial affects noted in our laboratory might simply be that this type of albumin and its fractions improved the solvent nature of the culture media so that it is more similar to that found in the microenvironment within the oviduct. Since this supplement is less defined we have implemented a very strict quality control program to reduce the lot-to-lot variations that can be inherent when using these products.

Conclusion

The addition of growth factors to culture media has the potential to improve the development of zygotes to the blastocyst stage when used in conjunction with the culture media systems available today. These factors might mimic the autocrine and paracrine factors that are evident during in vivo development. During in vivo development, expression of growth factor ligands by either the oviduct and/or uterus coupled with the presence of receptor sites on the embryo indicates a paracrine relationship with maternal growth factors. The addition of these growth factors might represent the most important biological substances that could improve current in vitro human embryo culture methodologies. The important aspect to distinguish when considering these substances is the temporal expression of these factors and the fact that we do not know what the actual bioavailability is during the development in an ever changing reproductive tract. For example how would one determine how to establish concentrations of these factors in our current static culture systems? Perhaps the use of microfluidic culture systems would be more applicable here. There is a possibility that these factors could override checkpoints within the embryo that might cause premature gene expression within the embryo. Signaling pathways within the embryo could be modified leading to altered imprinting. Much research and controlled studies are required before these co-factors can be routinely used to support human embryos prior to replacement.

References

1. Wiemer KE, Cohen J, Tucker MJ, Godke RA. The application of co-culture in assisted reproduction: 10 years of experience with human embryos. In: Dale, B, eds. Development of the Human Embryo in vitro. *Hum Reprod* 1998;**13**(suppl 4);226–38.
2. Sharkey AM, Dellow K, Blayney M, *et al.* Stage-specific expression of cytokine and receptor messenger ribonucleic acids in human embryos. *Biol Reprod* 1995;**53**: 955–62.
3. Kimber SJ, Sneddon SJ, Bloor DJ, *et al.* Expression of genes involved in early cell fate decisions in human embryos and their regulation by growth factors. *Reproduction* 2008;**135**:635–47.
4. Daliri M, Appa Rao KBC, Kaur G, *et al.* Expression of growth factor ligand and receptor genes in preimplantation stage water buffalo (*Bubalus bubalis*) embryos and oviduct epithelial cells. *J Reprod Fertil* 1999;**117**:61–70.
5. Hardy K, Spanos S. Growth factor expression and function in the human and mouse preimplantation. *J Endocrinol* 2002;**172**:221–236.

Chapter 27

Metabolomics

Denny Sakkas and David K. Gardner

Introduction

A steady improvement in ART delivery rates, better access to care, and the relative ineffectiveness of other treatment options has made ART the mainstay of infertility treatment. At the current time, more than 1% of all children born in the USA, Europe and Australia are from ART-related conceptions.

A major advance in infertility treatment was the ability to perform controlled ovarian superovulation in the patient. This resulted in the availability of numerous embryos per treatment cycle and the transfer of multiple embryos in an attempt to increase pregnancy rates. However, the price for this is the subsequent potential for a multiple pregnancy.

The risks related to multiple gestations are well documented and include preterm delivery, low birth weight, and even a dramatic increase in the relative risk for cerebral palsy. Decreasing the prevalence of multiple gestations, while maintaining (or preferably improving) overall pregnancy rates, remains the most significant contemporary goal of infertility research [1].

Single embryo transfer

In numerous countries, the dangers associated with multiple pregnancies have been allayed by legal restrictions on the number of embryos that can be transferred in a single IVF cycle. For example, in a number of northern European countries the government has set a legal limit of only one embryo to be transferred per cycle for specific patient groups, i.e., single embryo transfer (SET). In other parts of the world, where no legal restrictions exist, the onus is on the individual clinic (as well as the patient) to decrease the number of embryos transferred so that an acceptable balance can be achieved between the risks associated with multiple gestations and "acceptable" pregnancy rates. This approach has worked well in countries such as Finland and Australia which enjoy remarkably high rates of SET.

Implementing SET in the laboratory

A major issue impacting the number of embryos transferred is an apparent inability to accurately estimate the reproductive potential of an individual embryo within a cohort of embryos. Over the past 30 years morphological assessment has proven to be a stalwart procedure for embryologists to use to select which embryo(s) to replace. Since the early years of IVF it was noted that embryos cleaving faster and those of better morphological

How to Improve Your ART Success Rates, ed. Gab Kovacs. Published by Cambridge University Press.

appearance were more likely to lead to a pregnancy. Morphological grading systems have evolved over the past decade and in addition to the classical parameters of cell number and fragmentation, numerous other characteristics have been examined including: pronuclear morphology, early cleavage to the two-cell stage, multinucleation, the ability to grade independently the inner cell mass and trophectoderm of the blastocyst, all of which can be combined in some form of sequential assessment.

Faced with the scenario that the worldwide IVF community will in the future have to select only one or two embryos for transfer, we will be forced to make certain changes. The first may be to rely on less aggressive stimulation protocols hence generating a lower number of eggs at collection. The second is to improve the selection process for defining the quality of individual embryos so that the ones chosen for transfer are more likely to implant.

Assessing the embryo for transfer

Criteria for adopting non-invasive embryo assessment in the laboratory

The inherent ease of laboratory assessment of various morphological markers makes it the preferred assessment technique of embryo transfer. Even with the adoption of more complex forms of assessment it will remain as one of the main tools available for embryo selection. For a new assessment procedure to be acceptable in an IVF laboratory setting it must satisfy a number of criteria. It should be able to measure:

1. a difference in predicting embryo viability without harming the embryo;
2. the difference quickly; and,
3. the difference consistently and accurately.

Non-invasive assessment of embryo culture media

In two retrospective studies on different animal models it was established that a relationship exists between metabolic parameters and embryo viability. In 1980, it was observed that day 10 cattle blastocysts which had an elevated glucose uptake developed better, both in culture and in vivo after transfer than those blastocysts with a lower glucose uptake. Subsequently, in 1987, it was determined that glucose uptake by individual day 4 mouse blastocysts prior to transfer to recipient females was significantly higher in those embryos that went to term compared to those embryos that failed to develop after transfer. More importantly, it has been shown in the mouse model that the metabolic activity of blastocysts can be used prospectively to select embryos for transfer. Those embryos which had a metabolic profile similar to that of embryos developed in vivo, had the highest viability. Of interest those blastocysts which had lost control of their metabolism had almost no developmental potential. Such data provide compelling evidence that metabolic function is linked to embryo viability and is reviewed in [2].

Human embryo studies assessing metabolism

A limited number of studies have been performed on nutrient uptake and the subsequent viability of the human embryo [2]. In a retrospective analysis Conaghan and colleagues observed an inverse relationship between pyruvate uptake by two- to eight-cell embryos and subsequent pregnancy. More recently, Gardner and colleagues have determined that the greater the glucose uptake by day 4 and day 5 human embryos the more likely it is that the blastocyst will implant [3]. Gardner and colleagues had previously determined that glucose consumption on day 4 by human embryos was twice as high in those embryos that went on to form blastocysts [2]. In studies on amino acid turnover by human embryos, Houghton *et al.* [4] determined that alanine release into the surrounding medium on day 2 and day 3 was highest in those embryos that did not form blastocysts. Brison *et al.* [5] have reported changes in concentration of amino acids in the spent medium of human zygotes cultured for 24 h in an embryo culture medium containing a mixture of amino acids analysed using high performance liquid chromotography. They found that aspargine, glycine and leucine were all significantly associated with clinical pregnancy and live birth.

Other non-invasive assessment techniques

Other techniques have also been reported to measure metabolic parameters in culture media; however, they are yet to be tested in a clinical IVF setting. These include the measure of oxygen consumption of developing embryos using a microsensor system. Recently, more emphasis has been placed on the relationship between reactive oxygen species (ROS) levels in culture media to the outcome of in vitro fertilization cycles. In a recent study, in the human, by Bedaiwy *et al.* [6], it was found that increasing levels of ROS generation in day 3 in vitro embryo culture media may have a detrimental effect on in vitro embryo growth parameters, as well as clinical pregnancy rates in IVF and ICSI cycles.

Metabolomics

The complete array of small-molecule metabolites that are found within a biological system constitutes the metabolome, which can be considered to reflect the functional phenotype. Metabolomics is the systematic study of this dynamic inventory of metabolites, rather than the analysis of a few chosen nutrients and their metabolic end products. Consequently, taking a metabolomic-based approach will generate algorithms based on many parameters, which should theoretically increase the power of the selection criteria. Using various forms of spectral and analytical approaches, metabolomics attempts to determine metabolites associated with physiologic and pathologic states. Certainly it appears that embryos which result in pregnancy are different in their metabolomic profile compared to embryos that do not lead to pregnancies corroborating previous data on embryo metabolic activity [2, 7].

Investigation of the metabolome of embryos, by analysis of the culture media they grow in, using targeted spectroscopic analysis and bioinformatics, will plausibly assist in identifying the most viable embryo(s) within a cohort. Seli and colleagues [7] established that these differences are detectable in the culture media using both Raman and near infrared (NIR) spectroscopy. In their initial work, a total of 69 day 3 spent embryo culture media samples from 30 patients with known outcome (0 or 100% sustained implantation rates) were evaluated using Raman and/or NIR spectroscopy. A regression formula was developed to calculate a relative "embryo viability score" – relating to embryo reproductive potential – which correlated implantation outcome to both Raman and NIR spectral metabolomic profiles. Both Raman and NIR spectroscopic analysis of the spent culture media of embryos with proven reproductive potential demonstrated significantly higher viability scores than those that failed to implant. Interestingly, when human embryos of similar morphology are examined using the same NIR spectral profile, their viability scores vary remarkably in relation to morphology indicating that the metabolome of embryos that look similar differ

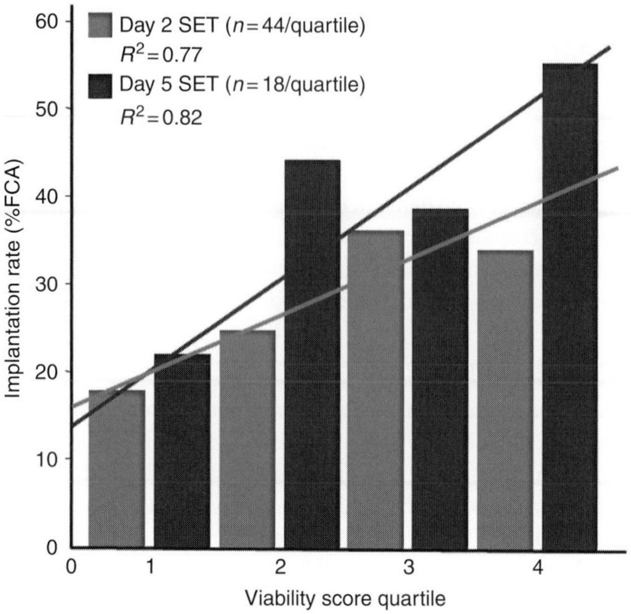

Figure 27.1 Blinded prediction of implantation in relation to increasing viability scores after analysis of day 2 and 5 embryo culture media by near infrared (NIR) Spectroscopy. Implantation rate = Number of foetal cardiac activity (FCA)+/Total number of single embryo transfers (SETs). (Molecular Biometrics Inc. Unpublished Data.)

significantly. This observation is in agreement with the study of Katz-Jaffe *et al.* [8], and Gardner *et al.* [3], who revealed that the proteome and glucose uptake respectively, of individual human blastocysts of the same grade differed between embryos, again indicating that embryo morphology is not completely linked to its physiology.

The algorithm established by Seli was subsequently used to predict the likelihood of pregnancy from blinded embryo culture media samples. When the algorithm developed was used to blindly test a subgroup of 16 day 3 embryo samples collected at different centers and cultured using a different type of commercial media, viability scores of embryos with proven reproductive potential were significantly higher compared to embryos that failed to implant. A larger analysis of single embryo transfer cycles has also been undertaken whereby NIR spectral analysis of frozen day 2 and 3 embryo culture media samples was performed blinded to outcome. Individual metabolic profiles were established from 7 μl of the samples with each measurement taking less than one minute. Statistical analysis performed on the metabolic profiles established a viability score (as generated above) that was significantly different ($p < 0.001$) between the pregnant and non-pregnant patients. A cut-off value for predicting pregnancy was taken at > 0.3. When this cut-off was used to examine embryos of excellent and good morphology that underwent single embryo transfer a significant difference was found in the establishment of pregnancy.

More recent data have used a semi-quantitative approach to apply this technology. A series of studies have been undertaken whereby algorithms for predicting outcomes of day 2, 3 and 5 SETs have been developed and tested blindly against samples unrelated to those used to develop the algorithms. The data have confirmed that as the Viability Scores™ generated by the algorithms increase the tendency for the assessed embryo to implant and display foetal cardiac activity (FCA) also increases (Figure 27.1). Subsequent data have also shown that this pattern is independent of morphology as the ability of the Viability Score™ to relate to FCA is maintained within groups of embryos with the same morphology.

Conclusion

Numerous technologies are progressing towards providing a non-invasive assessment of embryo culture media to aid in the prediction of embryo viability. In addition to predicting embryo viability a strong possibility exists that similar technologies will be able to "non-invasively" determine more subtle embryo characteristics including aneuploidy and sex [3, 10]. In the near future it is highly likely that a rapid metabolic or metabolomic assessment tool will be part of the routine procedure used to select an embryo for transfer.

References

1. Adashi EY, Barri PN, Berkowitz R, *et al.* Infertility therapy-associated multiple pregnancies (births): an ongoing epidemic. *Reprod Biomed Online* 2003;**7**:515–42.
2. Sakkas D and Gardner DK. Noninvasive methods to assess embryo quality. *Current Opin Obstet Gyn* 2005;**17**:283–288.
3. Gardner DK, Wale PL, Collins R, Lane M. Glucose consumption of single post-compaction human embryos is predictive of embryo sex and live-birth outcome. *Hum Reprod* 2011; in press.
4. Houghton FD, Hawkhead JA, Humpherson PG, *et al.* Non-invasive amino acid turnover predicts human embryo developmental capacity. *Human Reprod* 2002;**17**:999–1005.
5. Brison DR, Houghton FD, Falconer D, *et al.* Identification of viable embryos in IVF by non-invasive measurement of amino acid turnover. *Hum Reprod* 2004;**19**:2319–24.
6. Bedaiwy MA, Mahfouz RZ, Goldberg JM, *et al.* Relationship of reactive oxygen species levels in day 3 culture media to the outcome of in vitro fertilization/intracytoplasmic sperm injection cycles. *Fertil Steril* 2010;**94**:2037–42.
7. Botros L, Sakkas D, Seli E. Metabolomics and its application for non-invasive embryo assessment in IVF. *Mol Hum Reprod* 2008;**14**:679–90.
8. Katz-Jaffe MG, Gardner DK, Schoolcraft WB. Proteomic analysis of individual human embryos to identify novel biomarkers of development and viability. *Fertil Steril* 2006;**85**:101–7.
9. Picton HM, Elder K, Houghton FD, *et al.* Association between amino acid turnover and chromosome aneuploidy during human preimplantation embryo development in vitro. *Mol Hum Reprod* 2010;**16**:557–69.
10. Gardner DK, Larman MG, Thouas GA. Sex-related physiology of the preimplantation embryo. *Mol Hum Reprod* 2010;**16**:539–47.

Chapter 28

Role of preimplantation genetic diagnosis

Anver Kuliev

Introduction

Preimplantation genetic diagnosis (PGD) was introduced 20 years ago as an option to avoid the birth of affected offspring with inherited disorders without facing pregnancy termination (for review see [1]). However, its wider application was associated with the possibility of detecting and avoiding the transfer of embryos with chromosomal abnormalities, destined to be lost during implantation or post-implantation development. So PGD provides the possibility for pre-selection of the embryos with higher developmental potential, as an important alternative to the traditional selection of the embryos based on morphologic criteria in IVF, because despite possible correlation between normal morphology and euploidy, many morphologically normal embryos may still be found to have chromosomal abnormalities [1–3].

Because of the above potential improvements PGD has been applied in dozens of thousands of poor prognosis IVF cycles. However, there is still a controversy in the utility of PGD, which is mainly due to the need for improving the accuracy of PGD technology for aneuploidy testing [3]. On one hand, current testing has been available for only a limited number of chromosomes, and on the other, the widespread use of cleavage stage biopsy appeared to be insufficiently reliable for detection of chromosomal status of the embryo. However, there is currently progress in each of these areas, with the recent introduction of the techniques for testing all 24 chromosomes, and combining polar body sampling with embryo biopsy.

An obvious impact has been observed in PGD for chromosomal rearrangements, which has already become an established procedure for carriers of balanced translocations [1, 2]. So the present chapter describes the progress in the above areas, demonstrating that PGD may soon become a genuine addition to assisted reproduction in the effort of choosing the embryos with improved potential to result in viable pregnancy.

Chromosomal abnormalities in oocytes and embryos

The usefulness of PGD in assisted reproduction is obvious from the data on the prevalence of chromosomal abnormalities in oocytes and embryos. We performed 3064 PGD cycles, using FISH analysis of 20 986 oocytes, showing that as many as 9812 (46.8%) of these oocytes were aneuploid, originating comparably from the first and second meiotic divisions: 31.1% from meiosis I, represented by gain or loss of chromsome/chromatids in PB1, and 33.7 % from meiosis II, represented by gain or loss of chromatid in PB2. Only meiosis I errors were found in 30.4% of abnormal oocytes and only meiosis II errors in 39.8%, as was evident from

How to Improve Your ART Success Rates, ed. Gab Kovacs. Published by Cambridge University Press. © Cambridge University Press 2011.

chromsome/chromatid errors either in PB1 or PB2, the remaining 29.8% being with sequential meiosis I and meiosis II errors, represented by oocytes with both PB1 and PB2 abnormal [4].

These results are of clinical significance, as the genotype of the resulting zygotes cannot be predicted without testing the outcome of both meiotic divisions. For example, testing of meiosis I errors alone should reduce the aneuploidy rate in embryos at least by two-thirds. Despite the fact that, approximately one-third of these oocytes will be aneuploid following the second meiotic division, PB1 testing could still sufficiently improve the implantation and pregnancy rates in poor prognosis IVF or intracytoplasmic sperm injection (ICSI) patients, by applying ICSI selectively to the oocytes with aneuploidy-free PB1. On the other hand, only half of the abnormalities deriving from second meiotic division may be detected by PB1 analysis, so to avoid the transfer of all the embryos resulting from aneuploid oocytes, testing of both PB1 and PB2 will still be required. As PB1 and PB2 have no biological significance in pre- and post-implantation development, their removal and testing may become a useful tool in assisted reproduction practices to identify the aneuploidy-free oocytes, which should help preselecting the oocytes with the highest potential for establishing viable pregnancy and improving the IVF efficiency.

The above overall rates of aneuploidies in oocytes are comparable to those detected in PGD for aneuploidies at the cleavage stage [3], taking into consideration additional fertilization-related abnormalities and paternally derived meiotic errors, which could also have been detected at this stage. However, the types of anomalies in oocytes and embryos are different, which is attributable mainly to a high frequency of mosaicism, comprising up to a half of the chromosomal abnormalities at the cleavage stage.

So the most accurate pre-selection of embryos for transfer may be performed by a sequential testing of meiosis I, meiosis II, and mitotic errors, through sequential PB1 and PB2 followed by blastomere or blastocyst sampling. This may allow avoidance of the transfer of embryos with prezygotic chromosomal errors, which seem to be the major source of chromosomal abnormalities, and also detection of possible mitotic errors in embryos resulting from euploid zygotes, some of which may not be of clinical significance.

However, there is still a need for the development of methods for full karyotyping of oocytes and embryos, which presently includes the use of microarray technology. These may enable the detection and exclusion from transfer of the aneuploid embryos, of which a certain proportion could have been misdiagnosed as normal by the commercially available FISH probes, although there are still important limitations of these highly labour intensive procedures.

Even with possible progress in full karyotyping, the accuracy of PGD for aneuploidies will depend on avoiding misdiagnosis due to mosaicism at the cleavage stage. Assuming that every second embryo may be mosaic at the cleavage or blastocyst stage, it will be of importance to obtain the meiosis information for each embryo, so that false negative diagnosis may be avoided.

PGD impact on reproductive outcome

The above data provide the background for clinical application of aneuploidy testing, making obvious that the recent controversy about PGD application in IVF is not about its utility, as the transfer of chromosomally abnormal embryos should clearly be avoided, but concerns the accuracy and reliability of the testing. The high aneuploidy prevalence in oocytes and embryos makes obvious, that without the detection and avoidance of chromosomally abnormal embryos, there is a 50% chance of transferring abnormal embryos, destined to be lost during implantation or post-implantation development. So in addition to the clear benefit of avoiding transfer of aneuploid embryos, which contributes to the improvement of the pregnancy outcome of poor prognosis IVF patients, this should improve the overall standard of medical practice, upgrading the current selection of embryos by morphological criteria to include testing for aneuploidy. It may be expected that, in future, no IVF center without such an upgrade will be sufficiently competitive, as informed patients will not opt for transfer of embryos with 50% risk of chromosomal abnormality. The majority of these chromosomally abnormal embryos seem to be eliminated before implantation, as only one in ten of recognized pregnancies are chromosomally abnormal.

Incidental transfer of aneuploid embryos in the absence of chromosomal testing is likely to lead to failures of implantation and pregnancy failures in poor prognosis IVF patients, or may compromise the pregnancy outcome by leading to spontaneous abortions. A clinical impact of aneuploidy testing, in terms of the improved outcome of pregnancies through the reduction of spontaneous abortions, has been observed not only for IVF patients with advanced reproductive age, but also those with repeated IVF failures and repeated spontaneous abortions [3]. Although randomized controlled studies will still be required to further quantify the clinical impact of pre-selection of aneuploidy-free zygotes for embryo transfer, the available results suggest the clinical relevance of the preselection of these oocytes and embryos. On the other hand, PGD is still a highly sophisticated procedure, involving biopsy of the oocyte and/or embryo, which may have detrimental effect on embryo development if not performed to the highest standard. Likewise, the FISH technique applied to single cells, also requires sufficient training and experience due to its present limitations.

So the failure of observing the positive effect of aneuploidy testing on reproductive outcome in some recent reports may be due to possible methodological shortcomings [3]. This is mainly due to potential detrimental effect of two blastomere removal in some of these reports, which definitely reduced the implantation potential of the biopsied embryos to the extent that could not be bridged even by preselection of aneuploidy-free embryos. Without taking into consideration these technical details, the data may be misinterpreted as showing a lack of PGD impact on pregnancy outcome, although even the absence of the differences between PGD and non-PGD groups in these studies may have suggested the beneficial effect of preselection of aneuploidy-free embryos, in terms of compensating a detrimental effect of two cell biopsy at the day 3. The failure to detect the positive effect may be also due to exclusion from testing a few key chromosomes, or poor efficiency of aneuploidy testing with over 10% failed results, that have affected the appropriate pre-selection of embryos, resulting in exclusion of potentially normal embryos from transfer.

Because of the above methodological shortcomings, the data should not be misinterpreted in favor of transferring embryos without aneuploidy testing, which suggests an alternative of incidental transferring of chromosomally abnormal embryos, being a major cause of a low implantation rate in poor prognosis IVF patients, and explaining a high fetal loss rate in these patients without PGD. This has been demonstrated by testing of products of conception from poor prognosis non-PGD IVF patients, which confirmed the high prevalence of chromosomal aneuploidy in the absence of PGD.

So the accumulated experience makes it obvious that in order to achieve the expected benefit, the testing should first of all not damage the embryo viability and be performed accurately according to the available standards [2, 5]. In other words, there seems to be actually no controversy in the usefulness of aneuploidy testing, the major issue being its safety and reliability, which will no doubt be further improved in the near future.

In the absence of sufficient data from well-designed randomized controlled studies, the beneficial impact of PGD has also been demonstrated by the comparison of reproductive outcome in the same patients with and without PGD, with the assumption that the previous reproductive experience of the patients may serve as an appropriate control for PGD impact. In two large series, overall comprising over 500 couples, implantation, spontaneous abortions, and 'take home baby' rates were analyzed before and after PGD, demonstrating significant improvement after PGD [1, 6]. This included an almost five-fold improvement in implantation rate, and three-fold reduction of spontaneous abortion rate, which contributed to more than a two-fold increase of take home baby rate after PGD, suggesting the obvious clinical usefulness of aneuploidy testing for IVF patients with poor reproductive performance.

The impact was even higher in translocation patients, with implantation rate after PGD being as high as 61.6%. The comparison of spontaneous abortion rates before and after PGD revealed an almost six-fold reduction of spontaneous abortion rate (87.8% before and 15.6% after PGD). The take home baby rate in these patients was only 11.5% before PGD, reaching 79.4% after PGD application.

Conclusion

In the light of these data, the current IVF practice of selection of embryos for transfer based on morphologic criteria may hardly be an acceptable procedure for poor prognosis IVF patients. In addition to an extremely high risk of establishing an affected pregnancy from the onset, this will significantly compromise the very poor chances of these patients to become pregnant, especially with the current tendency of limiting the number of transferred embryos to only two, leaving only a single embryo on average with a potential chance of reaching the term.

It may, therefore, be predicted that, with in future improvement safety and accuracy PGD will definitely contribute to improving the overall standards of assisted reproduction practices, by substituting the present practice of selecting embryos for transfer using morphologic parameters by pre-selection of chromosomally normal embryos with the higher potential to result in pregnancy.

References

1. Verlinsky Y, Kuliev A. *Practical Preimplantation Genetic Diagnosis*. London: Springer Verlag, 2006.
2. Verlinsky Y, Kuliev A. *Atlas of Preimplantation Genetic Diagnosis-Second Edition*. London: Taylor & Francis, 2005.
3. Munne S, Wells D, Cohen J. Technology requirements for preimplantation genetic diagnosis to improve assisted reproduction outcomes. *Fertil Steril* 2010;**92**:408–30.
4. Kuliev A, Zlatopolski Z, Kirillova I, Cieslak-Jansen J. Meiosis errors in over 20,000 oocytes in practice of preimplantation aneuploidy testing. *Reprod BioMed Online* 2010;**22**:2–8.
5. Preimplantation Genetic Diagnosis International Society (PGDIS). Guidelines for good practice in PGD. *Reprod BioMed Online* 2008;**16**:134–47.
6. Gianaroli L, Magli MC, Ferraretti A. The beneficial effects of PGD for aneuploidy support extensive clinical application. *Reprod BioMed Online* 2004;**10**:633–40.

Chapter 29

Assisted hatching

S. Das and M. W. Seif

Introduction

The World Health Organization estimates that one in six couples experience some delay in conception. An increasing number of these couples require treatment by assisted reproduction technology (ART) procedures of IVF or intracytoplasmic sperm injection (ICSI).

Implantation rate of embryos resulting from IVF cycles is generally less than 20% [1], culminating in a generally low 'take home baby' rate. This may be the result of poor embryo quality, poor endometrial receptivity, and observed lower rate of hatching of cultured embryos due to hardening of the zona pellucida. Recently, failure of the embryonic zona pellucida to rupture following blastocyst expansion has been suggested as a possible contributing factor in implantation failure.

Structure and physiology of the zona pellucida

The human embryo is surrounded by an outer sulphated glycoprotein coat known as the zona pellucida which comprises of three main constituents: ZP1, ZP2, and ZP3. ZP1 provides the structural integrity to the embryo while ZP2 and ZP3 are known to have biological functions. ZP3 is responsible for initiating the acrosome reaction of the bound spermatozoa. ZP2 activity prevents polyspermy and penetration by sperm of other species. After fertilization, the zona maintains the three-dimensional integrity of the uncompacted embryo and facilitates free passage of the compacted embryo through the fallopian tube into the uterus and protects the embryo from microorganisms and immune cells. The blastocyst-stage embryo eventually hatches out of this protective coat six days after fertilization just before implantation.

Hardening of the zona pellucida is thought to be influenced by suboptimal culture of embryos in vitro, advancing age in vivo, duration of hormonal stimulation during IVF/ICSI, and smoking. This is thought to occur as a result of cross-linking of its constituent glycoproteins. In the absence of measurable qualitative criteria to ascertain "hardening" of the zona, thickness of more than 15 μm is thought to reflect a degree of hardness that can affect implantation negatively. About 15% of embryos display thickening of zona more than 15 μm.

Rationale and indications for assisted hatching

Local thinning of the zona is observed only in embryos that actively cleave unlike embryos that do not undergo cleavage. Embryos demonstrating uniform zonae are less likely to implant as compared with those showing local thinning. It has also been suggested that the

How to Improve Your ART Success Rates, ed. Gab Kovacs. Published by Cambridge

inability to implant appears to be associated with the resilience of the zona rather than its actual thickness.

Drilling a hole in the zona is thought to facilitate the release of the embryo and subsequent implantation irrespective of the underlying cause – be it thickening/hardening of zona or lack of resilience.

Zona manipulation of some form has been offered to:

- Older women (>35 years of age);
- Women with high FSH levels;
- Those with high risk of zona hardening – in vitro oocyte maturation;
- Prior to replacement of frozen thawed embryos; and
- Following recurrent implantation failure [2].

Assisted hatching methods

Artificially disrupting the zona pellucida is known as assisted hatching (AH) and was first suggested in the 1980s. It was subsequently observed in women undergoing embryo biopsy for pre-implantation genetic diagnosis. There is some evidence that embryos that have undergone zona manipulation for AH tend to implant one day earlier than unhatched embryos. A variety of techniques have since been employed to assist embryo hatching:

- Mechanical zona dissection
- Chemical drilling/thinning of zona using acid Tyrode's
- Laser photoablation
- Piezo micromanipulation
- Mechanical expansion with hydrostatic pressure

The mechanical method was one of the first methods described to achieve thinning/slitting of the zona in order to create a defect to facilitate embryo hatching. It involves holding the embryo in position by gentle suction from the holding pipette. The microneedle is then passed through the zona pellucida at the largest perivitelline space and advanced tangentially. The embryo is then released from the holding pipette and held by the microneedle. The microneedle is brought to the bottom of the holding pipette and the embryo is gently rubbed against until a cut is made. The embryo is then rotated until the slit is visible at the 12 o'clock position. The embryo is firmly held by the holding pipette and the zona is cut in a similar manner creating a cross-shaped slit. This method is hugely dependent on operator expertise and also subject to great variation in the degree of zona thinning between embryos.

Chemical-assisted hatching involves stabilizing the embryo with a holding pipette. A 10 μm pipette containing acid Tyrode's solution is oriented next to an area of empty perivitelline space and a defect is created in the zona using a mouth-controlled delivery system to blow the acid Tyrode over the external surface of the zona. Embryos are then rinsed several times to wash the excess acid Tyrode before returning to the standard culture media until transfer.

Mechanical and chemical methods require extensive technical skill to produce standardized and uniform defect in the zona.

Laser-assisted hatching involves the use of a 1480 nm diode laser attached to the objective turret of the microscope. The Laser Assisted Hatching software is designed for easy positioning, focus and measurement of embryos and simple alignment of the laser. The laser has three preset energy intensities of low (35 mW), medium (45 mW), and high (55 mW) that can be delivered in a single 25 ms pulse with a single click of the mouse controller. Low power is used for perforating very thin (< 10 μm) zona or to minimize exposure, medium power for drilling the zona of most embryos (10–15 μm), and high power for perforating thick (> 15 μm) or hard zona pellucida. This method therefore, has the advantage of providing computer controlled, touch-free, precise, and uniform thinning of the zona. It has been shown to produce no thermal, mutagenic, or mechanical effect on the embryo.

The use of vibrations from piezoelectric pulse to produce a precise and controlled zonal defect without any toxicity to the embryo has also been described.

Very recently, mechanical distension of the zona with hydrostatic pressure has been described. This method involves injection of the HTF-HEPES culture medium into the perivitelline space. The authors have described abrupt expansion immediately following injection which is only maintained for about 30 seconds. They hypothesize that this transient expansion brings about ultrastructural changes in the zona which facilitates hatching. The preliminary trial has shown higher pregnancy rates in the study group as compared with the control group [3].

The zona may be thinned, breached to its full thickness or completely removed. A study comparing varying degrees of laser-assisted hatching showed significant negative impact of full thickness breach of zona at one point on embryo implantation. However, partial/quarter laser zona thinning significantly improves implantation in poor prognosis groups of patients [4]. Another retrospective study comparing implantation rates following the use of mechanical, chemical, and laser-assisted hatching techniques showed universal improvement in pregnancy rate in poor prognosis patients with no inter-method differences [5].

The site of zona manipulation has been the subject of debate. Historically and logically, manipulation has always been performed at a site away from the inner cell mass to minimize damage to the embryo. However, in their preliminary report from a recent prospective randomized study, Miyata *et al.* have demonstrated that AH is more successful when manipulation was done near the site of the inner cell mass as compared with those done at the site opposite to it, clear evidence of the distinct polarity of the embryo during the hatching process [6]. These findings and newer techniques like hydrostatic distension could change the way AH is performed in the future.

However, there remains considerable uncertainty over whether assisted hatching significantly improves IVF/ICSI success rates or whether it is associated with negative consequences.

Assisted hatching and pregnancy outcomes

Our group conducted a Cochrane review in 2003 which was updated in 2007 [7] to determine whether assisted hatching of embryos following assisted conception improved live birth and clinical pregnancy rates. The primary outcome measure was live birth rate per woman randomized, as this reflects the 'take home baby' rate that is crucial to any ART.

Twenty-eight randomized controlled trials involving assisted hatching conducted on embryos of 1876 women were included in the metanalyses and various subgroups were analysed. Although the measure of live birth rate was considered to be the moot question in evaluation of any outcome related to AH technique, only 25% of the studies that fulfilled the inclusion criteria reported it. Based on the available data, the evidence suggests that there is no effect of AH on live birth rate in all the analysed subgroups.

Metanalyses showed significant improvement in the odds of clinical pregnancy rate after AH (OR 1.29, 95% CI 1.12–1.49). The significance was attenuated when the analysis was limited to more robust trials and was in fact eliminated when analysis was limited to trials reporting live birth rates.

Clinical pregnancy rate appears to improve in women with poor prognostic characteristics (OR 1.04, 95% CI 0.82–1.33). Those with good prognostic features did not appear to benefit from AH.

Clinical pregnancy rate was improved following chemical and laser methods of AH (OR 1.38, 95% CI 1.11–1.73; OR 1.27, 95% CI 1.03–1.56 respectively). Mechanical method of AH does not appear to confer any benefit. This could be due to fewer studies based on the technique and therefore significantly small numbers in this category. Significant improvement in clinical pregnancy rate was seen independent of the degree of assisted hatching, be it thinning, drilling a small hole in the zona or complete zona removal (OR 1.33, 95% CI 1.04–1.72; OR 1.23, 95% CI 1.01–1.50 and OR 1.93, 95% CI 1.21–3.09, respectively).

The type of ART–IVF or ICSI, transfer of fresh or frozen embryos, undergoing the first or repeat cycle of ART does not appear to influence clinical pregnancy rates when AH is used.

No significant difference in miscarriage rates was seen following AH (OR 1.13, 95% CI 0.74–1.73). Assisted hatching appears to be associated with significant increase in multiple pregnancy rates (OR 1.67, 95% CI 1.24–2.26) with a 0.8% higher chance of monozygotic twinning with AH regardless of the technique employed.

Conclusion

Current evidence provides insufficient data to investigate the impact of assisted hatching on several important outcomes including monozygotic twinning, embryo damage, congenital and chromosomal abnormalities, and in vitro blastocyst development. From the few studies that report, there appears to be no high risk of the occurrence of ectopic pregnancy, congenital/chromosomal anomalies, or embryo damage following AH.

Overall, the quality of evidence evaluating the benefits and risks of AH is mixed. It appears to be a safe procedure and could be used in selected patient groups. There is insufficient evidence to determine the positive effect of AH on live birth rate. The cost implication of the procedure needs to be evaluated with respect to "take home baby" rate before routine inclusion of AH in assisted reproduction services. Currently, the application of AH is more technologically driven rather than evidence based.

References

1. Gardner DK, Lane M, Schoolcraft WB. Culture and transfer of viable blastocysts: a feasible proposition for human IVF. *Hum Reprod* 2000;**15** Suppl 6: 9–23.

2. Al-Nuaim LA, Jenkins JM. Assisted hatching in assisted reproduction. *Br J Obstet Gynaecol* 2002;**109**:856–62.

3. Fang C, Li T, Miao B, Zhuang G, Zhou C. Mechanically expanding the zona pellucida of human frozen thawed embryos: a new method of assisted hatching. *Fertil Steril* 2010;**94**:1302–07.

4. Mantoudis E, Podsaidly BT, Gorgy A, Venkat G, Craft IL. A comparison between quarter, partial and total laser hatching in selected infertility patients. *Hum Reprod* 2001;**16**:2182–86.

5. Balaban B, Urman B, Alatas C, *et al.* A comparison of four different techniques of assisted hatching. *Hum Reprod* 2002;**17**:1239–43.

6. Miyata H, Matsubayashi H, Fukutomi N, *et al.* Relevance of the site of assisted hatching in thawed human blastocysts: a preliminary report. *Fertil Steril* 2010;**94**:2444–7.

7. Das S, Blake D, Farquhar C, Hooper L, Seif MW. Assisted hatching on assisted conception (IVF and ICSI). *Cochrane Database Syst Rev* 2006: CD001894.

Chapter 30

The role of ultrasound in embryo transfer

Hakan E. Duran and Bradley J. Van Voorhis

Introduction

Atraumatic, "easy" embryo transfer (ET) to the uterus undoubtedly contributes to improved embryo implantation rates and pregnancy rates with IVF. Multiple studies suggest that the overall ease of the ET is strongly correlated to cycle outcome. One large study found a 1.7-fold higher pregnancy rate after easy transfers as compared to difficult ET (reviewed in [1]). The presence of blood on the catheter following ET reflects a traumatic transfer and has been associated with a lower pregnancy rate after IVF. Although the mechanism for the reduced pregnancy rate is not known, it is possible that endometrial injury creates a hostile environment to the embryo. In addition, prostaglandin release caused by contact between the uterine fundus and the transfer catheter may stimulate uterine contractions which, in turn, could lead to expulsion of the transferred embryo.

Preparation for ET

In most clinics, difficulty with the ET is anticipated by performing a trial or "mock" transfer (see Chapter 31). The uterine cavity is sounded by passing the catheter to the uterine fundus to measure the full length of the uterine cavity and cervical canal. The cervical canal is "mapped" and notes are made about the type of speculum required, type of catheter used, need for a tenaculum, as well as the direction and curve of the catheter required to successfully guide the catheter to the uterine fundus. If difficulty is encountered, steps can be taken to improve the likelihood that the actual ET goes smoothly. If cervical stenosis is encountered, the cervix can by dilated by a number of techniques including mechanical dilation, use of an osmotic dilator such as a laminaria, placement of a Malecot catheter, and even hysteroscopic "shaving" of the cervical canal. In cases of cervical stenosis, reduced pregnancy rates are reported when cervical dilatation is done within five days of ET, whereas dilatation done several weeks before ET appears to improve pregnancy rates. Therefore the mock transfer should be performed before the start of the IVF cycle, if possible.

In addition to cervical stenosis, sometimes an extremely flexed uterus can make an ET difficult. When this is noted during the mock transfer, steps can be taken to help ensure an atraumatic ET. In the case of a very anteflexed uterus, having a full bladder at the time of the ET can straighten the uterus, facilitating ET. In addition, the need for a tenaculum can be anticipated for use in straightening the uterus at the time of the ET. Because placement of a tenaculum can be painful and cause uterine contractions, in cases where the need for uterine

How to Improve Your ART Success Rates, ed. Gab Kovacs. Published by Cambridge University Press.

manipulation is anticipated, we will place a loosely tied stitch into the cervix for use in traction during the ET. The stitch can then be easily removed following ET.

Performance of the ET

The ET procedure starts by placing a speculum in the vagina to visualize the cervix which is then cleansed with a saline solution or with culture media. Some recommend aspirating or flushing excess cervical mucus, in an attempt to reduce the likelihood that the transfer catheter is plugged. After confirmation of patient identity, the transfer catheter is loaded with the embryo(s). The catheter is then inserted through the cervical canal and into the endometrial cavity where the embryos are deposited. The catheter is then withdrawn and handed back to the embryologist to check for retained embryos.

Clinical touch technique

This is the traditional ET technique which relies on the dexterity, tactile ability, and the personal experience of the clinician who performs the ET blindly while trying to accomplish an atraumatic ET. If a mock transfer has been performed, the clinician is aided by knowledge of the distance to the uterine fundus as well as any curves in the catheter that may be required. The classical clinical touch technique relied on advancement of the catheter through the uterine cavity until the tip was perceived to make contact with the uterine fundus. The catheter was then withdrawn 5–10 mm and the embryo(s) injected. With the recognition that contact with the uterine fundus could incite bleeding as well as uterine contractions, a modified technique was developed which made use of the knowledge of the uterine length from the mock transfer. In this case, the catheter is advanced to within 1–2 cm of the total distance between the cervix and the fundus, thus avoiding contact with the fundus. Today, most clinicians using the clinical touch technique for ET utilize this modified approach.

Ultrasound-guided ET

Ultrasound (U/S) guidance has been suggested as an aid to optimize ET [2], as it may facilitate an atraumatic insertion of the catheter and ensure correct location in the uterine cavity before depositing the embryo(s). When transabdominal U/S is used, the bladder should be full to aid in visualization. A number of commercially-available catheters are echogenic which improves visualization allowing for real-time feedback about the location of the catheter during ET. Ultrasound guidance is typically done using a 3.5–5 MHz 2-D transabdominal sector transducer from a mid-sagittal or oblique plane of the uterus and cervix. In our experience, scanning through an oblique sagittal plane is superior to a mid-sagittal plane since interference of the U/S waves by the upper blade of the speculum is avoided. The direction of the U/S probe in relation to the patient's abdomen when the best image is obtained may assist in "aiming" the catheter in the right direction.

Although most ETs are performed easily and quickly with either the clinical touch or with ultrasound-guided techniques, proponents of U/S guidance list several possible advantages. If a mock transfer is done prior to the stimulation, measurements and anticipated uterine position may change after ovarian stimulation due to hormonal differences and enlarged ovaries. This may lead to placement of embryos at "suboptimal" depths with the clinical touch technique. Several studies suggest a distance between 10 and 20 mm from the uterine fundus is optimal for ET, although others have found similar pregnancy rates when ET is performed at greater than 2 cm from the fundus. Therefore, this advantage of U/S guidance remains theoretical at this time. Ultrasound guidance may be helpful in uteri distorted by fibroids or those with cesarean section scar defects in which the catheter may get misdirected. The full bladder required for abdominal U/S may help to straighten the cervico-uterine angle and facilitate entry of the catheter, particularly for a strongly anteverted uterus. Ultrasound guidance can be particularly helpful in training institutions as the image provides real-time feedback to both the trainee and instructor. We have screens for patients to watch the ET and many find great comfort in visualizing this final step of a long and arduous treatment cycle.

Disadvantages of U/S guidance include the need for a second operator in the room as well as the time and discomfort of ensuring a full bladder. Sometimes visualization is poor, particularly in obese patients, and the operator may need to move the catheter to enhance detection. This movement could disrupt the endometrium. This movement is seldom required with new echogenic catheters.

Transvaginal U/S provides better visualization of the cervical canal and uterine cavity than transabdominal scanning and some have studied this approach for ET [3]. One advantage is that transvaginal U/S does not require a full bladder. However technical difficulties have been reported in advancing a loaded ET catheter next to a transvaginal U/S probe in the vagina due to space constraints. One prospective randomized trial has failed to show any advantage of the transvaginal U/S guidance compared to transabdominal U/S. Nevertheless, in the setting of an acutely retroflexed uterus, transvaginal U/S guidance may be particularly helpful. Perhaps development of vaginal U/S probes with thinner caliber, specifically designed to be used for ET while the speculum is still in place may increase the use of this technique.

Another promising technology to improve ET technique may be the real-time 3D U/S, i.e., 4D ultrasonography [4]. It allows a real-time constructed coronal section of the uterine cavity to be obtained instead of a 2D sagittal view. There are currently a few studies in the literature suggesting improved visualization of catheter location and embryo disposal by using 3D and/or 4D ultrasonography technique. Obtaining a coronal section of the uterus will improve the mid-line placement of the ET catheter and help avoid lateral disposition of embryo(s). However, for 4D ultrasonography to be utilized more commonly for ET purposes, better graphical processors providing a closer-to-real-time experience need to be developed. Another hurdle in adoption of this technique may be its application in an obese woman, where the quality of the image may be compromised more significantly than a 2D image, especially when acquired transabdominally.

Ultrasound-guided ET versus clinical touch – What is the evidence?

A total of 17 randomized clinical trials have been conducted comparing U/S guidance with clinical touch. A 2010 Cochrane review noted that, while all of the studies reported clinical pregnancy (defined as intrauterine pregnancy with visualization of fetal heart beat via U/S), only seven of them reported ongoing pregnancy (intrauterine pregnancy beyond 12 weeks after ET) and only three studies reported live birth; the latter two were the main outcome measures of the analysis [5]. Clinical pregnancy rate was about 30% higher for US guided ET (OR 1.31, 95% CI 1.18–1.46) when compared to clinical touch method. Ongoing pregnancy rate was also higher for U/S guidance (OR 1.38, 95% CI 1.16–1.64). There was no statistically significant difference between live birth rates between the two ET techniques in the few studies that reported this outcome (OR 1.14, 95% CI 0.93–1.39). Three other meta-analyses have had similar conclusions. Considering the relative paucity of live birth data reported, more studies addressing this outcome are warranted before reaching a final conclusion on the impact of U/S guidance on ET outcome. However, current data certainly favors U/S guidance. In addition, U/S guidance has been associated with fewer ectopic pregnancies following ET in some, but not all studies.

In our center, we have been performing ultrasound-guided ET for many years and it has become an integral part of our practice. We find it an indispensible tool for improving our ET technique as well as a fundamental requisite for clinical training. We also find that allowing the patient to visualize the transfer helps to engage the patient/couple in the process and contributes to their confidence and overall satisfaction. It would be very difficult for our team to go back to the clinical touch method without a sense of losing one's candle in the dark.

Conclusion

Embryo transfer remains to be an important, yet inefficient step in IVF cycle. Ultrasound guidance is a means to improve the efficiency of ET in terms of implantation, clinical pregnancy and, probably, live birth rates, although this outcome requires further study. An increase in implantation rate may also encourage a higher rate of single embryo transfer, reducing multiple pregnancy rates after IVF cycles. Transvaginal and/or 3D/4D ultrasonography are promising techniques to be utilized for ET procedures, although some optimization and further study is needed.

References

1. Mains L, Van Voorhis BJ. Optimizing the technique of embryo transfer. *Fertil Steril* 2010;**94**:785–90.
2. Strickler RC, Christianson C, Crane JP, *et al.* Ultrasound guidance for human embryo transfer. *Fertil Steril* 1985;**43**: 54–61.
3. Porat N, Boehnlein LM, Schouweiler CM, Kang J, Lindheim SR. Interim analysis of a randomized clinical trial comparing abdominal versus transvaginal ultrasound-guided embryo transfer. *J Obstet Gynaecol Res* 2010;**36**:384–392.
4. Letterie GS. Three-dimensional ultrasound-guided embryo transfer: a preliminary study. *Am J Obstet Gynecol* 2005;**192**:1983–7;discussion 1987–8.
5. Brown J, Buckingham K, Abou-Setta AM, Buckett W. Ultrasound versus 'clinical touch' for catheter guidance during embryo transfer in women. *Cochrane Database Syst Rev* 2010 **20**;(1):CD006107.

Chapter 31

Does dummy embryo transfer help?

Ragaa Mansour

Dummy embryo transfer

Embryo transfer (ET) is the final, yet crucial step of IVF. To most clinicians, ET would appear to be a straightforward procedure: only the simple task of inserting the embryo transfer catheter in the uterine cavity and ejecting the embryo(s). Unfortunately, the reality is not as simple as it may appear.

Extra time and attention should be given to the procedure of embryo transfer. Meldrum *et al.* [1] recognized that meticulous embryo transfer technique is essential for IVF success. This final step in assisted reproduction will determine the outcome of a long process and great effort; from ovulation induction and oocyte retrieval, to the tedious high technology procedures in the laboratory, not to mention the high hopes of infertile couples.

A rehearsal, i.e., the dummy embryo transfer before the actual one, has been shown to improve the pregnancy rates [2]. This procedure is important to evaluate the length and direction of the uterine cavity and cervical canal as well as the cervico-uterine angulations. Dummy ET also helps in choosing the most suitable kind of catheter to be used. Another advantage of the dummy ET is to discover any unanticipated difficulty in introducing the catheter such as pin-point external os, the presence of cervical polyps or fibroids, or anatomical distortion of the cervix from previous surgery or congenital anomaly. The procedure of dummy ET is usually performed one to two months prior to the start of the IVF cycle or immediately before the actual ET. However it is recommended to perform both. It is performed as follows: the patient is put in the lithotomy position and the cervix is visualized using the vaginal speculum. The cervix is wiped using sterile gauze to remove excess mucus. A sterile soft ET catheter is introduced through the cervical canal into the uterine cavity. If the soft catheter does not pass, a more rigid, but malleable one can be used. Choosing the most suitable catheter for each patient should be done before the actual ET to avoid harshly navigating the cervical canal with the ET catheter loaded with embryos.

The uterine length and the degree of the angle between the cervix and uterine body should also be noted.

Dificulties in introducing the ET catheter

One must note that various difficulties may arise while performing the embryo transfer.

One cause for the failure of the catheter to pass the internal os is the unnoticed coiling and bending of the catheter inside the cervical canal, which can be misleading, especially with soft

How to Improve Your ART Success Rates, ed. Gab Kovacs. Published by Cambridge University Press.

catheters. This can be discovered by experienced practitioners and by doing a simple test of rotating the catheter 360°. If it recoils, it means it is coiled inside the cervical canal.

Another significant cause for the failure of the catheter to pass the internal cervical os is simply a lack of achieving proper alignment between the ET catheter (straight) and the utero-cervical angle (curved or acutely angulated). A situation in which you need to curve the catheter while you have the embryos already loaded should be completely avoided. Proper evaluation of the cervico-uterine angle and determining how much curvature is needed for the catheter should be done before loading the embryos. That is why it is important to perform a dummy ET right before the actual one and revise the previously performed ultrasound picture of the uterus.

It has been demonstrated that curving the ET catheter according to the cervico-uterine angle improves the clinical pregnancy rate. Straightening the utero-cervical angle can be achieved by a full bladder before ET [3]. This effect is achieved indirectly by performing ET under ultrasound guidance.

Another method to facilitate introduction of the catheter is simply by gentle maneuvering of the vaginal speculum (the degree of opening and how far it is pushed inside).

The use of a more rigid catheter is sometimes needed in order to pass the internal os. It is advantageous that these rigid catheters be malleable. Malleability is essential to allow making the required curve, which will overcome the acute cervico-uterine angulations. Using a malleable stylet to place the outer sheath correctly and negotiate the cervical canal before introducing the soft catheter was found to have no negative impact on implantation and delivery rates. The use of a special introducer designed to overcome difficulties in selected patients in passing the ET catheter was described.

The effect of cervical traction with a tenaculum on the utero-cervical angle was studied using a radio-opaque guide-wire [4]. The authors found that moderate cervical traction straightens the uterus. It was concluded that the routine use of the tenaculum theoretically makes the passage of an embryo transfer catheter easier and less traumatic. On the other hand it should be remembered that holding the cervix with a volsellum initiates uterine contractions. Moreover, holding the cervix with a volsellum is painful and should be done under general anesthesia or local anesthetic.

In extremely rare cases it is very difficult or even impossible to pass the catheter inside the uterine cavity. It may be due to anatomical distortion of the cervix by previous surgery or fibroid or due to congenital anomaly. Scarring of the lower uterine segment or distorted endometrial cavity creates difficulty in catheter introduction.

Yanushpolosky and colleagues [5] demonstrated that hysteroscopic evaluation and/or correction of the endocervix, followed by transcervical placements of a Malecot catheter, for an average of 10 days, allowed easier entry through the cervical canal in patients in whom previous ET has been difficult. Cervical dilatation may be resorted to in cases of cervical stenosis. However, a short interval between dilatation and ET is not recommended. Very low pregnancy rates were reported when cervical dilatation was done during oocyte pick-up or two days before ET. It is also helpful to place a laminaria approximately one month before starting the IVF cycle as reported by Glatstein in 1997 [6] or to place hygroscopic rods in the cervix prior to ovarian stimulation [7]. The standard method of dilatation with successively larger dilators may be difficult and traumatic in some tortuous or stenotic cervical canals.

In conclusion it is crucial that the ET catheter must pass the internal os and enter the uterine cavity, otherwise the whole IVF cycle will be a total failure. Performing a rehearsal or the dummy ET is important: (1) to determine the most suitable kind of ET catheter for each patient, (2) to determine the degree of cervico-uterine angle, and (3) to measure the uterine cavity length. It can be done 1–2 months before the IVF cycle, or immediately before the actual ET. It is recommended to perform both. It has been shown that dummy ET significantly improved pregnancy rates [2].

References

1. Meldrum, DR, Chetkowski, R, Steingol, KA, *et al.* Evolution of a highly successful in vitro fertilization-embryo transfer program. *Fertil Steril* 1987;**48**:86–93.
2. Mansour, R, Aboulghar, M, Serour, G. Dummy embryo transfer: a technique that minimizes the problems of embryo transfer and improves the pregnancy rate in human in-vitro fertilization. *Fertil Steril* 1990;**54**:678–81.
3. Sharif, K, Afnan, M, Lenton, W. Mock embryo transfer with a full-bladder immediately before the real transfer for in-vitro fertilization treatment: the Birmingham experience of 113 cases. *Hum Reprod* 1995;**10**:1715–8.
4. Johnson, N and Bromham DR. Effect of cervical traction with a tenaculum on the uterocervical angle. *Br J Obstet Gynaecol* 1991;**98**:309–12.
5. Yanushpolsky EH, Ginsburg ES, Fox JH, Stewart EA. Transcervical placement of a Malecot catheter after hysteroscopic evaluation provides for easier entry into the endometrial cavity for women with histories of difficult intrauterine inseminations and/or embryo transfers: a prospective case series. *Fertil Steril* 2000;**73**:402–5.
6. Glatstein IZ, Pang SC, McShane PM. Successful pregnancies with the use of laminaria tents before embryo transfer for refractory cervical stenosis. *Fertil Steril* 1997;**67**:1172–4.
7. Serhal P, Ranieri DM, Khadum I, Wakim RA. Cervical dilatation with hygroscopic rods prior to ovarian stimulation facilitates embryo transfer. *Hum Reprod* 2003;**18**:2618–20.

Chapter 32

Embryo transfer: Does position matter?

Wendy S. Vitek and Sandra A. Carson

Introduction

In recognition of the importance of embryo transfer in the success of IVF, research has focused on optimizing the technical aspects of the technique. Suboptimal technique can compromise implantation rates by disrupting the endometrium, inducing uterine contractions, and depositing the embryos in suboptimal locations for implantation. Successful embryo transfers result from the atraumatic delivery of embryos to the mid-portion of the uterus, a location associated with maximal implantation potential. Evidence supports minimizing endometrial trauma with soft catheters (see Chapter 33), optimizing the "ease" of transfers through trial transfers (see Chapter 31) and techniques that minimize uterine contractions and ultrasound (U/S) guidance (see Chapter 30) to target ideal embryo deposition. Therefore, the position of the uterus, as it relates to difficult transfers, and the position of the transfer catheter at embryo deposition are important factors that impact the success of embryo transfers. The aim of this chapter is to review the evidence regarding uterine position and catheter position on embryo transfer outcomes and to discuss techniques that optimize these factors.

Difficult transfers and uterine position

Although the impact of difficult transfers on implantation rates and pregnancy rates has been debated, a meta-analysis of nine controlled trials found an association between "ease" of embryo transfer and pregnancy outcomes [1]. Patients with difficult transfers experienced significantly lower implantation rates (11.7% versus 18.7%, OR 0.64, 95% CI 0.52–0.77) and pregnancy rates (22.3% versus 31.6%, OR 0.74, 95% CI 0.64–0.87). Difficult transfers were generally classified as embryo transfers that required cervical or uterine manipulation, increased force and/or were accompanied by trauma. Difficult transfers can be encountered with cervical stenosis or extreme uterine positions, such as sharply anteverted, retroverted, anteflexed, or retroflexed uteri. While cervical manipulation with a tenaculum may aid in navigating a stenotic cervix or a sharp cervico-uterine angle, it can lead to the release of oxytocin and prostaglandins, resulting in uterine junctional zone contractions or endometrial wavelike movements. Lensy *et al.* documented a significant increase in opposing and random cervico-fundal contractions captured through digitized transvaginal U/S images in all 20 patients undergoing mock transfers with the aid of a tenaculum [2]. Franchin *et al.* quantified the frequency of uterine contractions at the time of embryo transfer and found that fewer than three uterine contractions/minutes was associated with a clinical pregnancy

How to Improve Your ART Success Rates, ed. Gab Kovacs. Published by Cambridge

rate of 53%, while more than five uterine contractions/minute was associated with a decreased clinical pregnancy rate of 14% (p <0.001) possibly due to expulsion of the embryos [3]. In addition to increased uterine contractions, difficult transfers can lead to endometrial trauma. An indirect marker of endometrial trauma is the presence of blood on the outside of the transfer catheter. This finding has been associated with lower pregnancy rates and a higher incidence of retained embryos [4]. While firm catheters may aid in catheter placement with difficult transfers, the increased force and rigidity of the catheter may induce endometrial trauma. A meta-analysis found that firm catheters are associated with lower pregnancy rates than soft catheters [5].

Trial transfers and uterine position

In order to minimize difficult transfers, trial transfers can be preformed. This was discussed in detail in Chapter 31. In summary, trial transfers prior to ovarian stimulation map the cervical angle and the uterine depth. Mansour *et al.* randomized 335 patients to trial transfer prior to ovarian stimulation or no trial transfer [6]. No difficult transfers occurred in the group randomized to trial transfer, while 50 (29.8%) difficult transfers were encountered in the group randomized to no trial transfer. The implantation rates and pregnancy rates were 13.1% and 4.4% respectively in the group randomized to no trial transfer, compared to 22.8% and 7.2% in the group randomized to trial transfer. The low implantation rates in this study have been criticised, but no further randomized trials have been reported, nor have randomized trials examining timing of trial transfers been reported.

Trial transfers can be performed prior to ovarian stimulation or at the time of embryo transfer. Performing trial transfers prior to ovarian stimulation allows for advance planning to prevent difficult transfers due to cervical stenosis or extreme uterine positions. In the event of cervical stenosis, cervical dilation can be performed prior to ovarian stimulation to allow sufficient time for the endometrium to recover from the trauma associated with dilation. Placement of laminaria or a Malecot catheter have been described as effective alternatives to mechanical dilation. Extreme uterine positions can often be straightened with techniques that minimize cervical manipulation. A full bladder at the time of embryo transfer can straighten a sharply anteverted uterus. A long cervical stitch, placed at the time of oocyte retrieval, can be used to straighten a sharply retroverted uterus with less manipulation than a tenaculum.

Alternatively, trial transfers can be performed at the time of embryo transfer, which may avoid unnecessary preparation as stimulated ovaries in the posterior cul-de-sac may convert a retroverted uterus into an anteverted uterus. The empty trial catheter should be advanced to the level of the internal os in order to map the cervical angle, while avoiding disruption of the endometrium. If the cervix is easily traversed, the transfer catheter can be loaded with embryos and the transfer can be performed. If persistent cervical stenosis or sharp cervico-uterine angles are encountered, a malleable outer sheath can be used to cannulate the cervix to the level of the internal os, in order to facilitate the introduction of a soft catheter for transfer while minimizing endometrial trauma. This approach may minimize the time the embryos spend in the catheter.

In rare cases when a transcervical transfer cannot be accomplished, a transmyometrial transfer, referred to as the Towako method, can be performed while maintaining high pregnancy rates [7]. The Towako method introduces the transfer catheter through a needle attached to an endovaginal U/S probe.

Ultrasound guidance and catheter position

Varying position of the catheter at the time of embryo deposition is associated with differences in pregnancy rates and ectopic pregnancy rates. Early IVF successes were accomplished with the tip of the transfer catheter placed 5–10 mm from the uterine fundus using a "clinical touch" technique. Woolcott *et al.* found that blind catheter placement results in abutment of the catheter tip with the fundus or tubal ostia in more than 25% of cases [8]. Fundal contact may trigger uterine contractions and induce more endometrial disruption. The introduction of transabdominal ultrasound-guided embryo transfers has enabled precise catheter placement and is associated with improved outcomes. This has been reviewed in Chapter 30. A recent Cochrane review of 17 randomized controlled trials found that ultrasound-guided embryo transfers increased clinical pregnancy rates over the "clinical touch" technique (OR 1.38, 95% CI 1.16–1.64) [9]. Ultrasound-guided embryo transfers have also provided insight into variables that affect the success of transfers, such as the optimal location for embryo deposition. Baba *et al.* utilized 3D U/S to examine the relationship between the location of embryo-transfer-associated air bubbles and the resultant gestational sac and found that 80% of embryos implant in the areas to which they are initially transferred [10]. Given that embryos implant near the site of deposition, investigators have aimed to pinpoint the location for transfer that is associated with the highest implantation rates.

Coroleu *et al.* randomized 180 patients undergoing ultrasound-guided embryo transfers to varied distances (10 +/− 1.5 mm; 15 +/− 1.5 mm; or 20 +/− 1.5 mm) between the tip of the catheter and uterine fundus at the time of embryo deposition. Implantation rates were significantly higher with placement of the catheter tip 15–20 mm from the fundus as compared to 10 mm from the fundus (33.3% versus 20.6%, $p < 0.05$) [11]. Given the wide variation observed in uterine cavity lengths, Frankfurter *et al.* compared deposition in the middle to lower uterine segment and the fundal region, instead of a fixed distance from the uterine fundus (Figure 32.1). In this prospective cohort study, pregnancy rates were improved with lower and mid-portion transfers compared to fundal transfers (39.6% versus 31.2%, $p<0.005$) [12]. With the introduction of 3D U/S, the site for optimal embryo deposition has been further refined. Gergely *et al.* utilized 3D/4D U/S to define the maximal implantation potential point, which is the intersection of a line drawn from each fallopian tube in the mid-portion of the uterus (Figure 32.2) [13]. These investigators hypothesize that natural pregnancies implant in the posterior aspect of the mid-portion of the uterus in a trajectory with the ostia of the fallopian tubes and that the maximal implantation potential point is an approximation of this location. A cohort study of over 5000 patients, utilizing 3D/4D U/S to target the maximal implantation potential point was associated with a 10% increase in pregnancy rate [14]. Avoiding fundal embryo transfers not only improves pregnancy rates, but also appears to decrease the rate of ectopic pregnancy. Transfers performed with the catheter tip less than 5 mm from the fundus are associated with an increased rate of ectopic pregnancy [15]. Gergely *et al.* also found that targeting the maximum implantation potential point significantly reduced the ectopic pregnancy rate from 1.82% to 0.49% ($p = 0.003$).

Conclusion

In conclusion, uterine position and catheter position are important factors that influence the ability to deliver embryos to the mid-portion of the uterus in an atraumatic fashion. Randomized controlled trials have demonstrated that pregnancy rates are significantly

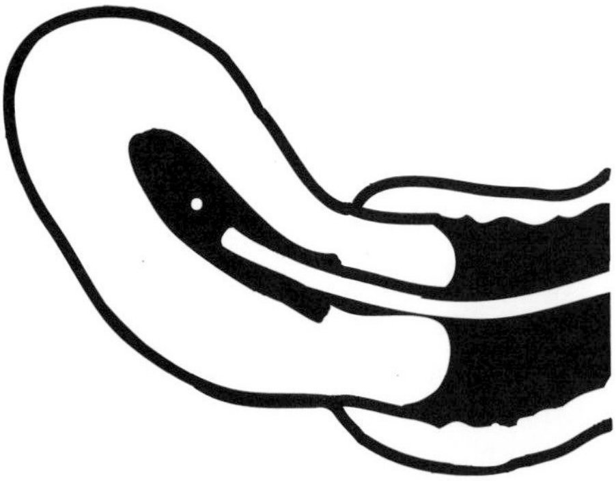

Figure 32.1 Sagittal view of embryo transfer at the mid-fundus.

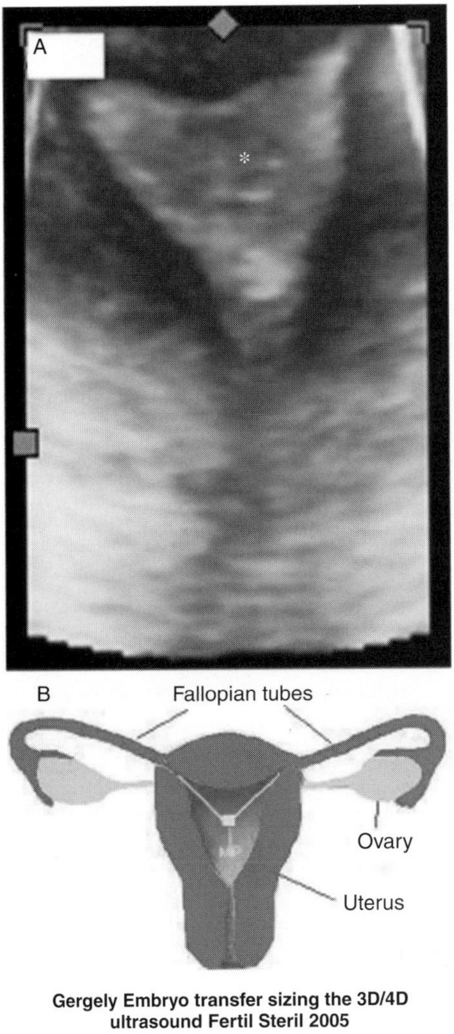

Figure 32.2 (A) Three-dimensional ultrasound image with the maximal implantation potential (MIP) point marked with an asterisk. (B) Anatomic diagram demonstrating the MIP point. Reprinted from *Fertility and Sterility*, **84**(2), Gergely RZ, DeUgarte CM, Danzer H, Surrey M, Hill D, DeCherney A, Three dimensional/four dimensional ultrasound-guided embryo transfer using the maximal implantation potential point, pg 501, Copyright 2005, with permission from Elsevier.

increased by minimizing difficult transfers through trial transfers and by depositing embryos in the mid-portion of the uterus under ultrasound guidance. Advances in ultrasound technology have allowed further refinement of the maximal implantation potential point in an attempt to deliver embryos to the precise location that natural pregnancies implant.

References

1. Sallam H, Sameh S, Sadek S, Agameya A. Does a difficult embryo transfer affect the results of IVF and ICSI? A meta-analysis of controlled studies. *Fertil Steril* 2003;**80** (3 Suppl):127.
2. Lesny P, Killick SR, Robinson J, Raven G, Maguiness SD. Junctional zone contractions and embryo transfer: is it safe to use a tenaculum? *Hum Reprod* 1999;**14**:2367–70.
3. Fanchin R, Righini C, Olivennes F, *et al.* Uterine contractions at the time of embryo transfer alter pregnancy rates after in-vitro fertilization. *Hum Reprod* 1998;**13**:1968–74.
4. Goudas VT, Hammitt DG, Damario MA, *et al.* Blood on the embryo transfer catheter is associated with decreased rates of embryo implantation and clinical pregnancy with the use of in vitro fertilization-embryo transfer. *Fertil Steril* 1998;**70**:878–82.
5. Abou-Setta AM, Al-Inany HG, Mansour RT, Serour GI, Aboulghar MA. Soft versus firm embryo transfer catheters for assisted reproduction: a systematic review and meta-analysis. *Hum Reprod* 2005;**20**:3114–21.
6. Mansour R, Aboulghar M, Serour G. Dummy embryo transfer: a technique that minimizes the problems of embryo transfer and improves the pregnancy rates in human in vitro fertilization. *Fertil Steril* 1990;**54**:678–81.
7. Kato O, Takatsuka R, Asch RH. Transvaginal-transmyometrial embryo transfer: the Towako method; experiences of 104 cases. *Fertil Steril* 1993;**59**;51–3.
8. Wolcott R, Stanger J. Potentially important variables identified by transvaginal ultrasound-guided embryo transfer. *Hum Reprod* 1997;**12**:963–9.
9. Brown JA, Buckingham K, About-Setta A, Buckett W. Ultrasound versus "clinical touch" for catheter guidance during embryo transfer in women. *Cochrane Database System Rev* 2010; **20**:CD006107.
10. Baba K, Ishihara O, Hayashi N, *et al.* Where does the embryo implant after embryo transfer in humans? *Fertil Steril* 2000;**73**:123–5.
11. Coroleu B, Barri PN, Carreras O, *et al.* The influence of the depth of embryo replacement into the uterine cavity on implantation rates after IVF: a controlled, ultrasound-guided study. *Hum Reprod* 2002;**17**:341–6.
12. Frankfurter D, Trimarchi JB, Silva CP, Keefe DL. Middle to lower uterine segment embryo transfer improves implantation and pregnancy rates compared with fundal embryo transfer. *Fertil Steril* 2004;**81**:1273–37.
13. Gergely RZ, DeUgarte CM, Danzer H, *et al.* Three dimensional/four dimensional ultrasound-guided embryo transfer. *Fertil Steril* 2005;**84**:500–3.
14. Nazari A, Askari HA, Check JH, O'Shaughnessy A. Embryo transfer technique as a cause of ectopic pregnancy in in vitro fertilization. *Fertil Steril* 1993;**60**:919–21.
15. Gergely R. 3D/4D ultrasound-guided embryo transfer targeting maximal implantation potential (MIP) point increases pregnancy rates and reduces ectopic pregnancies. *Human Reprod* 2010;**25**(suppl 1):i87.

Chapter 33

Embryo transfer catheters

Amr Wahba, Ahmed Abou-Setta,
Ragaa Mansour and Hesham Al-Inany

Introduction

Embryo transfer (ET) is the final critical step in IVF treatment. Despite its apparent simplicity, ET remains the rate limiting step in the success of IVF owing to the high rate of implantation failure. It is still an enigma why transfer is the most inefficient step. The main factors that affect the embryo implantation are uterine receptivity, embryo quality, and efficiency of the ET procedure. Among the few essential steps of ET, catheter technology emerges as one crucial factor which has gained recent attention. The ET catheter, being the vehicle that carries and transfers the precious products of IVF, may play a pivotal role in the success of this decisive step, with the clinician acting as the vehicle driver whose meticulous mission is to transfer these embryos with a high degree of reliability into the uterine cavity in the safest and least traumatic way. The choice of ET catheter has been reported to be the third most important variable in the success of IVF .This chapter will explore the essential features of ET catheters that may have an impact on the success of IVF in an evidence-based approach.

Description of embryo transfer catheters

Embryo transfer catheters are sterile devices used for the introduction of embryos into the uterine cavity following IVF. All ET catheters available are mainly composed of non-embryo toxic plastics and/or metal. Variations in the ET catheter design include variations in length, caliber, location of distal opening (end or side opening), degree of stiffness, and malleability, presence or absence of an outer sheath, presence or absence of internal stylet or obturator, echodensity, quality of materials, and finish.

The so-called double lumen catheter is a single lumen ET catheter equipped with an outer sheath which acts as an introducer or a guiding catheter while the inner catheter acts as the transfer catheter. These type of catheters are of variable lengths, usually between 18 and 23 cm, the inner transfer cannula may be soft or firm with an end opening and a detachable outer sheath that is attached to the inner catheter by a Luer taper.

Soft catheters are less traumatic but have a higher failure rate to negotiate the cervix. Firm catheters, use of an internal stylet or a rigid outer sheath make catheter placement easier, but may cause more bleeding, trauma, mucus plugging, and stimulation of uterine contractions.

How to Improve Your ART Success Rates, ed. Gab Kovacs. Published by Cambridge University Press.

Table 33.1 Some examples of ET catheters

		Features
Soft ET catheters	Cook® Soft-Trans	Consists of 12.5 cm firm proximal part and a 4.0 cm soft distal part
	Gynetics® Delphin	21 cm long, uses a combination of a soft, flexible intrauterine catheter and a solid cervix catheter, but is softer than Gynetics® Emtrac-A ET catheter
	Frydman®	Outer catheter: firm, made of polypropylene, 14.5 cm long, 2.2 mm OD. Inner catheter: soft, made of polyurethane, 23 cm long, 1.53 mm OD, open ended.
	Edwards-Wallace®	Outer catheter: firm, made of Teflon Inner catheter: 18 or 23 cm long, made of polyethylene, with an open end, 1.6®mm OD
	Cook® Sydney IVF	Outer catheter: 19 cm long, has a polycarbonate hub, a bulb tip and the distal end is angled. Inner catheter: 23 cm long and the tip is 2.8 French size.
Firm ET catheters	Gynetics® Emtrac-A	21 cm long, consists of a soft, flexible intrauterine catheter and a solid cervix catheter
	Tom Cat®	11.5 cm long, made of polyethylene, 1 mm OD, 0.3 mm ID
	Erlangen®	Consists of an introducing metal cannula (fitted with an obturator), 2 mm OD, its tip is olive-shaped with a diameter of 3 mm. The silicon movable collar is usually placed 2–3 cm from the tip and an insertion catheter. The instrument has a length of 25 cm
	T.D.T.™(Tight Difficult Transfer)	Consists of a single lumen 18 cm long, polyethylene/polyprene cannula (Frydman 4.5) and a partly polyethylene, partly metal transfer catheter. The cannula is as a standard, equipped with a malleable metal obturator, enabling its bending into the required curve necessary for passage through the cervical canal
	Rocket® Embryon	18 cm long. The inner transfer catheter is made of polyurethane and the outer sheath is made of white polythene.

Types of embryo transfer catheters

Embryo transfer catheters can be subdivided mainly on the basis of the material they are made of and whether they are equipped with, or without, an introducing cannula that facilitates the transfer procedure. Some of the commercially available ET catheters are shown in Table 33.1.

Features of embryo transfer catheters affecting the outcome of embryo transfer

Despite the wide variations in the design of ET catheters, the main features that have been studied and found to have a possible influence on the success of ET procedure include flexibility, with or without outer sheath, and echodensity.

Flexibility and rigidity of embryo transfer catheters

A systematic review comparing soft and firm ET catheters revealed that the soft ET catheters overall, had superior performance. This was apparent in the implantation, clinical pregnancy, and 'take-home baby' rate [1]. One theory why the softer catheters produce better results is built on decreasing the trauma to the endometrium. The softer the materials used, the lesser the chance of damage to the endometrium and the lesser the chance of uterine contractions that causes expulsion of the transferred embryos. Soft transfer catheters follow the natural curvature of the uterine cavity better than the firmer catheters, possibly reducing the risk of burrowing into the posterior endometrium in the anteflexed uterus.

Since blood on the tip of the catheter or actual bleeding occurring during ET has been reported to be associated with decreased rate of embryo implantation and clinical pregnancy rate, it seems that the least traumatic and the smoothest transfers are the ones associated with better pregnancy rates. Despite the observation that soft catheters were associated with a higher degree of failure to negotiate the cervix and they had a higher rate of blood, mucus, and retained embryos at the tip of the ET catheter, this did not seem to alter the implantation or pregnancy rates [1]. The role of retained embryos in decreasing the pregnancy rate is controversial.

A more recent systematic review and meta-analysis comparing soft (Cook or Wallace) catheters with hard (TDT, Frydman, Tomcat, Rocket) catheters demonstrated an increased chance of clinical pregnancy when soft ET catheters were used. The TDT catheter was compared against both soft catheters and other hard catheters, showing a decreased chance of clinical pregnancy when the TDT catheter was used. In the same review, a meta-analysis of six prospective trials comparing the Cook and Wallace soft catheters showed no demonstrable difference in clinical pregnancy rates [2]. In a review of firm catheters, TDT catheters were shown to have poorer clinical outcomes compared to other firm catheters.

With or without a sheath

When double lumen soft ET catheters were compared with single lumen firm ET catheters in a randomized controlled trial, a 50% increase in pregnancy rate was noted. The soft inner catheter within a stiff outer sheath obviates the need for transferring embryos through the more rigid catheters in case of difficult transfers. Stiffer outer sheaths stabilize the softer inner cannula, which carries the embryos and actually enters the endometrial cavity for ET. However, it is important to mention that in order to benefit from the advantages of the softness of the catheter, the outer rigid sheath should be minimally used just to stop short of the internal cervical os, otherwise contractions can be initiated, which are probably mediated by the release of prostaglandins .

Among other factors that might contribute to the better results of the double lumen catheter is that the tip of the transfer catheter is protected within the guiding catheter when contact is made with the cervix, potentially reducing contamination of embryos by the cervical flora. Contamination of the catheter tip has been reported to yield lower pregnancy rates. The live birth rate after IVF is influenced by the presence of bacteria in the catheter tip. In addition, the guiding catheter may protect the embryos from physical trauma during passage through the cervical canal.

Echodensity and visibility with ultrasonography

The use of ultrasound (U/S) guidance to facilitate ET has proven useful in women with a previously difficult transfer. Recent meta-analyses provided robust evidence indicating that ultrasound-guided ET using transabdominal U/S is significantly more effective than ET by clinical touch alone [4].

A study that compared the visibility of the Rocket transfer catheter under U/S guidance with that of the Wallace catheter showed that the Rocket transfer catheter was clearly seen in significantly more transfers than the Wallace catheter. Interestingly, there was not a concomitant statistically significant difference in implantation or pregnancy rate between catheters [5].

It has been postulated that new echodense catheters which are more readily detectable by U/S may refine transfer techniques even more, thus improving IVF outcome by fulfilling the goals of atraumatic ET with precise embryo deposition. Some catheters already on the market have this feature, due to an echodense tip (Cook Echo-Tip catheter, Cook Ob/Gyn, Spencer, IN, USA; a modification of the soft-tip Wallace catheter in that the catheter has an echogenic stainless steel band at the tip of the inner sheath) or echogenicity extending along the whole length of the catheter (SureView Wallace embryo replacement catheter). It was hypothesized that these echogenic catheters would be easily tracked during their passage through the uterine cavity. This would minimize the to-and-fro motion necessary to identify the catheter tip which, in turn, would minimize disruption of the endometrium with improvement in implantation rates. However, despite the advantage of enhanced visualization of the new echogenic catheters which has simplified the procedure of ET, studies have not shown any significant improvement regarding pregnancy rates compared to the standard catheters [6]. The use of the new catheter was associated in one study with a significant increase in the number of twin pregnancies.

Yet, Aboul Foutouh *et al.* [7] argued that under U/S guidance, individual catheter choice does not statistically significantly affect the clinical pregnancy rate in a modern clinical IVF practice. This may be explained by the decrease in the incidence of difficult transfers and endometrial injury with ET under U/S guidance.

Conclusion

Evidence has shown that the type of ET catheter can have an influence on the success of IVF. The ideal ET catheter should be soft enough to avoid any trauma to the endocervix or endometrium, malleable enough to be able to negotiate the cervical canal, protected from bacterial contamination, and easily visualized and guided by U/S.

References

1. Abou-Setta AM, Al-Inany HG, Mansour RT, Serour GI, Aboulghar MA. Soft versus firm embryo transfer catheters for assisted reproduction: a systematic review and metaanalysis. *Hum Reprod* 2005;**20**: 3114–21.

2. Buckett WM. A review and meta-analysis of prospective trials comparing different catheters used for embryo transfer. *Fertil Steril* 2006;**85**:728–34.

3. Abou-Setta AM. Firm embryo transfer catheters for assisted reproduction: a systematic review and meta-analysis using direct and adjusted indirect comparisons. *Reprod Biomed Online* 2006;**12**:191–8.

4. Abou-Setta AM, Mansour RT, Al-Inany HG, *et al.* Among women undergoing embryo transfer, is the probability of pregnancy and live birth improved with ultrasound guidance over clinical touch alone? A systemic review and meta-analysis of prospective randomized trials. *Fertil Steril* 2007;**88**:333–41.

5. El Shawarby SA, Ravhon A, Skull J, *et al.* A prospective randomized controlled trial of Wallace and Rocket embryo transfer catheters. *Reprod Biomed Online* 2008;**17**: 549–52.

6. Karande V, Hazlett D, Vietzke M, Gleicher N. A prospective randomized comparison of the Wallace catheter and the Cook Echo

Tip® catheter for ultrasound-guided embryo transfer. *Fertil Steril* 2002;77:826–30.

7. Aboulfotouh I, Abou-Setta AM, Khattab S, *et al.* Firm versus soft embryo transfer catheters under ultrasound guidance: does catheter choice really influence the pregnancy rates? *Fertil Steril* 2008;**89**:1261–2.

Chapter 34

Bed rest after embryo transfer

Giuseppe Botta and Gedis Grudzinskas

Introduction

If there is any added value from evidence-based medicine, it is to provide a source of courage for fertility practitioners and doctors to replace what they feel in their hearts with facts which often serve to dispel the mythology that has hitherto been a feature of modern medicine. Behavior before, during and after embryo transfer (ET) has largely escaped rigorous scientific scrutiny as it continues to be the last or perhaps only element of IVF-ET procedures which is considered to be a "green-finger" technique beyond the scope/ability of hard-line and insensitive scientific enquiring minds.

What will happen when I stand up? This is a question often asked, or worse, not asked by women undergoing either intra-uterine insemination or embryo transfer. In the absence of evidence the tendency had been to advise women to remain horizontal for a short period or for longer intervals to full bed rest for 24 hours.

Is there sufficient anecdotal evidence that remaining horizontal for some time may be helpful, a matter which to some unjustifiably fuels anxiety of women and their husbands/partners?

Evidence that uterine contractility is highest in the peri-ovulatory phase is sound and interpreted as facilitating rapid sperm transit to the oocyte in the natural setting. What is its relevance in ART?

This short review examined the evidence as to whether rest after ET will improve live birth rates, reaching the conclusion that there is no evidence that it does. Should we now in all circumstances advise all our patients immediately after ET to rise and behave as usual?

Bed rest after embryo transfer: the data

The notion that bed rest following embryo transfer should be the norm, presumably was based on conservative medical dogma that rest facilitates the recovery process, notably recovery from the then more invasive open surgical techniques of oocyte retrieval, the speedy recovery from which should ipso facto, facilitate implantation in the early days of IVF. Given the social mores of the time and the pioneering nature of this fertility treatment, this advice was likely to have been religiously followed. After all how else was one to address the little understood processes of implantation of human embryos especially in the context of the low implantation and live birth rates of the time. Such was the concern, that if a couple had the financial means, women were not only advised to rest but to do so in a hospital facility. In

How to Improve Your ART Success Rates, ed. Gab Kovacs. Published by Cambridge

some societies this was directed at taking women out of their busy domestic existence, whilst in others, away from their husbands and families where often doctors had a fear of the effects of "heavy" conjugal responsibilities. Thus to rest became the norm for many years, and if not possible was considered a possible reason for failure of the procedure, provoking feelings of avoidable guilt or inadequacy. As techniques of oocyte retrieval and methods of anaesthesia and analgesia became less invasive women and others began to question the need for such a hard-line position on restriction of almost all activity after ET for at least a day. Well-intentioned, though this approach may have been, it soon began to be challenged as more women became pregnant following ET not having been on full bed rest because they would not or simply could not afford to be immobilized either at home or in a hospital bed. Thus in accord with many other changes in medical and surgical practice, not just in ART, the impact of such conservative approaches began to be questioned and to some degree subjected to scientific scrutiny.

We have shown that resting for 24 hours following ET is not associated with a better outcome than a bed rest of 20 minutes [1]. We stated: "Women, a few minutes after embryo transfer, can stand, empty their bladder and return home with no apparent risk to the process of implantation. No restriction of the routine activity of the patients need be advised after the transfer. This observation has some important economic implications: a short bed rest following embryo transfer avoids an extra day of recovery in the clinic and its related costs. Moreover, the early return of the patient to her daily activities allows an immediate return to work with no loss in productivity." As one of the earliest randomized control trials (RCTs) on this subject challenging the received wisdom, it was difficult to assess quite what impact if any our report had. One may speculate that our conclusion provided reassurance for some women who, of necessity needed to be immediately ambulant, to being ignored by the profession at large. Nevertheless, some women instinctively feel that rest is helpful, for emotional reasons if nothing else. Subsequent studies, typically observational, confirmed our findings, and as the efficiency of ART improved with most centers reporting 2–3 fold increases in live birth rates to those seen in the 1980s, more robust study designs were used to address the benefits or otherwise of immobilization/bed rest after ET.

The UK National Institute of Clinical Excellence (NICE) in 2004 issued the NICE Clinical Guidelines 011 for Fertility [2], which included the following recommendation:

> 1.11.9.4 Women should be informed that bed rest of more than 20 minutes' duration following embryo transfer does not improve the outcome of in vitro fertilisation treatment. Citing Grade A as the strength of evidence for this recommendation, being at least one RCT.

Data from other robust studies have been in accord, as well as recommending that bed rest after ET is useless [3].

Abou-Setta *et al.* [4] on behalf of the Cochrane Library performed screening and selection of 2436 possible trial citations independently by two review authors. Four prospective, truly randomized trials met the inclusion criteria. The trials compared two competing post ET interventions or an intervention versus no treatment in women undergoing IVF and intracytoplasmic sperm injection (ICSI). With respect to bed rest after ET, the primary outcome, live birth rate, was not reported in any of the included trials and the ongoing pregnancy rate was only available for one trial that compared immediate ambulation with 30 minute bed rest, with no evidence of an effect with bed rest (OR 1.00; 95% CI 0.54–1.85). Secondary outcomes were sporadically reported with the exception of clinical pregnancy rate, which was reported in all of the included trials. There was no significant difference between less bed rest and more rest (OR 1.13; 95% CI 0.77–1.67).

Taking the embryo for a walk?

Kucuk and colleagues [5] have added novel evidence of the beneficial effects of moderate levels of exercise for women undergoing ART, reporting substantially higher implantation and live birth rates than if there was a low level of exercise. Given that ART involves minor surgery for the oocyte retrieval, it is not a surprise that women do not have high levels of activity, but their data indicate that immobilization or reduced physical activity should not be advised. It is notable that none of the women undergoing ART had a high level of activity, so an enquiry about physical activity and reinforcing/advising women to maintain their normal moderate level of activity makes complete sense. We are not, after all, conducting an intervention, and whether the benefits come from exercise-induced benefits acting directly on the implantation process or via complex neuroendocrine pathways is of secondary relevance if any.

Conclusion

So if rather than having a nap, taking the embryo for regular walks or other forms of moderate exercise will lead to a higher chance of live birth then women should be encouraged to do so.

References

1. Botta G, Grudzinskas G. Is a prolonged bed rest following embryo transfer useful? *Human Reproduction* 1997;**12**:2489–92.
2. The UK National Institute of Clinical Excellence (NICE). NICE *Clinical Guidelines 011 for Fertility* 2004:112–14.
3. Lambers MJ, Lambalk CB, Schats R, Hompes PG. Ultrasonographic evidence that bedrest after embryo transfer is useless. *Gynecol Obstet Invest* 2009;**68**: 122–6.
4. Abou-Setta AM, D'Angelo A, Sallam HN, Hart RJ, Al-Inany HG. Post-embryo transfer interventions for in vitro fertilization and intracytoplasmic sperm injection patients. *Cochrane Database Syst Rev* 2009;7:CD006567.
5. Kucuk M, Doymaz F, Urman B. Effect of energy expenditure and physical activity on the outcomes of assisted reproduction treatment. *Reprod Biomed Online* 2010;**20**:274–9.

Chapter 35

Intercourse around the time of embryo transfer

Kelton P. Tremellen

Introduction

In vitro fertilization treatment breaks the normal nexus between sexual intercourse and conception. Many couples abstain from intercourse around the time of embryo transfer as they fear that uterine contractions at orgasm or pressure created by penile contact with the cervix may dislodge the embryo. Furthermore, many doctors actively discourage their patients from having intercourse around the time of embryo transfer as they are concerned that it may produce painful rupture of ovarian follicles or super-fecundity related to natural and IVF conception [1]. Despite these concerns, there is a substantial body of evidence supporting the need for exposure of the female reproductive tract to semen/seminal plasma around the time of embryo implantation in order to maximize reproductive efficiency. Several animal studies have identified that components of seminal plasma have the ability to improve embryo development and implantation rates in vivo [2]. For example, removal of the seminal plasma producing male accessory sex glands of rodents does not preclude natural conception but does result in impaired blastocyst development and pregnancy outcomes [3]. Therefore, it is apparent that a policy of abstinence around the time of embryo transfer may not only be unnecessary but potentially detrimental. This chapter will examine the evidence suggesting why intercourse around the time of embryo transfer is beneficial to IVF outcomes.

Clinical studies examining the effect of intercourse on IVF conception

Only one study to date has examined if intercourse around the time of embryo transfer effects IVF implantation rates [4], while several studies have looked at the effect of artificial insemination with whole semen or seminal plasma on IVF conception rates [5–7]. In the largest of these studies couples undergoing stimulated IVF treatment (400 cycles) or frozen embryo transfers (200 cycles) were randomly allocated to either abstain or have intercourse in the two days before and after embryo transfer, with all embryo transfers occurring at the cleavage stage of development [4]. The clinical implantation rate in the group who did have intercourse was significantly improved by 50% compared to the abstaining group, suggesting that intercourse does aid implantation.

Three studies have examined if artificial exposure to whole semen or seminal plasma at the time of oocyte retrieval may alter IVF implantation rates. The first study of this kind

How to Improve Your ART Success Rates, ed. Gab Kovacs. Published by Cambridge

randomized 113 women to either high-vaginal artificial insemination with their partner's untreated semen or no insemination and found a two-fold improvement in pregnancy rates in the inseminated group [5]. Interestingly, this improvement in pregnancy rates was observed even in the group with tubal factor infertility, excluding a natural artificial insemination related conception effect. A second study using artificial insemination at the time of oocyte retrieval found no significant effect but this study was weakened by improper randomization as many couples originally allocated to the insemination arm of the trial were moved to the control group when there was an inadequate volume of semen available for insemination [6]. Furthermore, these investigators made no comment on whether couples were instructed to abstain around the time of oocyte retrieval, thereby raising the possibility of exposure of the control "no insemination" group to semen through intercourse. The final randomized control trial allocated patients to high-vaginal insemination with either their partner's seminal plasma or a saline placebo at the time of oocyte retrieval [7]. This study of 168 patients reported a 45% relative increase in implantation rates in the seminal plasma exposed group which did not reach statistical significance. Therefore, the vast majority of evidence suggests that exposure of the female reproductive tract to sperm/seminal plasma through either artificial "insemination" or intercourse positively, not negatively, influences IVF outcomes.

Mechanisms by which intercourse in the peri-transfer period may assist IVF conception

Overall it is clear from the available evidence that intercourse around the time of embryo transfer is not harmful to IVF conception but may actually assist successful implantation. The observations that improvements in IVF pregnancy rates were seen in both women with tubal factor infertility undergoing artificial insemination using whole semen [5] or sperm-free seminal plasma [7] suggests that the mechanism for action is not simply natural conception but rather a beneficial effect on embryo development or endometrial receptivity. Evidence from animal studies suggests that exposure to semen at the time of intercourse may produce an "immunological priming" reaction that benefits conception [2, 8]. In the rodent model exposure of the female to semen produces an inflammatory reaction within the endometrium with the release of cytokines such as granulocyte macrophage colony-stimulating-factor (GM-CSF) that are known to have positive effects on embryo development [8]. While intercourse and artificial exposure to seminal plasma has been show to produce an inflammatory reaction in the human cervix and to up-regulate endometrial cytokine production in human endometrial cultures [9], it is uncertain if seminal plasma can enter the uterine cavity in sufficient quantities to initiate an endometrial cytokine response that may benefit embryo development. However, a post-coital cervical inflammatory reaction may assist in maternal sperm antigen uptake, with seminal plasma immunosuppressive factors such as TGFβ and prostaglandin E_1 helping create a beneficial "tolerant" immune response that prevents the mother's immune system from rejecting the semi-allogenic (immunologically foreign) embryo [8]. Furthermore, the influx of neutrophils and macrophages into the cervix within hours of intercourse may help reduce the bacterial load within the external cervical os, thereby reducing the chances that passage of the embryo transfer catheter will inoculate the endometrial cavity with bacteria capable of producing an embryo toxic endometritis.

Conclusion

A solitary large randomized control trial suggests that intercourse around the time of embryo transfer has the ability to improve IVF implantation rates. Two smaller randomized control studies suggest that exposure to semen or seminal plasma before embryo transfer may assist IVF conception. While the mechanism for this improvement is not fully understood, it is likely to involve the ability of semen/seminal plasma to induce an immune reaction within the female reproductive tract that augments embryo development and endometrial receptivity. On the negative aspect, it has been suggested that intercourse around the time of embryo transfer may pose a risk to the woman since enlarged hyper-stimulated ovaries containing multiple fragile corpora lutea are vulnerable to rupture during intercourse, resulting in pain or significant intra-peritoneal haemorrhage. Therefore, we would advocate that intercourse around the time of embryo transfer should be encouraged to augment IVF conception, except in the small sub-set of women experiencing pelvic discomfort related to an exaggerated hyperstimulation response.

References

1. Cahill DJ, Jenkins JM, Soothill PW, Whitelaw A, Wardle PG. Quadruplet pregnancy following transfer of two embryos: Case report. *Hum Reprod* 2003;**18**:441–3.
2. Robertson SA. Seminal fluid signalling in the female reproductive tract: lessons from rodents and pigs. *J Anim Sci* 2007;**85** (13 Suppl): 36–44.
3. Wong CL, Lee KH, Lo KM, *et al.* Ablation of paternal accessory sex glands imparts physical and behavioural abnormalities to the progeny: an in vivo study in the golden hamster. *Theriogenology* 2007;**68**:654–62.
4. Tremellen KP, Valbuena D, Landeras J, *et al.* The effect of intercourse on pregnancy rates during assisted human reproduction. *Hum Reprod* 2000;**15**:2653–8.
5. Bellinge BS, Copeland CM, Thomas TD, *et al.* The influence of patient insemination on the implantation rate in an in vitro fertilization and embryo transfer program. *Fertil Steril* 1986 **46**:252–6.
6. Fishel S, Webster J, Jackson P, Faratian B. Evaluation of high vaginal insemination at oocyte recovery in patients undergoing in vitro fertilization. *Fertil Steril* 1989;**51**:135–8.
7. von Wolff M, Rösner S, Thöne C, *et al.* Intravaginal and intracervical application of seminal plasma in in vitro fertilization or intracytoplasmic sperm injection treatment cycles – a double-blind, placebo-controlled, randomized pilot study. *Fertil Steril* 2009;**91**:167–72.
8. Robertson SA, Guerin LR, Moldenhauer LM, Hayball JD. Activating T regulatory cells for tolerance in early pregnancy – the contribution of seminal fluid. *J Reprod Immunol* 2009;**83**:109–16.
9. Gutsche S, von Wolff M, Strowitzki T, Thaler CJ. Seminal plasma induces mRNA expression of IL-1beta, IL-6 and LIF in endometrial epithelial cells in vitro. *Mol Hum Reprod* 2003;**9**:785–91.

Chapter 36

Heparin and aspirin as an adjunctive treatment in women undergoing IVF

Rodney D. Franklin and William H. Kutteh

Pharmacology of and rationale for heparin

Heparin is a polymer of acidic sulfated disaccharides, derived from porcine mucosa. The length of the polysaccharide chain determines the properties of the molecule – shorter chains are low molecular weight heparins and longer chains are high molecular weight (or unfractionated) heparins. Heparin binds to and potentiates the action of antithrombin, inducing a conformational change. Unfractionated heparin simultaneously binds thrombin and antithrombin, facilitating the inactivation of thrombin. The conformational change in antithrombin induced by heparin allows the molecule to bind to and inactivate factors involved in the clotting cascade. Low molecular weight heparins are more selective inhibitors of factors IXa and Xa than unfractionated heparin. The use of unfractionated heparin to improve pregnancy outcomes in infertile women has inspired interest in low molecular weight heparin because of several potential advantages. Low molecular weight heparin has been advocated because of its presumed mechanism of action against thrombosis, the absence of frequent monitoring during pregnancy, and the potential for once-a-day administration based on its longer half-life. Further, its safety profile is similar to unfractionated heparin, which has a low incidence of severe bleeding episodes, thrombocytopenia, or bone loss (Table 36.1). In contrast, low molecular weight heparin is only partially reversible with protamine sulfate.

Several mechanisms of action have been proposed to understand the potential therapeutic effect of heparin toward decreasing implantation failure. Heparin could act in vivo to: (1) immunomodulate cell-mediated or humoral events to prevent production or alter the action of antiphospholipid antibodies (aPL), (2) produce an antithrombotic effect independent of aPL that overrides aPL action, (3) block the action of aPL directly or indirectly, or (4) facilitate the elimination and clearance of aPL from the body. Antiphospholipid antibodies, a group of autoantibodies that bind to negatively charged phospholipids, are thought to have clinical significance because of their association with thromboembolic events and adverse pregnancy outcomes. The rationale for heparin use has been that the anticoagulant activity overrides the thrombotic action caused by aPL binding to phospholipids, ß-2 glycoprotein, or other cross-reactive substances. Recent studies have indicated that defective endovascular

How to Improve Your ART Success Rates, ed. Gab Kovacs. Published by Cambridge University Press.

Table 36.1 Prophylactic unfractionated heparin compared to low molecular weight heparin

Characteristic	Unfractionated	Low molecular weight
Source	Porcine mucosa	Porcine mucosa
Structure	Glycosaminogylcan	Glycosaminogylcan
Size in Daltons	~ 15,000	~ 5,000
Mechanism of action	Thrombin-AT → ↓Xa	AT → ↓ Xa
Crosses placenta	No	No
Administration frequency	Twice daily	Once daily
T ½, subcutaneously	~ 2 hours	~ 3 to 6 hours
Protamine sulfate reversal	100%	~ 50%
Cost per week prophylaxis	$46 dollars (US)	$532 dollars (US) $372 generic
Hemorrhage, severe	< 1%	< 1%
Thrombocytopenia (HIT)	< < 1%	< 1%
Osteoporosis	Rare	Rare
Bleed with abdominal surgery	3%	4%
Bleed with DVT treatment	3%	4%
Ecchymosis, severe	0	0
Anemia	< 1%	< 1%
Epidural hematoma	Low	Increased

AT = antithrombin; Xa = factor Xa; HIT = heparin induced thrombocytopenia; DVT = deep vein thrombosis. Source: Sanofi-Aventis product insert information for FDA approval of enoxaparin sodium.

trophoblastic invasion rather than excessive intervillous thrombosis is the most frequent histological abnormality in aPL-associated recurrent pregnancy loss. Antiphospholipid antibodies have been shown to inhibit trophoblastic differentiation, proliferation, and migrations, and these effects have been proposed to cause recurrent implantation failure. Additionally, aPL may exact their action on the trophoblast by interference with membrane surface antigens resulting in altered cell activity. All of the effects of aPL can be mediated by complement and induce cell injury, inflammatory reactions, and microvascular thrombosis. In vitro studies have shown that unfractionated heparin enhanced the differentiation of extra villous trophoblasts into giant multinuclear cells. Moreover, unfractionated heparin has been shown to inhibit aPL binding to cardiolipin and phosphatidlyserine in vitro at lower doses than low molecular weight heparin.

Pharmacology of and rationale for low-dose aspirin

Low-dose aspirin (81–100 mg) is a quick, irreversible inhibitor of cyclo-oxygenase in platelets, which prevents the conversion of arachidonic acid to thromboxane A_2, a potent vasoconstrictor and stimulator of platelet aggregation. Daily doses of low-dose aspirin promote a shift from thromboxane A_2 and towards prostacyclin which inhibits the platelet aggregation that leads to vasodilatation and increased blood perfusion. Theoretically, the antithromboxane effects of aspirin on inhibition of platelet aggregation are thought to work in concert with heparin to promote and enhance implantation. Higher doses of aspirin would be counter-productive as both thromboxane and prostacyclin production is inhibited at higher doses.

It has been proposed that low-dose aspirin may improve implantation rates by enhancing uterine blood flow. Some studies of patients with implantation failure suggest that impaired uterine blood flow may decrease uterine receptivity for the embryo. In contrast, other studies indicate that low-dose aspirin may increase uterine perfusion based on Doppler flow ultrasonography.

Prevalence of aPL and IVF outcomes

In an attempt to evaluate the association of different immunologic factors, including aPL, with diagnostic subpopulations of patients with reproductive failure, Buckingham and Chamley reviewed the literature and found that aPL are not predictive of adverse outcomes from IVF [1]. They identified over 100 relevant articles published between 1984 and 2007 and found 27 published reports characterizing aPL in infertile women undergoing IVF. The prevalence of aPL in infertile women averaged 22.2% among the 4617 women studied. The studies reported a wide range of aPL positivity (0 to 66%); however, the authors criticized the variations across studies in aPL epitopes assayed, assay techniques used among laboratories for aPL and lupus anticoagulant, and thresholds for aPL positivity.

Ten studies evaluated aPL status and related pregnancy and birth outcomes in women undergoing IVF (Table 36.2). Gleicher *et al.* retrospectively reviewed studies of aPL positive patients with one or more phospholipids and found no significant differences in the clinical pregnancy rates or live birth rates between the antibody positive and negative groups. A larger prospective study by Sher *et al.* found no significant differences in the clinical pregnancy rates between the aPL negative and positive groups (16.0% and 27.5%, respectively). Subsequently, Kutteh *et al.*, using more stringent criteria to define aPL positivity, found no significant differences in the clinical pregnancy rates or live birth rates. Only one study, by Lee *et al.*, found statistically lower live birth rates in aPL positive versus aPL negative women. In summary, these studies demonstrated that aPL had no effect on the outcome of IVF when considering pregnancy rates or live birth rates. Based on growing evidence of non-effect, in 2008, the Practice Committee of the American Society of Reproductive Medicine issued a statement advocating against the practice of testing for and treating aPL in this population.

Safety measures with heparin and aspirin during IVF

When using heparin, it recommended that the clinician obtain a baseline activated partial thromboplastin time and platelet counts prior to cycle initiation. Some women with aPL will have the lupus anticoagulant which may result in a prolonged activated partial thromboplastin time. Moreover, most cases of heparin-induced thrombocytopenia are not induced by prophylactic doses of heparin but would have been diagnosed as thrombocytopenia or low platelets prior to the initiation of heparin. Platelet counts will decline by approximately 50 000 per cc during normal pregnancy.

There is no indication for treatment with heparin before ovum retrieval in women without a history of thrombosis but who have tested positive for aPL. In women who are

Table 36.2 Summary of studies (*n*> 50) reporting IVF outcomes in women with antiphospholipid antibodies

Name, year	Type of cohort	*n*	% CPR aPL-positive	% CPR aPL-negative	% LBR aPL-positive	% LBR aPL-negative	*p*-value
Gleicher, 1994	Retrospective	105	32.8%	23.9%	26.3%	15.8%	NS
Sher, 1994	Prospective	196	16.0%	27.5%			NS
Birdsall, 1996	Prospective	240	38.9%	36.1%	27.9%	25.5%	NS
Kutteh, 1997	Prospective	191	35.3%	39.7%			NS
Kowalik, 1997	Prospective	525	57.7%	46.2%	49.7%	43.8%	NS
Denis, 1997	Retrospective	793	65.7%	55.3%	67.8%	57.0%	NS
Chilcott, 2000	Prospective	380	9.0%	9.0%	12.4%	12.0%	NS
Buckingham, 2006	Prospective	99	31.6%	15.8%	36.3%	23.8%	NS
Lee, 2007	Prospective	54	20.5%	37.5%	17.6%	80.0%	<0.05
Sanmarco, 2007	Prospective	101	27.5%	19.7%	22.5%	13.1%	NS

CPR, clinical pregnancy rate; LBR, live birth rate.

aPL positive and have an indication for prophylaxis but do not have history of thrombosis, prophylactic doses of heparin should start from the time of embryo transfer to reduce the risk of thrombosis, which increases from the beginning of the luteal phase [2]. Alternatively, some clinicians will wait until a positive pregnancy test to start prophylaxis based on the increased risk of thrombosis associated with pregnancy. Women with aPL and a history of thrombosis should discontinue oral anticoagulation therapy and switch to therapeutic doses of heparin for ovulation induction. Bleeding complications are reduced by discontinuing heparin 12–24 hours prior to ovum retrieval and resuming 6 hours later when the risk of bleeding is minimal and the patient is clinically stable. Low-dose aspirin may be added, but should be interrupted 5–7 days before oocyte retrieval to avoid bleeding.

Pharmacologic therapy and IVF outcomes

Historically investigators believed that aPL and recurrent pregnancy loss were connected and that treatment with heparin combined with low-dose aspirin was safe and efficacious. A review of the evidence reveals conflicting findings. A meta-analysis by Gelbaya *et al.* included six studies and over 2500 patients and found no significant difference between women who received low-dose aspirin or placebo (RR 1.09, 95% CI 0.92–1.29) [3]. In the same year, Banerjee *et al.* concluded that no significant difference in low-dose aspirin versus placebo in their meta-analysis of over 1200 women undergoing IVF when considering live birth rate (RR 0.94, 95% CI 0.64–1.39). Roupp *et al.* in 2008 analyzed ten studies with over 2800 patients in their meta-analysis comparing low-dose aspirin to placebo in women undergoing IVF and

Table 36.3 Use of aspirin in prospective trials of IVF treatment

Name, year	No. pregnant/ total TX		Odds ratio	Lower limit	Upper limit	Relative weight
	Low dose aspirin	Control				
Weckstein, 1997	9/15	4/13	3.37	0.70	16.17	0.69
Check, 1998*	2/18	6/10	0.08	0.01	0.58	0.45
Rubinstein, 1999*	67/149	42/149	2.08	1.29	3.37	7.36
Urman,2000	55/139	59/136	0.85	0.53	1.38	7.40
Bordes, 2003*	27/69	15/69	2.31	1.09	4.89	3.04
Lentini, 2003	13/42	10/42	1.43	0.55	3.77	1.83
Van Doreen, 2004	31/85	29/85	1.11	0.59	2.08	4.30
Waldenstrom,2004*	249/703	203/677	1.28	1.02	1.60	33.49
Pakkila, 2005	44/186	48/175	0.82	0.51	1.32	7.59
Frattarelli, 2008	116/417	250/833	0.90	0.69	1.17	25.14
Dirckx, 2009	31/97	30/96	1.03	0.56	1.90	4.63
Lambers, 2009	28/84	26/85	1.13	0.59	2.17	4.07
Summary	672/2004	722/2370	1.13	0.99	1.29	--

* Denotes studies that reached statistical significance. The 95% confidence intervals of most meta-analyses (shown above as the lower and upper limits) include the number 1.00 therefore they are not considered statistically significant.
Total TX = total (women) treated or number of embryo transfer procedures.

reported a slight improvement in clinical pregnancy rate (RR 1.15, 95% CI 1.03–1.27). Our updated meta-analysis (Table 36.3) includes twelve studies with 4374 women undergoing IVF and suggests a slight but not significant benefit for low-dose aspirin over placebo (RR 1.13, 95% CI 0.99–1.29). Based on these meta-analyses, it appears that any benefit of low-dose aspirin may be minimal at best.

Exogenous heparin has been shown to inhibit binding of aPL with phospholipids and endogenous heparin manufactured by trophoblasts should function in the same fashion. Few studies have investigated the role of heparin and low-dose aspirin in aPL positive women undergoing IVF. In 1997 Schenk *et al.* and Kutteh *et al.* independently reported no significant differences in implantation and pregnancy rates in aPL-positive women undergoing IVF with or without heparin therapy. Stern *et al.* [5] prospectively randomized 143 women who were aPL-positive or antinuclear antibody positive and had previously failed pregnancy after the transfer of at least ten embryos. Implantation rates and pregnancy rates were the same in those treated with heparin 5000 units twice daily plus aspirin 100 mg daily or those treated with placebo. A systematic review by Nelson and Greer 2008 in women with definitive antiphospholipid syndrome or repeated IVF failure suggested that the use of low molecular weight heparin and aspirin started at the time of ovulation induction improved the pregnancy rate in subsequent IVF cycles. In 2009, the Policy and Practice Committee of the British Fertility Society reported that pragmatic treatment with low molecular weight heparin and low-dose aspirin of women undergoing IVF diagnosed with definitive antiphospholipid syndrome and in those with repeated implantation failure was justified [4]. However, the Committee noted that the level of evidence was weak (Grade C) and that the recommendation was made in the absence of directly applicable clinical studies of good quality.

Practice recommendations and conclusion

Antiphospholipid antibodies do not affect IVF success, thus routine testing for aPL before IVF is not warranted. The idea of improved implantation with low-dose aspirin seems practical, but our best evidence suggests that low-dose aspirin would provide minimal benefit as adjunctive therapy for women undergoing IVF. Mechanisms of heparin influence on aPL induced changes and implantation are not well understood. The best randomized controlled trials do not support the use of heparin and aspirin in aPL positive patients with IVF failure [5]. The prospective, randomized trial of treatment with heparin and aspirin in women with aPL and IVF implantation failure demonstrated no benefit of treatment. Because of the controversy between IVF success and the presence of aPL, the American Society of Reproductive Medicine issued a practice committee report on this issue. An evidence-based literature search using aPL and IVF as identifiers was conducted. The published data were combined, and the clinical pregnancy and live birth rates were 57% and 46%, respectively, in the aPL-positive patients, as compared with 49.2% and 42.9%, respectively, in the aPL-negative patients. That report concluded that aPL testing is not warranted in patients undergoing IVF, and treatment is not indicated in positive patients in the absence of other risk factors for thrombosis.

References

1. Buckingham KL, Chamley LW. A critical assessment of the role of antiphospholipid antibodies in infertility. *J Reprod Immunol* 2009;**80**:132–45.
2. Bellver J, Pellicer A. Ovarian stimulation for ovulation induction and in vitro fertilization in patients with systemic lupus erythematosus and antiphospholipid syndrome. *Fertil Steril* 2009;**92**: 1803–10.
3. Gelbaya TA, Kyrgiou M, Li TC, Stern C, Nardo LG. Low-dose aspirin for in vitro fertilization: a systematic review and meta-analysis. *Hum Reprod Update* 2007;**13**:357–64.
4. Nardo LG, Granne I, Stewart J. Policy & Practice Committee of the British Fertility Society. Medical adjuncts in IVF: evidence for clinical practice. *Hum Fertil (Camb)* 2009;**12**:1–13.
5. Stern C, Chamley L, Norris H, Hale L, Baker HW. A randomized, double-blind, placebo-controlled trial of heparin and aspirin for women with in vitro fertilization implantation failure and antiphospholipid or antinuclear antibodies. *Fertil Steril* 2003;**80**:376–83.

Chapter 37

Place of oestrogen supplements in luteal phase after embryo transfer

Francisco J. Ruiz Flores and Juan A. Garcia-Velasco

Introduction

As early as 1980, it was suggested that there seems to exist a luteal phase defect resulting from ovarian stimulation, and that this could represent a potential cause for an unsuccessful IVF cycle.

The use of gonadotropin releasing hormone (GnRH) agonists in IVF cycles causes suppression of pituitary luteinizing hormone (LH) secretion for as long as ten days after the last dose of agonist. At the same time, the supraphysiological secretion of steroids induced during the ovarian hyperstimulation is going to strongly suppress LH concentrations. The corpus luteum may be dysfunctional without the LH signal, and subsequent oestrogen (E2) and progesterone (P4) secretion may be abnormal. Without proper E2 or P4 stimulation, endometrial receptivity may be compromised, leading to decreased implantation and pregnancy rates. Because the luteal phase characteristics appear to be similar between GnRH agonist and antagonist cycles, it could be assumed that the supplementation regimen would be the same in both agonist and antagonist protocols.

The recognition of this problem led practitioners to employ luteal phase supplementation initially with human chorionic gonadotropin (hCG). Its administration during this phase aimed at maintaining stimulation of the corpus luteum to produce sufficient E2 and P4 levels in order to allow implantation of the developing embryo. Serum E2 and P4 often drop to low levels later in the luteal phase of an IVF cycle resulting in reduced implantation and pregnancy rates, unless hormonal support is provided. It is well accepted that luteal phase supplementation is crucial from the time of clearance of exogenous hCG (given for final oocyte maturation) until the rise of endogenous hCG during the initial stages of implantation.

The administration of hCG for luteal phase supplementation presented a higher risk of ovarian hyperstimulation syndrome and this was sufficient reason to switch to a different protocol with P4 supplementation in stimulated cycles, which is the most used luteal phase support to date. The role of P4 as luteal support in stimulated cycles is now well established.

Because the corpus luteum produces not only P4 but also E2 and other steroid hormones, it has been questioned whether adding E2 to P4 could further improve implantation rates. It was then described by some investigators that there is a significant difference in serum E2 concentrations between conception and non-conception cycles in fertile women undergoing donor insemination. The decline of E2 in unsuccessful cycles raised speculations that peri-implantation endometrial development may be compromised. The role of E2 in the

How to Improve Your ART Success Rates, ed. Gab Kovacs. Published by Cambridge

follicular phase of the menstrual cycle is well established, as it is essential for endometrial priming, but it is also responsible for proliferation of uterine surface epithelium, glands, stroma, and blood vessels. The role of E2 in the luteal phase remains unclear, and its depletion in the human luteal phase does not appear to adversely affect the morphological developmental capacity of the endometrium. It has been shown that the high E2 level during the early luteal phase of an IVF cycle induces a strong negative feedback on the pituitary, decreasing LH secretion to very low levels. However, early luteal phase administration of high-dose E2 does not induce premature luteolysis in regularly cycling women, suggesting that other factors may be responsible for the luteal phase defect observed after a stimulated cycle. The benefit of additional supplementation with E2 is still controversial and a matter of much debate, with some reports favoring the use of E2, and many others failing to observe any potential benefit.

Available evidence

A meta-analysis of the available randomized trials published by Pritts and Atwood [1] in 2002, attempted to evaluate whether luteal phase supplementation conferred any benefit in fertility outcomes for women undergoing IVF cycles. The addition of E2 to a standard P4 treatment in the luteal phase was evaluated in three trials. The luteal support varied in the three trials, lasting from 2 weeks total, to 3 weeks total or until 12 weeks gestation. The E2 doses ranged from 2 to 6 mg daily orally with progesterone being given both by the vaginal and intra-muscular routes. They concluded that adding E2 to P4 might increase implantation rates (IR) in long and short agonist protocols and suggesting the beneficial effect of E2 might be related to the dose in which it is administered.

In 2005, Lukaszuk [2] and collaborators showed significantly better support of the luteal phase when oral E2 was added to P4, suggesting that E2 supplementation could help embryos that insufficiently stimulate E2 production, or where there is a weak maternal reaction. There seemed to be a higher pregnancy rate per patient in a 6 mg E2 supplement group but not in a 2 mg group, when compared both with no E2 group.

A randomized controlled trial (RCT) [3] in 2006 evaluated the addition of E2 to P4 for luteal phase supplementation in GnRH antagonist cycles, as most of the previous studies had been carried upon GnRH agonist cycles. The authors did not find any evidence that might favour the addition of 4 mg E2 to P4 in order to increase the probability of pregnancy.

Another RCT [4] in 2008 performed by our group tried also to evaluate the benefit of adding E2 to standard P4 luteal phase supplementation in patients undergoing IVF/intra-cytoplasmic sperm injection (ICSI) cycles with GnRH agonists or antagonists. Patients were randomized to receive either vaginal P4 or a combination of vaginal P4 plus transdermal E2 as luteal support. We found no difference between supporting the luteal phase with or without E2. We concluded that in IVF/ICSI cycles adding E2 to P4 does not seem to improve cycle outcome.

Gelbaya and collaborators [5] reported in 2008 in a systematic review and meta-analysis that the addition of E2 to P4 for luteal phase support in IVF/ICSI cycles had no beneficial effect on pregnancy rates.

Also in 2008, Kolibianakis and his team [6] published a systematic review and meta-analysis, comparing the effectiveness of the combination of E2 and P4 administration for luteal phase support versus P4 only administration, in terms of positive beta hCG, pregnancy, and live birth rates in IVF cycles. They concluded that the currently available evidence suggested that the addition of E2 to the luteal phase supplementation protocol does not increase the probability of pregnancy.

A more recent meta-analysis in 2010 by Jee and collaborators [7] aimed to clarify whether the addition of E2 to standard P4 supplementation was beneficial in both GnRH agonist and antagonist IVF cycles. They included seven studies in their work. The combined data they presented suggests that the addition of E2 to the standard supplementation protocol does not improve IVF outcomes in GnRH agonist and antagonist cycles. In this meta-analysis data from 2 mg and 6 mg E2 supplement groups were combined, resulting in "no difference" between study and control group. This is in contrast to the conclusion drawn from the previous described study by Lukaszuk.

Most of the published clinical trials are underpowered, so this is why meta-analyses may help interpret the results in a more correct fashion than the published evidence on the hypothetic benefit of E2 supplementation in the luteal phase. It should also be stressed that the maximum number of patients analyzed in the eligible trials or even the maximum number of patients analyzed in the sensitivity analyses performed is far below the ideal sample size required to definitely answer the question. Thus, there is an obvious need for further RCTs that will assess, in a more robust way, the effect of adding E2 supplementation to P4 during the luteal phase on the chances of pregnancy.

Conclusion

The results of the various meta-analyses previously described indicate that the addition of E2 to P4 supplementation in the luteal phase does not improve IVF outcomes.

Even though routine E2 supplementation appears to have an insignificant role proven by all the meta-analyses, it still remains to be determined whether adding E2 is beneficial to a particular group of IVF patients. The subgroup of patients that may benefit from additional E2 supplementation needs to be further clarified, along with the optimal dose of E2, when exactly it should be started, and when exactly it should be ended. How to administer E2 is still debatable, although historically oral E2 valerate has been the preferred choice, there are alternative routes of administration, such as vaginal or transdermal. These have been described to avoid first passing through the liver and to facilitate treatment compliance. Interestingly, the vaginal route is more physiologic, as it has been demonstrated that there is a first uterine pass, where E2 is absorbed from the vaginal mucosa directly into the endometrium. It is still unclear whether the effect of E2 supplementation is dependent on the dosage or even the route of administration. In order to avoid the heterogeneity of current studies, future trials should address the effect of E2 supplementation in patients undergoing GnRH antagonists – an issue less studied than the agonist protocol – as well as different routes of administration. Similarly, the end point of future trials should be live birth rate, as it reflects clearly the impact on the cycle much better than biochemical or clinical pregnancy rates.

In conclusion, the role of luteal E2 supplementation for successful embryo implantation in humans awaits further studies. Although the findings of the meta-analyses demonstrate no beneficial effect of E2 supplementation in the luteal phase of IVF cycles, the actual evidence remains rather scarce, with limited and heterogeneous trials, precluding the extraction of clear and definite conclusions. A large, properly designed, and adequately powered RCT, that would further clarify the role of luteal E2 supplementation in IVF that would consider the optimal regimen (dose and route) is still needed.

On the basis of the currently best available evidence, routine use of E2 supplementation during P4 supported luteal phase in IVF cycles is not yet justified.

References

1. Pritts EA, Atwood AK. Luteal phase support in infertility treatment: a meta-analysis of the randomized trials. *Hum Reprod* 2002;**17**:2287–99.
2. Lukaszuk K, Liss J, Lukaszuk M, Maj B. Optimization of estradiol supplementation during the luteal phase improves the pregnancy rate in women undergoing in vitro fertilization–embryo transfer cycles. *Fertil Steril* 2005;**83**:1372–6.
3. Fatemi HM, Kolibianakis EM, Camus M, *et al.* Addition of estradiol to progesterone for luteal supplementation in patients stimulated with GnRH antagonist/rFSH for IVF: a randomized controlled trial. *Hum Reprod* 2006;**21**:2628–32.
4. Serna J, Cholquevilque JL, Cela V, *et al.* Estradiol supplementation during the luteal phase of IVF-ICSI patients: a randomized, controlled trial. *Fertil Steril* 2008;**90**:2190–5.
5. Gelbaya TA, Kyrgiou M, Tsoumpou I, Nardo LG. The use of estradiol for luteal phase support in in vitro fertilization/intracytoplasmic sperm injection cycles: a systematic review and meta-analysis. *Fertil Steril* 2008;**90**:2116–25.
6. Kolibianakis EM, Venetis CA, Papanikolaou EG, *et al.* Estrogen addition to progesterone for luteal phase support in cycles stimulated with GnRH analogues and gonadotrophins for IVF: a systematic review and meta-analysis. *Hum Reprod* 2008;**23**:1346–54.
7. Jee BC, Suh CS, Kim SH, Kim YB, Moon SY. Effects of estradiol supplementation during the luteal phase of in vitro fertilization cycles: a meta-analysis. *Fertil Steril* 2010;**93**:428–36.

Chapter 38

Progesterone supplementation

Luciano G. Nardo and Lamiya Mohiyiddeen

Progesterone has a pivotal role in human reproduction. It is secreted by the corpus luteum during the second half of the menstrual cycle in normal ovulating women. Progesterone induces transformation of the uterine glands, increases vascularity of the endometrial lining, and stabilizes the endometrium in preparation for implantation of the embryo. Progesterone has also been shown to interact with progesterone receptors on gamma/delta T cells leading to the expression of progesterone-induced blocking factor that may inhibit destructive function of natural killer (NK) cells on the endometrium. Treatment with progesterone has been found to improve pregnancy rates in menstruating women with luteal phase defect.

Justification of luteal phase support in IVF cycles

It has been shown that the use of gonadotropin releasing hormone (GnRH) agonists or antagonists used to prevent premature ovarian luteinizing hormone (LH) surge may have an adverse effect on corpus luteal function. Meta analyses of luteal phase support for IVF cycles have found higher live birth rates with supplement progesterone compared to placebo [1, 2]. Impairment of endogenous gonadotropin secretion caused by persistent pituitary suppression in the luteal phase may be responsible for the premature luteolysis that occurs during controlled ovarian stimulation.

Gonadotropin-releasing hormone antagonists cause less sustained pituitary suppression than GnRH agonists, and so it seems plausible that the luteal phase in antagonist cycles would be less compromised than in agonist cycles. However, Beckers *et al.* [3] demonstrated that the luteal phase was deficient in patients who received GnRH antagonist during stimulation and were not given luteal phase support (LPS).

Luteal phase support is considered essential to counter any luteal insufficiency that may have a negative impact on early pregnancy establishment and maintenance. Progesterone, human chorionic gonadotropin (hCG), oestrogen (E_2), or a combination of these hormones are used for LPS in IVF cycles.

Routes of administation of natural progesterone

Progesterone is usually well tolerated. The side effects will depend on route of administration. Parenteral intramuscular (IM) progesterone has been used for the treatment of infertility and miscarriage for over 45 years. It is rapidly absorbed and has a slow clearance when administered in an oil vehicle – peanut oil, olive oil, or ethyl oleate. Intramuscular progesterone

How to Improve Your ART Success Rates, ed. Gab Kovacs. Published by Cambridge

administation is associated with some side effects including allergic reaction, sterile abscesses, bleeding into the muscle, and pain at the injection site. There are reported cases of acute eosinophilic pneumonia following use of IM progesterone.

Oral progesterone, available in the USA in preparations of 100 mg and 200 mg tablets, is rendered ineffective by the rapid clearance by first pass metabolism. Although the drug produces good serum levels of progesterone the concentration is not very high in the endometrium [4]. Thus, oral progesterone is considered less effective than IM or vaginal progesterone. The side effects secondary to metabolites of oral progesterone include light-headedness, vertigo, drowsiness, and gastric discomfort. In Europe the oral progesterone commonly used includes dydrogestrone.

Vaginal route of progesterone supplementation has gained wide application mainly due to patient comfort and effectiveness. Vaginal route results in prolonged bioavailability due to the local effect and as a result uterine tissue is found to have higher than expected progesterone level despite low serum progesterone level. Vaginal preparations are shown to achieve similar histologic changes on the endometrium as those after an IM injection.

Compounded progesterone vaginal suppositories have been used for over two decades. A dose of 300 mg to 600 mg is frequently used, spread over two to three dosages. They can result in a significant vaginal build up causing vaginal irritation. Recently there have been various attempts to improve the efficacy and reduce the side effects of vaginal progesterone.

Vaginal progesterone gel, crinone, achieves lower serum levels of progesterone but attains higher levels in the endometrium tissue than IM progesterone. A dose of 90 mg once daily application results in progesterone levels equivalent to that of 400–600 mg compounded vaginal suppositories. The main side effect of crinone is vaginal irritation but to a lesser extent compared to vaginal suppositories rendering it more tolerable.

Endometrin vaginal tablets are the newest progesterone vaginal tablets. The main advantage over the suppositories is that the tablets absorb the vaginal secretions and disintegrate into an adhesive powder that adheres to the vaginal epithelium facilitating absorption. A study found that 200 mg of endometrin is able to produce the same serum levels after six days compared to 800 mg cyclogest. Also endometrin caused less irritation compared to cyclogest. In a large multicenter randomized study, comparing the use of crinone vaginal gel 8% and endometrin twice or three times a day, the clinical pregnancy rate was comparable. Also there was no significant difference in ongoing pregnancy rates with IM progesterone and endometrin.

There is a registered multicenter trial using novel progesterone ring in the luteal phase of IVF cycles. The progesterone ring may prove to be the best tolerated of all progesterone preparations as the preliminary data suggest equal efficacy.

Progesterone versus hCG for luteal phase support

It is believed that use of hCG may rescue the function of the failing corpus luteum in IVF cycles. The administration of hCG leads to an increased production of oestrogen and progesterone by the corpus luteum. In a prospective randomized study [5] that compared the efficacy of LPS using either hCG, hCG in combination with daily vaginal progesterone or vaginal progesterone only, there were no statistically significant differences in the clinical ongoing pregnancy rate between the three groups. When a standardized discomfort scale was used, the fewest complaints were within the progesterone only groups. It was shown that progesterone only for LPS leads to the same clinical ongoing pregnancy rate as hCG, with minimal impact on the patient comfort.

Several studies have compared vaginal progesterone with hCG. The clinical pregnancy rates were similar in both groups. Meta-analyses investigating the effectiveness of IM progesterone versus hCG showed no difference in pregnancy rates but an increased risk of ovarian hyperstimulation syndrome (OHSS) after hCG administration. The risk of OHSS in the group receiving hCG was estimated to be twice compared to the progesterone group.

Few trials assessed whether hCG and progesterone are superior to progesterone alone in women with previous failed cycles. The combination was found to be superior in women with low mid-luteal E_2 levels. Other trials that looked at the combination of vaginal progesterone and hCG versus vaginal progesterone only did not show any difference in pregnancy rates in both groups.

Addition of E_2 to progesterone in luteal phase support

Although the role of progesterone in luteal support is well established, it is not yet clearly demonstrated whether additional supplementation of E_2 in stimulated IVF cycles may be beneficial.

Some of the randomized studies evaluating micronized E_2 in patients using long GnRH-agonist protocol showed an increase in implantation rates and pregnancy rates with addition of 6 mg of E_2 daily. Other reports concluded that the ongoing pregnancy rate was similar when patients were randomized to receive either 600 mg of micronized progesterone vaginally or 600 mg of micronized progesterone and 4 mg of E_2 valerate orally.

A recent trial evaluating the addition of E_2 to vaginal progesterone in GnRH antagonist cycles showed that the endocrine profile was similar in the group that received progesterone and E_2 or progesterone alone. The authors concluded that the addition of E_2 in GnRH-antagonist cycles is unlikely to affect pregnancy rates. The addition of E_2 to progesterone for LPS in IVF cycles showed no beneficial effect on pregnancy rates in a systematic review and meta-analysis including 10 trials [6]. Oestrogen supplements are discussed in detail in Chapter 37.

Addition of GnRH agonists as luteal phase supplement in GnRH agonist and antagonist stimulated cycles

GnRH agonists have been proposed for ovulation trigger in patients who are stimulated with a GnRH-antagonist and at risk for OHSS. The total amount of gonadotropins released during the surge is significantly lower when GnRH agonist is used to trigger ovulation as compared with the natural cycle and when the standard dose of hCG is used to trigger final oocyte maturation. There may be possible benefits to the use of GnRH agonist to trigger ovulation as it induces surge of FSH as well as LH and results in significantly higher number of metaphase II oocytes [7].

Two randomized prospective studies comparing GnRH agonist with hCG showed lower pregnancy rate in patients receiving the GnRH-agonist to trigger ovulation [7]. Both groups received vaginal progesterone supplementation for luteal support. It was hypothesized that the lower pregnancy rates were due to luteal phase defect rather than adverse effects on the number of mature oocytes collected, fertilization rate, and embryo quality. This was further confirmed in a study that randomized oocyte donors to receive either GnRH agonist or hCG and found no difference in pregnancy rates in the recipients.

A study reported significantly higher pregnancy, implantation, and live birth rates when 0.1 mg of GnRH analogues were added to 400 mg progesterone and 4 mg E_2 compared the group that received progesterone and E_2 only [8]. Another study that tested the novel approach of using a GnRH agonist for support throughout the luteal phase found that the pregnancy rate was higher in the group that received daily supplementation of agonist.

In a recent randomized controlled trial, ovulation induction was performed with either 10 000 IU hCG or 0.5 mg GnRHa (buserelin) supplemented with 1500 IU hCG on the day of oocyte retrieval [9]. Both groups received progesterone luteal supplementation. One bolus of hCG injection resulted in significant decrease in early pregnancy loss compared to just giving GnRH agonists for ovulation trigger. It is believed that administration of one bolus of low dose hCG in addition to progesterone in the luteal support rescues the corpus luteum and results in higher clinical pregnancy and live birth rates.

Timing of luteal phase support

Timing of LPS is poorly reported in the literature. In vitro fertilization units around the world continue luteal phase support for different periods of time as demonstrated by a published survey from 21 centers worldwide [10]. Most fertility physicians start progesterone after the oocyte retrieval and continue until 8–10 weeks of gestation. Few randomized studies have addressed the time of start of LPS.

In a randomized trial all women were treated with long protocol using GnRH agonist and luteal support with vaginal progesterone from the day of embryo transfer until the day of positive hCG test. The study group withdrew progesterone from the day of positive hCG while the control group continued administration of vaginal progesterone during the next three weeks of pregnancy. It was concluded that prolongation of progesterone supplementation in early pregnancy had no influence on the miscarriage rate and live birth rate. Therefore progesterone supplementation could be withdrawn safely at the time of positive pregnancy test.

Studies have not shown any difference when LPS was started at oocyte retrieval compared with starting at embryo transfer. In another study there was no significant difference on ongoing pregnancy rate when LPS was started on the day of hCG administration, the day of oocyte retrieval or the day of embryo transfer. From published studies it is evident that the timing of LPS should not be later than three days after oocyte retrieval.

The increase in endogenous hCG levels during early pregnancy makes up for possible lack of endogenous LH that has been caused by stimulated IVF cycles. Prolongation of LPS to first trimester may delay a miscarriage but it does not improve live birth rates.

Conclusion

There is a general agreement that progesterone is the first drug of choice for luteal phase support. Vaginal and IM progesterone seem to have comparable implantation and clinical pregnancy rates with patient preference for vaginal progesterone. There are no significant differences in success rates with progesterone supplementation alone, progesterone and E_2, progesterone and hCG, and hCG alone. The use of hCG to support the luteal phase increases the risk of OHSS. The use of GnRH agonist in the luteal phase especially in patients on GnRH antagonist protocol appears to be beneficial.

Supplementation is usually started after oocyte retrieval and before embryo transfer, and there is no evidence to support luteal phase support beyond the first positive hCG result or upto the time of viability scan.

References

1. Daya S, Gunby J. Luteal phase support in assisted reproduction cycles. Cochrane Database Syst Rev 2004:CD004830.
2. Nosarka S, Kruger T, Siebert I, *et al.* Luteal phase support in in-vitro fertilization: meta-analysis of randomized trials. *Gynecol Obstet Invest* 2005; **60**: 67–74.
3. Beckers N, Macklon N, Eijkemans M, *et al.* Non-supplemented luteal phase characteristics after the administration of recombinant human chorionic gonadotropin, recombinant luteinizing hormone, or gonadotropin-releasing hormone (GnRH) agonist to induce final oocyte maturation in in vitro fertilization patients after ovarian stimulation with recombinant follicle stimulating hormone and GnRH antagonist cotreatment. *J Clin Endocrinol Metab* 2003; **88**: 4186–92.
4. McAuley JW, Kroboth FJ, Kroboth PD. Oral administration of micronized progesterone: a review and more experience. *Pharmacotherapy* 1996; **16**: 453–7.
5. Ludwig M, Finas A, Katalinic A, *et al.* Prospective, randomized study to evaluate the success rates using hCG, vaginal progesterone or a combination of both for luteal phase support. *Acta Obstet Gynecol Scand* 2001; **80**: 574–82.
6. Gelbaya TA, Kyrgiou M, Nardo LG. The use of estradiol for luteal phase support in in vitro fertilization/intracytoplasmic sperm injection cycles: a systematic review and meta-analysis. *Fertil Steril* 2008; **90**: 2116–25.
7. Humaidan P, Bredkjær HE, Bungum L, *et al.* GnRH agonist (buserelin) or hCG for ovulation induction in GnRH antagonist IVF/ICSI cycles: a prospective randomized study. *Hum Reprod* 2005; **20**: 1213–20.
8. Tesarik J, Hazout A, Mendoza-Tesarik R, *et al.* Beneficial effect of luteal-phase GnRH agonist administration on embryo implantation after ICSI in both GnRH agonist- and antagonist-treated ovarian stimulation cycles. *Hum Reprod* 2006; **21**: 2572–9.
9. Humaidan P, Bredkjaer HE, Westergaard LG, *et al.* 1500 IU human chorionic gonadotropin administered at oocyte retrieval rescues the luteal phase when gonadotropin-releasing hormone agonist is used for ovulation induction: a prospective, randomized, controlled study. *Fertil Steril* 2010; **93**: 847–54.
10. Aboulghar MA, Amin Y, Al-Inany H, *et al.* Prospective randomized study comparing luteal phase support for ICSI patients up to the first ultrasound compared with an additional three weeks. *Hum Reprod* 2008; **33**: 857–62.

Chapter 39

The place of corticosteroid cotreatment in IVF

Pedro N. Barri and Buenaventura Coroleu

Introduction

The use of corticosteroids in the luteal phase of IVF cycles has been a classic theme in clinical research. The rationale for their use is that the immunosuppression achieved with this treatment would reduce the presence of uterine lymphocytes and of peripheral immune cells, and of natural killer cells that could infiltrate and harm the preimplantation embryos. That means that endometrial inflammation would be avoided while also normalizing the cytokine expression profile.

Moreover, there seems to be no need to study the levels of antiphospholipid antibodies in search of an autoimmunity problem that could require complementary treatment with corticoids. In this regard, a recent review article showed that the presence of antiphospholipid antibodies does not correlate with the type of infertility diagnosis nor affect the outcome and therefore treatment is not indicated [2]. Nor is the opinion of the American Society of Reproductive Medicine favorable to systematic screening for autoimmune pathology in IVF patients with repeated implantation failures [1].

For this short review it is important to differentiate between the use of corticoids for normal IVF patients and their use in patients who have undergone assisted hatching of the zona pellucida of their embryos before transfer or in patients with autoimmunity problems. It is also important to distinguish between the studies that propose administering corticoids in the peri-implantation period combining them only with natural progesterone and those in which acetylsalicylic acid (ASA; aspirin) is also added. Finally, an important aspect is safety and the adverse effects that can arise from cotreatment with corticosteroids in the luteal phase of IVF cycles.

Since most published studies are insufficiently powered to draw conclusions as to efficacy and reveal inconsistent results, it is fundamental also to evaluate the systematic reviews and meta-analyses that have been published on the subject.

Medical treatment

Most works present great variability in the products and doses used, though the preparations used are, in order of frequency, prednisolone, dexamethasone, and hydrocortisone. The doses varied from 4 mg to 60 mg a day for prednisolone and 0.5 mg to 1 mg for dexamethasone while hydrocortisone was administered intravenously at doses of 100 mg. There is a study that refers to co-administration of low-dose ASA combined with prednisolone [4].

How to Improve Your ART Success Rates, ed. Gab Kovacs. Published by Cambridge University Press.

The treatment schedules also showed great variability but most studies started corticoid therapy from oocyte retrieval and kept it up for 14 days.

Clinical outcomes

It is important to mention that in assessing the studies we considered the following clinical outcomes:

- Live birth rate
- Pregnancy rate
- Implantation rate
- Adverse events

Live birth rate No study has shown a beneficial effect on the live birth rate when corticoid treatment has been applied to normal patients with no specific pathology.

Ongoing and pregnancy rates

Ongoing and pregnancy rates have been considered as primary outcomes for most of the studies and none of them has shown a significant improvement between intervention and control groups [3, 5].

In a group analysis according to the technique used, some studies showed significant borderline differences in favour of administering corticoids in conventional IVF cycles but not in cycles in which intracytoplasmic sperm injection (ICSI) has been carried out. No significant differences were observed for the aetiological factor of infertility, the dose of corticoids administered, or the application schedule.

Implantation rate

All the studies showed similar implantation rates with none of them suggesting that the administration of corticoids significantly improved the implantation rate. Miscarriage rates did not vary either whether or not corticoids were administered. However, the incidence of multiple pregnancy showed a non-significant trend towards a higher percentage of multiple pregnancy in the control groups of patients who were not receiving corticoids.

Adverse events

No differences were apparent in the incidence of ectopic pregnancy or ovarian hyperstimulation syndrome (OHSS), though in the study that used the combination of prednisolone and ASA the risk of OHSS was reduced significantly by the treatment received. There are no references to infectious complications or to fetal anomalies following administration of low-dose corticoids for a limited time.

Glucocorticoids for patients with autoantibodies

Controversy surrounds the possible relationship between the presence of autoantibodies and low reproductive outcome even with a worse result of an IVF cycle. There are reports that patients with autoantibodies have a higher risk of vasoconstriction and uteroplacental thrombosis and might benefit from corticoid therapy to suppress these antibodies.

A randomized controlled trial (RCT) showed that the low-dose administration of corticoids (prednisolone 5 mg/day) throughout the IVF cycle in patients with antinuclear or anticardiolipin antibodies, or were positive for lupus anticoagulant, were unable to lower the titers of autoantibodies but significantly improved the pregnancy rate. Another RCT carried out in patients with endometriosis who had non-organ specific autoantibodies showed that the administration of glucocorticoids was associated with significantly higher pregnancy rates.

In patients with antithyroid antibodies the administration of corticoids does not seem to improve pregnancy rates. However, some retrospective and non-controlled studies suggest that when patients with antiovarian antibodies were treated with prednisolone (0.5 mg/kg per day), they significantly reduced the titres of antibodies and improved the pregnancy rates. The authors speculated about a double effect on embryo quality and on endometrial receptivity. With regard to women with high titers of antisperm antibodies, there is an RCT that shows that treatment with high doses of corticoids during the first two weeks of the cycle achieved significant improvement in pregnancy rates [5].

Glucocorticoid treatment in IVF patients with assisted hatching

Classically, it was proposed that for patients with repeated implantation failure, making a small hole in the zona pellucida by means of laser or chemical substances allowed easier hatching of the embryo and better implantation. However, the micromanipulation of the zona might alter its protective capacity, and these small holes could spread as the embryo develops and allow the invasion of immune cells. In such cases the administration of glucocorticoids might reduce the concentration of immune cells around the embryo and thus enhance implantation.

A randomized study carried out in patients of advanced age and with FSH levels higher than 10 IU/L, who underwent embryo cryoreplacement and assisted hatching after thawing, showed that when they were administered an additional treatment with methylprednisolone (16 mg/day) and tetracycline for four days in the peri-implantation period their pregnancy rates improved.

For the same reason it would seem that since ICSI also involves piercing the zona pellucida these patients should be treated with corticoids. However, the only RCT that exists for this topic was unable to show any beneficial effect from applying this technique.

Glucocorticoids to improve ovarian response

The administration of corticoids has also been proposed to improve ovarian response to stimulation and the quality of the oocytes obtained. In this regard the literature shows that the preovulatory rise in intrafollicular cortisol levels could explain an effect of the corticoids in the final maturation of the oocytes. However, the studies show that the reduction in androgen levels secondary to corticoid administration might have an adverse effect on follicular physiology, which would raise doubts about any benefit that might be obtained from its administration in patients with a history of low response to ovarian stimulation.

From the clinical point of view, three RCTs treating patients with high androgen levels and a pattern of polycystic ovary with combinations of corticoids and gonadotropins could show no significant benefit.

Risks of glucocorticoid therapy

The large majority of the studies recommend administering low doses of corticoids (<10 mg/day of prednisolone) for a short period of time (4–7 days) in the preimplantation period. In these cases the secondary effects of the treatment are very uncommon and the treatment can be regarded as safe. It is a different matter in patients who receive high doses of corticoids (30–60 mg/day of prednisolone), who are subject to a greater risk of complications arising from the treatment. Complications range from minor skin bruising to infections, peptic ulceration, and impaired glycaemic control. For this reason patients with a previous history of peptic ulceration or diabetes mellitus must absolutely avoid glucocorticoid therapy.

It is important to bear in mind the risks of treatment with prednisolone or dexamethasone during pregnancy as these are drugs that cross the placenta barrier and reach the fetal circulation. A systematic review of several studies on the use of corticoids during pregnancy concluded that this strategy was associated with a greater risk of cleft palate. Another RCT in which the patients received a combination of ASA and prednisolone showed a significantly increased risk of hypertension, diabetes mellitus, and premature birth. Another study suggests that treatment with glucocorticoids might be associated with a higher incidence of growth-restricted fetuses and an intrauterine programming of cardiovascular, metabolic, and neuroendocrine disorders in adult life. The origin would be in the alteration that the corticoids exert on the development and the differentiation of the trophoblast, which would modify the invasion of the trophoblast in the decidua. For all of these reasons the continued use of glucocorticoids throughout the pregnancy is not recommended except when some severe maternal disease requires such therapeutic use.

Conclusion

While there is an extensive bibliography about the use of corticoids as cotreatment in infertile patients undergoing assisted reproduction techniques, there are not many quality, well-designed studies that allow clear conclusions to be drawn about a possible benefit of this pharmacological treatment.

From the review that we have made it does not seem that normal IVF patients significantly improve their chances of pregnancy when subjected to additional glucocorticoid treatment in the IVF cycle. I do not attach importance to the differences found between IVF and ICSI cycles that would favour the use of corticoids in conventional IVF cycles but not in ICSI cycles as in the latter the significant improvement derived from the corticoid treatment would disappear. Nor is it clear that this treatment is useful in improving ovarian response to stimulation in patients with a previous poor response. The additional benefit observed in patients who have undergone assisted hatching is of little clinical value as there are few indications for applying this technique, either routinely or in specific indications such as advanced patient age, high FSH levels, or repeated implantation failures.

However, it is a different matter in dealing with patients who present a previous autoimmune pathology and in whom it does seem that corticoid treatment might be beneficial. In these cases, though there are few well-designed studies, it seems sensible to consider treatment with low doses of corticoids over 4–6 days in the preimplantation period. Unless the patient is suffering from some systemic disease that requires continued corticoid treatment throughout the pregnancy, this treatment must be stopped as soon as an ongoing clinical pregnancy is diagnosed.

References

1. The Practice Committee of the American Society for Reproductive Medicine. Anti-phospholipid antibodies do not affect IVF success. *Fertil Steril* 2006;**86**: Suppl 4: 224–5.
2. Cervera R, Balasch J. Bidirectional effects on autoimmunity and reproduction. *Human Reprod Update* 2008;**14**: 359–66.
3. Boomsma CM, Keay SD, Macklon NS. Peri-implantation glucocorticoid administration for assisted reproductive technology cycles. *Cochrane Database Syst Rev* 2007:CD005996.
4. Revelli A, Dolfin E, Genarelli G, *et al.* Low-dose acetylsalicylic acid plus predisolone as an adjuvant treatment in IVF: a prospective, randomized study *Fertil Steril* 2008; **90**–5:1685–91.
5. Boomsma CM, Macklon NS. Does glucocorticoid therapy in the peri-implantation period have an impact on IVF outcomes. *Curr Opin Obstet Gynecol* 2008;**20**:249–56.

Chapter 40

Immunotherapy for IVF implantation failure: "just in case" or "just in time"?

Mohamed Taranissi and Tarek El-Toukhy

Introduction

Most IVF cycles fail at the implantation stage. Repeated implantation failure is a challenging dilemma for reproductive medicine specialists and infertile couples alike.

Broadly, the causes of recurrent implantation failure can be attributed to either embryonic or uterine (endometrial) factors. Extensive efforts have been devoted to improving the ability to select embryos with the highest chance of implantation for transfer, mainly through improvements in ovarian stimulation and extended embryo culture/blastocyst transfer. However, considerably fewer studies have focused on the different components of the uterine factor, namely anatomical, endocrinal, and immunological abnormalities. In particular, underlying immunological mechanisms in women with recurrent implantation failure remain an understudied area in the field of ART.

Abnormalities in immunological tolerance of the embryonic and fetal hemi-allograft have been suspected for a long time as possible causes for recurrent implantation failure. Two theories have gained popularity in recent years. Firstly, elevated peripheral blood natural killer (NK) cells (usually defined as a percentage of CD56+ CD16+/CD3- lymphocytes above 12%) and NK cell cytotoxicity has been implicated in the immunological basis of implantation failure after IVF treatment. Intravenous immunoglobulin (IVIG) is a fractionated blood product made from pooled human plasma and is used in the treatment of a variety of medical disorders. It is considered as a global immune suppressant, but its exact mechanism of action has not been completely understood. It down regulates in vivo and in vitro NK cell activity and modifies NK cell cytokine production profile. Its application in patients with recurrent implantation failure and those with recurrent pregnancy loss showing elevated NK cells has been associated with positive pregnancy outcomes [1, 5].

In addition, the importance of the balance of T-helper cells in pregnancy has been recognized. A shift in the T-helper type 1 and type 2 (Th1/Th2) cytokine profile towards a Th1 dominance has been suggested as having a significant role in repeated miscarriages and recurrent implantation failure. Consequently, therapeutic interventions aimed against Th1 cytokines, particularly tumour necrosis factor-α (TNF-α), have been proposed to restore the balance between Th1/Th2 ratio towards Th2 dominance and away from the cytotoxic Th1 dominant profile. Flow cytometric quantification of in vitro stimulated CD4+ T cells expressing TNF-α or interleukin 10 (IL-10) are commonly used to monitor Th1 bias. Adalimumab

How to Improve Your ART Success Rates, ed. Gab Kovacs. Published by Cambridge

(Humira, Abbott Laboratories, North Chicago, IL, USA), a TNF-α inhibitor, has been specifically studied in patients with previous implantation failure to improve IVF success rate.

Published literature

The available literature on the potential benefit of IVIG and Humira in recurrent implantation failure patients is not extensive and further studies are welcomed.

IVIG

Clark and colleagues [1] critically reviewed the literature on the value of IVIG in patients with recurrent IVF failure. The authors pooled the results of three randomized controlled trials and two (unpublished) cohort trials of IVIG in recurrent IVF failure and showed a significant increase in the live birth rate per woman ($p < 0.001$) after IVIG treatment with a small number needed to treat (NNT) to achieve an additional live birth of 3.7. This review was criticized because it combined unpublished observational (non-randomized) data with data from randomized trials. However, even when the analysis was limited to data from the three randomized trials only, the use of IVIG was still associated with a significantly higher live birth rate ($p = 0.012$) and a relatively low NNT of 6.

Van den Heuvel and colleagues [2] studied 31 women suffering from recurrent implantation failure or pregnancy loss and treated with IVIG and reported a significantly higher pregnancy rate in women with elevated NK cells after IVIG therapy compared with women with no evidence of NK cell elevation or autoimmunity ($p = 0.018$).

More recently, Heilmann and colleagues (2010) retrospectively reported the results of a cohort of 188 women with recurrent implantation failure who underwent 226 IVF cycles after IVIG therapy and showed a significantly higher live birth rate per patient compared with un-matched historical controls (42% versus 16.1%).

Humira

Compared to the literature on the application of IVIG in recurrent implantation failure patients, studies evaluating the use of the TNF-α blocker Humira are scarce. Winger and colleagues in 2009 reported the results of pre-IVF treatment of 75 women below the age of 38 years with elevated Th1/Th2 cytokine ratio using two 40 mg Humira injections separated by a two week interval with or without IVIG therapy [3]. The study showed a significantly higher implantation, pregnancy, and live birth rates in the treatment group compared with the control group, suggesting that the use of TNF-α blockers improves IVF outcomes in young women with recurrent implantation failure and Th1/Th2 cytokine ratio elevation.

Another study from the same group [4] involving 84 women demonstrating pre-treatment Th1/Th2 cytokine ratio elevation and undergoing IVF, showed a significant improvement in implantation, pregnancy, and live birth rates in the group treated with Humira and IVIG ($n = 76$) compared with an untreated control group ($n = 8$) irrespective of the degree of pre-treatment elevation in the cytokine profile. The two groups were comparable in baseline characteristics such as age, number of previous IVF attempts, and pregnancy history as well as their IVF cycle parameters. The results of this study suggest that correction of elevated Th1/Th2 cytokine ratio is associated with improvement in IVF outcome and led the authors to conclude that the beneficial effect of Humira could be either independent or additive to the IVIG benefit.

Limitations of current literature

Published studies suggest a favourable and promising role for immunotherapy in improving the success rate of IVF treatment in recurrent implantation failure patients.

Indeed, some of the studies have demonstrated an excitingly high success rate in this difficult group of patients. However, the optimum method to prove the efficacy of therapeutic interventions is through conducting adequately powered and well-designed randomized controlled trials. Most published studies on the use of IVIG and Humira in patients with recurrent implantation failure were limited by methodological inadequacies related to their retrospective design, non-standardized patient selection criteria, failure to exclude the presence of any concurrent evidence of autoimmune or thrombophilic conditions, the small number of women included in each study, heterogeneity in the prescribed dose and timing of immunotherapy intervention, and the lack of a sufficiently large control group or the use of unmatched historical controls. Furthermore, the identification of women eligible for the therapeutic intervention varied between the various published studies because of the inconsistent use and interpretation of diagnostic immunological tests and definition of at-risk women who might benefit from immunotherapy. In addition, the use of multiple interventions in the study group of more than one study renders it difficult to attribute the improvement in success rate to a specific intervention. Finally, although the safety profile of immunotherapy has been demonstrated in several uncontrolled studies, further and larger studies including cost-effectiveness evaluation of the proposed interventions will need to be carried out.

The future

Preliminary studies, as well as our own experience over a number of years, suggest a favorable role for immunotherapy using IVIG and Humira in improving the success rate of IVF treatment in women suffering from recurrent implantation failure. Further evidence, ideally from well-designed and adequately powered randomized trials or large case controlled studies, is urgently needed to substantiate that beneficial impact and propel immunotherapy with IVIG and TNF-α blockers into the realm of mainstream clinical practice. Such trials will need to target patients who are most likely to benefit from these interventions such as young women with intact ovarian reserve and unexplained recurrent implantation failure who exhibit Th1 cytokine bias or elevated NK cell level and/or cytotoxicity. These studies will require the adoption of accepted and easily reproducible inclusion and exclusion criteria, particularly laboratory parameters. They will also need to provide a clear framework regarding the dose, timing, and frequency of administering immunotherapy medication as guided by initial and follow up laboratory parameters, since in our experience this could be material in maximizing the benefit of the medication. Until these studies are concluded, controversy surrounding immunotherapy within the ART field will continue to occupy the interest of many IVF specialists and the potential role of this treatment will remain illusive.

References

1. Clark DA, Coulam CB, Stricker RB. Is intravenous immunoglobulins (IVIG) efficacious in early pregnancy failure? A critical review and meta-analysis for patients who fail in vitro fertilisation and embryo transfer (IVF). *J Assist Reprod Genetic* 2006;**23**:1–13.
2. Van Den Heuvel M, Peralta CG, Hatta K, Han VK, Clark DA. Decline in number of elevated blood CD3+ CD56+ NKT cells in response to intravenous immunoglobulin treatment correlates with successful pregnancy. *AJRI* 2007;**57**:447–59.

3. Winger EE, Reed JL, Ashoush S, Ahuja S, El-Toukhy T, Taranissi M. Treatment with adalimumab (Humira) and intravenous immunoglobulin improves pregnancy rates in women undergoing IVF. *Am J Reprod Immunol* 2009;**61**:113–20.

4. Winger EE, Reed JL, Ashoush S, El-Toukhy T, Ahuja S, Taranissi M. Degree of TNF-α/IL-10 cytokine elevation correlates With IVF success rates in women undergoing treatment with Adalimumab (Humira) and IVIG. *Am J Reprod Immunol* 2010; doi: 10.1111/j.1600–0897.2010.00946.x. [Epub ahead of print].

5. Hutton B, Sharma R, Fergusson D, Tinmouth A, *et al.* Use of intravenous immunoglobulin for treatment of recurrent miscarriage: a systematic review. *BJOG* 2007;**114**:134–42.

Chapter 41

Traditional Chinese medicine

Sheryl de Lacey and Caroline Smith

Introduction

The rising use of complementary medicines and therapies (CM) by patients in infertility care and treatment is controversial. Evidence is emerging that between 30–60% of infertility patients use CM whilst also engaged with assisted reproductive technology (ART) for treatment of infertility [1]. Women in particular, are reported to be turning to CM because of dissatisfaction with the approach of mainstream medicine, coupled with a desire for a more personalized approach in treatment. Others prefer the holistic philosophy of CM and/or a wish to take control of their healthcare decisions [2]. Increasingly, CM is being used in conjunction with mainstream medical treatment in a wide variety of health care settings. This combination may provide choice and complementary effects but may also potentially confound outcome measures for both therapies.

Across the world there is widespread use of CMs in consultation with naturopaths, acupuncturists, and other CM practitioners. But in many other cases, the use of CMs is self prescribed, and products are obtained from a variety of sources such as pharmacies, supermarkets, or health food shops. Complementary medicines and therapies include a range of modalities, one of which is known as traditional Chinese medicine (TCM). This consists of several different modalities including acupuncture, Chinese herbs, moxibustion, massage, dietary therapy, and exercise such as *tai chi* and *qi gong* for instance [3]. In this chapter we will leave aside the use and application of acupuncture since it is the focus of Chapter 43. Rather, we will focus in this chapter on the use and effectiveness of Chinese herbal medicine (CHM) in particular.

What is TCM and how does it approach health and fertility?

Whilst considered an alternative form of therapy in Western countries, TCM originated in China over 5000 years ago and is underpinned by theories derived from thousands of years of meticulous observation of the cosmos and the human body. It has remained a form of primary care throughout most Asian countries, and over time, has spread to almost all parts of the globe, so that nowadays TCM co-exists in Western countries alongside a range of mainstream health practices. This therapy can be applied to both chronic and acute health disorders, health maintenance, and health promotion, and has its own unique approach and philosophy. Like other CMs, TCM considers the health of the individual within a traditional understanding of the body as described in Daoism. Treatment is based on the diagnosis and

How to Improve Your ART Success Rates, ed. Gab Kovacs. Published by Cambridge

differentiation of syndromes which subsequently guide the implementation of treatment. The formula and doses of CHM prescribed for the individual are adjusted in response to signs and symptoms, tongue, and pulse diagnosis.

The TCM approach adopted by TCM practitioners working with men and women with infertility and using IVF has been influenced by the teaching and writings of TCM specialist Jane Lyttleton [4]. Lyttleton's approach gives emphasis to treating the individual with the purpose of producing healthier gametes. In practice the TCM practitioner provides herbal medicine and acupuncture, as well as advice about changes in lifestyle including diet, exercise, sleep, and stress management. Consequently, treatment which women may engage in prior to the commencement of ART has the aim of influencing the way in which the eggs are nourished and grow, and the environment in which they are released and travel down the fallopian tube. Traditional Chinese medicine may also improve the thickness and quality of the endometrium, and/or the health of the man's sperm [3]. Chinese herbal medicine is also sometimes used in the early stages of a pregnancy if there are signs of a threatened miscarriage or a weakening of the mother's body.

Studies of the effectiveness of CHM have tended to focus on gynecological conditions which impact on fertility such as polycystic ovarian syndrome, chronic pelvic inflammatory disease, hormonal irregularities, stress, immunological infertility, sperm motility, and endometriosis [3, 5]. Clinical studies published in Western journals are rare and consequently there is some scepticism about the use of CHM and their effectiveness. Nonetheless, patients increasingly engage with them and they express reluctance to disclose their CM use to mainstream medical practitioners [2]. Because of the potential for interaction between CHM and mainstream treatment approaches it is important to understand the scope of evidence concerning the use of CM and CHM in infertility. It is also vital to conduct open communication with patients about their use of it, its safety, and its effectiveness, and to distinguish between CHM administered by trained and experienced practitioners and patient self-prescribed/administered use of CHM.

Chinese herbs and their effectiveness in improving fertility and pregnancy

Literature exists in China which assesses the effectiveness of CHM in improving female fertility, and this is currently being evaluated in a Cochrane systematic review. Evidence available to date consists mainly of clinical studies rather than randomized clinical trials (RCTs); however, a Cochrane Systematic Review of CHM is discussed first below.

Flower *et al.* identified thirteen RCTs on the effectiveness of CHM and endometriosis published in Chinese literature between 1994 and 2000. Chinese herbal medicine is believed to regulate the endocrine and immune systems, and improve blood circulation and anti-inflammatory activity [5]. In this review Flower *et al.* identified 110 RCTs that were conducted in China and reported in Chinese. However, after being evaluated according to a protocol which included attention to selection, performance, attrition and detection bias, only two were able to be included in the review and only one trial reported on pregnancy outcomes. In this trial CHM was compared with Gestrinone for the treatment of endometriosis. The number of women with a confirmed pregnancy was 4 (at 3 months), 17 (at 4–6 months), 8 (at 7–12 months), 2 (at 13–24 months), and 1 (at over 24 months) in the CHM group; while the number of women with a confirmed pregnancy in the Gestrinone group was

0, 12, 12, 3, and 2, respectively. There was no significant difference between the two groups with regard to the total pregnancy rate (69.6% versus 59.1%; RR 1.18; 95% CI 0.87–1.59) or with regard to symptomatic relief. There were no significant adverse events in the CHM group, and there were fewer side-effects in the CHM group than in the Gestrinone group.

Clinical studies

The practice of TCM in Western countries is clinically represented by a prospective clinical cohort study which recruited 50 women with unexplained infertility [6]. During one menstrual cycle prior to treatment, women who participated were subjected to measures of endometrial thickness, serum FSH, follicular activity, serum progesterone, corpus luteum size, and pregnancy rate to establish a baseline. Women were then treated over three menstrual cycles using CHM that was individualized to the woman after traditional Chinese examination and assessment. The outcomes of this clinical study were encouraging. Significant differences over time were found with the size of the Graafian follicle, endometrium, levels of progesterone, size of corpus luteum, and vascularity. During the study period 56% of women had achieved a pregnancy, 7 women subsequently experienced a miscarriage, and 11 had given birth. No side-effects were reported. Further research is warranted however, since in this study there was no control group or randomization of the sample.

Chinese herbs are usually combined in formulas and given as teas, capsules, tinctures, or powders prescribed specifically for the individual, or in standardized formulas. In a review of CHM and infertility Huang and Chen report that Erzhi Tiangui Recipe (ETR) in combination with FSH was found to be effective in reducing the dosage of FSH required, improving ovarian reactivity and quality of oocytes, and increasing the pregnancy rate. Conversely, they report that the use of another CHM recipe used to promote blood circulation, resulted in decreased ovarian content. Combining CHM with intrauterine insemination (IUI) was reported to produce a better outcome for women with anti-sperm antibodies than those treated with TCM or IUI alone [3].

CHM as an adjunct to ART

There is limited clinical research which evaluates the role of CHM as an adjunct to ART. A recent Danish study compared associations between pregnancy and live birth rates between spontaneous CM users and non-users over a 12-month period of ART treatment. Data was gathered by questionnaire on two occasions and data was extracted from medical records about physiological responses such as ovarian response, embryo transfer, and treatment outcome. Women who used CM described using interventions such as acupuncture, reflexology, kinesiology, homeopathy, healing therapies, herbal supplements, and aromatherapy. The study findings indicated that CM use was associated with a lower ongoing pregnancy/live birth rate over the 12-month period despite CM users having undergone more IVF/intracytoplasmic sperm injection (ICSI) cycles and having had more embryos on average than non-CM users [1]. However, there were limitations to this study. First the type and combinations of CM and their associations with treatment outcome were unable to be determined since 40% of the women used more than one intervention. Further, it was not reported whether the women's use of CM was self-prescribed or administered by a trained practitioner in TCM. A further limitation in this study is that the direction of causality of treatment failure and CM use could not be determined. Therefore it remains unclear whether CM use caused treatment failure or whether poor prognosis led to CM use.

CHM and psychological outcomes

There is emerging evidence from qualitative studies of women's experiences of using TCM that suggest that this is an area requiring further attention and research. In the findings of a recent Australian study women reported using CHM to counter their perception of potential infertility due to their advanced age and concomitant declining fertility. But aside from CHM being used to boost fertility, women participants reported other purposes associated with its use. In addition, outcomes other than pregnancy were experienced as positive. Women reported increased well-being from individualized, holistic and health-focussed treatment options, combined with sensitive, supportive and non-paternalistic communication. Women also associated increased well-being and feelings of reduced stress with their perception of regaining control over their bodies and their decisions for treatment [2].

This study is limited by the small number of participants but nevertheless produced similar findings to qualitative studies involving participants with different health issues, thus increasing its credibility.

Issues of safety

Concern about safety is important. Many users and TCM practitioners consider CHM to be safe and well tolerated, yet few studies report on the effect of herbs on the mother and foetus in the short and long term. It is important to test CHM products for dosage and side-effects, and to provide evidence of the pharmacological consistency of each herb given the variation that may arise in response to its source of origin, harvest season, and the inevitable variation from batch to batch.

Conclusion

There continues to be increasing widespread use of CHM by infertile and sub-fertile couples in the community. There are some interesting effects suggested in the findings of clinical studies; however, most of these studies have occurred in China, are published in Chinese, and are therefore not easily accessible to Western health care practice. Despite the large number of clinical trials that have been conducted, robust RCTs, generally considered the gold standard in evidence of treatment effectiveness, are meager in this field. Clinical cohort studies are contradictory and troubled by confounding factors such as the use of a variety of combinations of CHMs, lack of clarity about whether CHM was self prescribed or administered by a qualified TCM practitioner, and small samples. Evidence describing safety and effectiveness remains sparse despite widespread mythology about its safety and efficacy, and widespread use in the community. It is therefore important that further research is undertaken and that future studies employ transparent, pragmatic, but meticulous clinical methods to provide more rigorous evidence [5].

References

1. Boivin J, Schmidt L. Use of complementary and alternative medicines associated with a 30% lower ongoing pregnancy/live birth rate during 12 months of fertility treatment. *Hum Reprod* 2009;**24**:1626–31.
2. Rayner J, McLachlan H, Forster D, Cramer R. Australian women's use of complementary and alternative medicines to enhance fertility: exploring the experiences of women and practitioners.

BMC Complement Altern Med 2009;**9**:52–61.

3. Huang S, Chen P. Traditional Chinese medicine and infertility. *Curr Opin Obst Gynecol* 2008;**20**: 211–15.
4. Lyttleton J. *Treatment of Infertility with Chinese Medicine*. London; Churchill-Livingstone, 2004.
5. Flower A, Liu J, Chen S, *et al*. Chinese herbal medicine for endometriosis: Review. 2009. *The Cochrane Collaboration Library* 3. http://www.thecochranelibrary.com.
6. Wing T, Sedlmeier E. Measuring the effectiveness of Chinese herbal medicine in improving female fertility. *J Chin Med* 2006;**80**:22–28.

Chapter 42

Adjuvant therapy to improve endometrial development – sildenafil and/or hyperbaric oxygen therapy

Mark Bowman

Adjuvant therapy to assist endometrial development can be considered in two circumstances. Firstly, a proportion of women have a thin endometrium on ultrasound monitoring, despite apparently appropriate estrogen/hormone priming during the assisted conception process. There is often no clear etiology (although repeated curettage may have an influential role), but the histology of the endometrium itself is quite normal. Secondly, endometrium may have been damaged in some way, for example following surgery or as a result of severe endometritis. In these circumstances adjuvant therapy may seek to either encourage endometrial healing or regrowth, beyond what steroid hormonal treatment can offer. Strategies that seek to either improve endometrial blood flow or to encourage healing or growth through increased oxygenation are the focus of this chapter.

From the outset, it should be recognized that there is no clear consensus as to whether a thin but otherwise histologically normal endometrium leads to a lower rate of implantation. De Geyter *et al.* [4] found no association between a thin endometrium per se and a reduced chance of success within IVF, Chen *et al.* [3] also found little negative impact of a thin endometrium when good quality blastocysts were transferred. Commonly, older women have a combination of reduced oocyte quality, a lower peak level of estradiol and a thin endometrium which is collectively associated with a low chance of success. Often these women have a high chance of conception with donor oocytes despite a persistently thin endometrium. However a focus on the thin endometrium and methods by which this can be addressed remains.

Sildenafil

Nitric oxide relaxes vascular smooth muscle through a cyclic GMP mediated pathway. Sildenafil citrate is a type 5 specific phosphodiesterase inhibitor which prevents the degradation of cyclic GMP and as a result causes vasodilatation including, it is reported, in uterine vasculature. As a result vaginal sidenafil has been postulated as a means of assisting endometrial development through enhancing the uterine artery blood flow.

Following an initial pilot study, Sher and Fisch reported on the use of sildenafil in 105 women who had prior unsuccessful IVF associated with a thin endometrium (which they defined as less than 9 mm). Many had a history of prior endometritis but 17% were said to

How to Improve Your ART Success Rates, ed. Gab Kovacs. Published by Cambridge University Press.

have no known cause for the thin endometrium. All patients underwent an OCP-based long down regulation cycle followed by follicle stimulating hormone (FSH) stimulation for IVF. Sildenafil 25 mg suppositories, especially formulated for vaginal administration, were given four times daily throughout the course of FSH stimulation [10].

The authors reported one group (70% of patients) who had an endometrium greater than 9 mm; this group had an ongoing pregnancy rate of 45%. In contrast, the group who had a persistently thin endometrium despite sildenafil (30% of the cohort) had no ongoing pregnancies. A majority of the poor outcome group had a history of prior endometritis.

In a subsequent communication to the publishing journal, Check and Graziano [1] pointed out a number of potential confounding variables that could have influenced Sher's findings. Many of the patients had only two failed cycles and it was by no means conclusive that a thin endometrium was the cause of the failures. Other potential causes of IVF failure were not addressed in the paper but could have been influential. The variable nature of many patients in their response to IVF stimulation suggests that many women could have developed an appropriate endometrium irrespective of sildenafil.

In their letter, the authors referred to their own study (subsequently published, Check *et al.* [2]) which failed to demonstrate a benefit from sildenafil. They randomized patients undergoing frozen embryo transfer to receive vaginal estrogen or sildenafil. No improvement in endometrial thickness was noted in the sildenafil group. They also noted that the pregnancy rate in women with thinner uterine linings was acceptable, particularly given most of that group had evidence of reduced ovarian reserve and other (ovarian derived) etiology for their infertility.

No subsequent randomized controlled trials have been undertaken to examine the effectiveness of sildenafil in leading either to a better developed endometrium or to an improved rate of embryo implantation. A recent study suggested a deceased incidence of natural killer cells in the endometrium of women with recurrent miscarriage as a result of sildenafil therapy, but the study was purely observational in nature [5]. At this point it is reasonable to conclude that adjuvant sildenafil for this purpose has no proven role within IVF treatment.

Hyperbaric oxygen

Commonly employed in the management of barotrauma that can result from undersea diving accidents, hyperbaric oxygen has also been used to promote healing in diseased or ischemic tissues. During hyperbaric oxygen treatment, the patient breathes high percentage oxygen under pressure within a specifically designed hyperbaric chamber.

Hyperbaric oxygen has been shown to lead to a number of physiological changes. Centrally, high pressures of oxygen tend to lead to decreased cardiac output by an increase in peripheral resistance and through a decrease in heart rate. This physiological response would seem to be counterproductive in terms of increasing oxygen tension at peripheral sites, although significant variations in regional/peripheral blood flow distribution can occur as a result of a number of factors [7]. The increased oxygen percentage inhaled, under pressure, is said to lead to increased delivery of oxygen to ischemic tissues, as well as promote new blood vessel formation. This observation has provided the rationale for the use of hyperbaric oxygen therapy for the treatment of chronic hypoxic wounds and as a result there is a rationale for also considering this treatment in women with endometrial scarring secondary to prior trauma.

From first principles, if prior damage has been so significant as to leave only dense fibrosis with effectively no residual viable endometrium, one would expect little prospect of hyperbaric oxygen to have an influential role in more appropriate endometrial development within IVF. However there are some circumstances where damage has led to diffuse fibrosis, but competent endometrial tissue persists. In these circumstances hyperbaric oxygen therapy might encourage new vessel formation and increase oxygenation, thereby leading to improved endometrial cell regeneration and development.

We reported a case of a successful pregnancy following hyperbaric oxygen therapy in a woman who had significant endometrial scarring secondary to packing of the uterine cavity. That procedure was necessary to achieve hemostasis during a significant post partum hemorrhage at the conclusion of her first pregnancy [6]. The patient subsequently experienced secondary infertility and had a number of unsuccessful IVF cycles before seeking a second opinion. Her penultimate cycle was undertaken using adjuvant sildenafil alone, without success.

A review hysteroscopy confirmed a universally scarred endometrium and a combination of hyperbaric oxygen and sildenafil was used in the next IVF cycle. Daily sessions in the treatment chamber were undertaken during the proliferative phase, each for 90 minutes. The patient conceived following embryo transfer and subsequently delivered a healthy baby by Caesarean section.

Given the known association between hyperbaric oxygen and increased peripheral vascular resistance, there is some rationale to consider concomitant sildenafil which could be expected to compensate for this resistance through its nitric oxide-mediated vasodilatory effect.

The use of hyperbaric oxygen therapy within IVF, predominantly for women with unexplained infertility, has been reported in a series of 32 women, with reportedly improved results [8]. However, personal experience of this therapy during IVF in patients with idiopathic thin endometrium has not shown an improvement in measurable thickness when measured by ultrasound.

Hyperbaric oxygen therapy could be properly evaluated in a randomized blinded trial, given sessions in a pressurized chamber could be a common variable between treatment and control groups. To date, however such a trial has not been undertaken. The logistic challenges in completing a trial of this nature include allocating appropriate chamber time to infertility patients, given the demand for treatment time using this expensive limited resource would compete with a number of other treatment groups (e.g., burns, infection, or cancer patients), would be significant.

Conclusion

At this point there is no high-level evidence that adjuvant therapy such as sildenafil or hyperbaric oxygen therapy improves either the observed endometrial thickness during IVF cycles or the ongoing pregnancy rate from IVF treatment. The concept that a thin yet histologically normal endometrium can be improved through vasodilatory strategies remains unproven, and many question whether there is any evidence at all to suggest that these patients have a problem of impaired implantation. For women with scarred endometrium, there is a rationale for considering adjuvant therapy although logically the presence of some competent endometrium would be required for treatment to be successful. There remains the opportunity for a more formal evaluation of the efficacy of hyperbaric oxygen therapy, possibly with concomitant sildenafil for this subset of patients.

References

1. Check J, Graziano V. Multiple confounders – measured with error? *Fertil Steril* 2003;**79**:1073–6.
2. Check J, Graziano V, Lee, G, *et al.* Neither sildenafil nor vaginal estradiol improves endometrial thickness in women with thin endometria after taking oral estradiol in graduating doses. *Clin Exp Obstet Gynecol* 2004;**31**:99–102.
3. Chen C, Zhang X, Confino E, Milad, M, Kazer, RR, *et al.* Thin endometrial strip does not predict poor IVF treatment outcome following embryo transfer on day 5. *Fertil Steril* **78**; Suppl 1: S120.
4. De Geyter C, Schmitter M, De Geyter M, *et al.* Prospective evaluation of the ultrasound appearance of the endometrium in a cohort of 1186 infertile women. *Fertil Steril* 2000;**73**:106–13.
5. Jerzak M, Kniotek, M, Mrozek J, *et al.* Sildenafil citrate decreased natural killer cell activity and enhanced chance of successful pregnancy in women with a history of recurrent miscarriage. *Fertil Steril* 2008;**90**:1848–53.
6. Leverment J, Turner, R, Bowman M, Cooke, CJ. Report on the use of hyperbaric oxygen therapy (HBO2) in an unusual case of secondary infertility. *Undersea Hyperb Med* 2004;**31**:245–50.
7. Mathieu D ed. *Handbook on Hyperbaric Medicine* Dordrecht: Springer, 2006.
8. Mitrović A, Nikolić B, Dragojević S, *et al.* Hyperbaric oxygen as a possible therapy of choice for infertility treatment. *Bosn J Basic Med Sci* 2006;**6**:21–4.
9. Neuman T, Thom S. *Physiology and Medicine of Hyperbaric Oxygen Therapy.* Philadelphia: Saunders Elsevier, 2008.
10. Sher G, Fisch J. Effect of vaginal sildenafil on the outcome of in vitro fertilization (IVF) after multiple IVF failures attributed to poor endometrial development. *Fertil Steril* 2002;**78**:1073–6.

Chapter 43

The role of acupuncture in IVF

Tarek El-Toukhy and Sesh Kamal Sunkara

Introduction

The majority of IVF cycles fail primarily because of low embryo implantation rates. Clinicians and patients are constantly seeking new treatment strategies to improve IVF results. One such treatment that has gained popularity in recent years is the use of acupuncture as an adjunctive treatment to improve the success rate of ART.

Acupuncture is part of ancient traditional Chinese medicine (TCM), which involves the insertion of needles in the skin at specific points to control the flow of energy (or Qi) through the body along specific channels called meridians. The role of acupuncture and its efficacy in reproductive medicine is far from clear. A scientific rationale for the use of acupuncture during IVF treatment is lacking, but theoretically focuses mainly on its potential role in enhancement of uterine receptivity through increased blood flow and quiescence. In addition, a perceived reduction in anxiety and stress after acupuncture has often been cited as an additional justification. However, convincing evidence to support these claims awaits clarification.

Published literature

Several randomized studies have reported treatment outcomes in women who had acupuncture during their IVF cycle. These studies were methodologically and clinically heterogeneous and unsurprisingly yielded conflicting results, rendering the clinical decision whether to recommend acupuncture during IVF treatment difficult to make. However, the use of acupuncture as an adjunct to IVF treatment has gained momentum after the publication of a systematic review by Manheimer and colleagues [3] and a Cochrane review by Cheong *et al.* [1], both of which reported a beneficial effect of acupuncture at the time of embryo transfer on the clinical pregnancy rate following IVF treatment. More recent publications by El-Toukhy and colleagues [2], Sunkara *et al.* [4], El-Toukhy and Khalaf [5], and Cheong and colleagues [6], have contradicted the results of these two reviews.

Analysis of evidence

Studies of acupuncture during IVF treatment have reported the use of acupuncture at the time of either oocyte retrieval or embryo transfer.

How to Improve Your ART Success Rates, ed. Gab Kovacs. Published by Cambridge University Press.

Acupuncture at the time of oocyte retrieval

Five randomized controlled trials (RCTs) have so far reported IVF outcome when acupuncture was performed at the time of oocyte retrieval. Four of these five studies were designed to assess the analgesic effect of acupuncture used at the time of oocyte retrieval compared to conventional analgesia and only one study reported pregnancy rate as a primary outcome. None of the five studies used placebo (sham acupuncture) in the control group.

Meta-analysis of two studies among the five that reported live birth rate as an outcome was reported in the recent review by Cheong *et al.* [6]. It showed no significant difference in live birth rates between the acupuncture and control groups (OR 0.87, 95% CI 0.59–1.29).

Pooling of results from all five studies ($n = 877$) in the review by El-Toukhy and Khalaf [8] for the outcome of clinical pregnancy rate showed no difference in the clinical pregnancy rate between the acupuncture and control groups (RR 1.06, 95% CI 0.82–1.37).

Meta-analysis of four out of the five studies in the review by Cheong *et al.* [6] that reported miscarriage as an outcome showed no significant difference between the acupuncture and control groups (OR 0.81, 95% CI 0.46–1.46).

Acupuncture around the time of embryo transfer

Ten RCTs have so far compared IVF treatment outcome when acupuncture was performed around the time of embryo transfer in the study group versus no or placebo (sham) acupuncture in the control group. These studies included in total over 2600 randomized women. Unlike the studies examining the effect of acupuncture at the time of oocyte retrieval, all these studies were designed with the aim of assessing the effect of acupuncture performed around the time of embryo transfer on the outcome of IVF treatment, mainly the clinical pregnancy rate per IVF cycle. Significant methodological and clinical heterogeneity existed among these ten studies with regard to the protocol of acupuncture used, the specific acupoints employed in each study, the experience of the clinician (acupuncturist) administering the acupuncture treatment, and the nature of the control intervention.

Studies involving acupuncture around the time of embryo transfer involved those that performed acupuncture only on the day of the embryo transfer and those that performed acupuncture on the day of embryo transfer and repeated again two to three days later. Cheong *et al.* [6] combined these studies separately in their meta-analysis. The authors reported no significant difference in the live birth rate between the study and control groups when acupuncture was performed only on the day of embryo transfer (OR 1.43, 95% CI 0.77–2.65). They also found no significant difference in the live birth rate when acupuncture was performed both on the day of embryo transfer and repeated two or three days later (OR 1.79 95% CI 0.93–3.44). Furthermore, the authors found no significant difference in the live birth rate when combining only those studies that used sham acupuncture (placebo) in the control group and acupuncture in the study group around the time of embryo transfer (OR 1.12, 95% CI 0.83–1.52).

In the review by El-Toukhy and Khalaf [5], meta-analysis of the nine RCTs of acupuncture around the time of embryo transfer showed no significant difference in the clinical pregnancy rate between the acupuncture and control groups (RR 1.16, 95% CI 0.91–1.48). The authors reported that five of the nine studies that were included in their review used sham acupuncture in the control group. Pooling of results from these five studies for the outcome of clinical pregnancy rate also showed no significant difference between the acupuncture and control groups in the clinical pregnancy rate (RR 1.18, 95% CI 0.85–1.62).

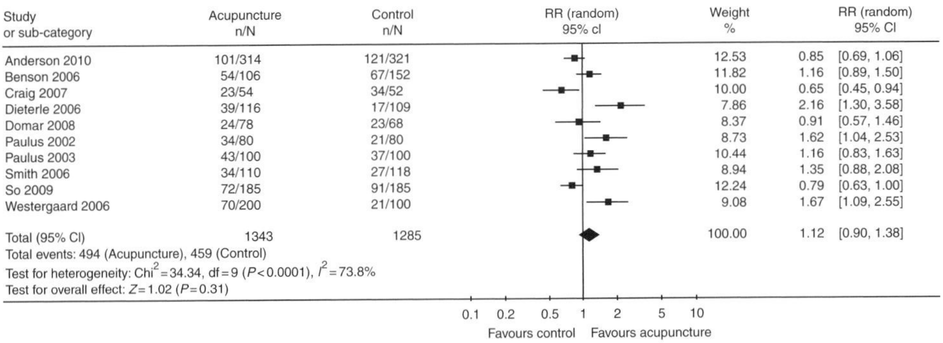
Study or sub-category
Acupuncture n/N
Control n/N
RR (random) 95% cl
Weight %
RR (random) 95% CI
Anderson 2010 101/314 121/321 12.53 0.85 [0.69, 1.06]
Benson 2006 54/106 67/152 11.82 1.16 [0.89, 1.50]
Craig 2007 23/54 34/52 10.00 0.65 [0.45, 0.94]
Dieterle 2006 39/116 17/109 7.86 2.16 [1.30, 3.58]
Domar 2008 24/78 23/68 8.37 0.91 [0.57, 1.46]
Paulus 2002 34/80 21/80 8.73 1.62 [1.04, 2.53]
Paulus 2003 43/100 37/100 10.44 1.16 [0.83, 1.63]
Smith 2006 34/110 27/118 8.94 1.35 [0.88, 2.08]
So 2009 72/185 91/185 12.24 0.79 [0.63, 1.00]
Westergaard 2006 70/200 21/100 9.08 1.67 [1.09, 2.55]
Total (95% CI) 1343 1285 100.00 1.12 [0.90, 1.38]
Total events: 494 (Acupuncture), 459 (Control)
Test for heterogeneity: Chi² = 34.34, df = 9 (P < 0.0001), I² = 73.8%
Test for overall effect: Z = 1.02 (P = 0.31)
0.1 0.2 0.5 1 2 5 10
Favours control
Favours acupuncture

Figure 43.1 Acupuncture versus control around the time of embryo transfer for outcome of clinical pregnancy.

The recently published randomized double-blinded placebo controlled trial by Anderson *et al.* [7] is the largest to date comparing acupuncture versus sham acupuncture at the time of embryo transfer in 635 women undergoing IVF treatment. This study showed no significant difference in the ongoing pregnancy and live birth rates between the study and control groups. The ongoing pregnancy rates were 27% (95% CI 22–32) and 32% (95% CI 27–37) and the live birth rates were 25% (95% CI 20–30) and 30% (95% CI 25–30) in the acupuncture and placebo groups, respectively. Including this study with the previous meta-analysis of the nine studies involving acupuncture around the time of embryo transfer showed no significant difference in the clinical pregnancy rate (RR 1.1, 95% CI 0.90–1.38) (Figure 43.1).

Conclusion

One of the pillars of modern western medicine is that proof of efficacy is required before an intervention is routinely applied in clinical practice. Acupuncture could be useful for other medical conditions, but the use of acupuncture to improve the success rate of IVF treatment cannot be recommended in light of the available evidence, including the recent evidence emerging from robustly conducted RCTs. Although acupuncture has the advantage of having no serious side-effects, women should be informed that there is no evidence of benefit to justify the added cost of having acupuncture to improve IVF treatment. Using the results of the largest study to date by Anderson *et al.* [7] to calculate its sample size, any future high-quality and sufficiently powered clinical trial examining the value of acupuncture in IVF will need to recruit over 4000 women to be able to detect a significant difference in the IVF clinical pregnancy rate related to the use of acupuncture. Undoubtedly, a larger sample size will be needed to detect a similar effect on the live birth rate. Given the considerable heterogeneity present among published studies, the lack of a standardized acupuncture protocol for IVF patients and an accepted placebo intervention, the prospect of such a study being conducted is unrealistic. Therefore, the advice that acupuncture in IVF treatment is not beneficial will remain valid for the foreseeable future. Moreover, the lack of a plausible biological rationale for any perceived benefit from the use of acupuncture in IVF makes it extremely difficult to justify its use in clinical practice [8].

References

1. Cheong YC, Hung Yu, Ng E, Ledger WL. Acupuncture and assisted conception. *Cochrane Database Syst Rev* 2008:**8**; CD006920.
2. El-Toukhy T, Sunkara SK, Khairy M, *et al.* A systematic review and meta-analysis of acupuncture in in vitro fertilisation. *Br J Obstet Gynaecol* 2008:**115**;1203–13.
3. Manheimer E, Zhang G, Udoff L, *et al.* Effects of acupuncture on the rates of pregnancy and live birth among women undergoing in vitro fertilisation: systematic review and meta-analysis. *BMJ* 2008:**336**;545–9.
4. Sunkara SK, Coomarasamy A, Khalaf Y, El-Toukhy T. Acupuncture and in vitro fertilization: updated meta-analysis. *Hum Reprod* 2009:**24**;2047–8.
5. El-Toukhy T, Khalaf Y. The impact of acupuncture on assisted reproductive technology outcome. *Curr Opin Obstet Gynecol* 2009:**21**;240–6.
6. Cheong Y, Nardo LG, Rutherford T, Ledger W. Acupuncture and herbal medicine in in vitro fertilisation: a review of the evidence for clinical practice. *Hum Fert* 2010:**13**:3–12.
7. Anderson D, Lossl K, Nyboe Anderson A, *et al.* Acupuncture on the day of embryo transfer: a randomized controlled trial of 635 patients. *Reprod BioMed Online* 2010:**21**;366–72.
8. El-Toukhy T, Khalaf Y. A new study of acupuncture in IVF: pointing in the right direction. *Reprod BioMed Online* 2010:**21**;278–9.

Chapter 44

Psychological perspectives on IVF treatment

Cora de Klerk and Nick Macklon

The experience of IVF treatment

Despite the relatively low chance of achieving a pregnancy in one IVF cycle, many women embarking on treatment have unrealistic expectations about treatment success. This is what Kalbian calls the "hope narrative" [1]: the childless woman strongly believes that the fertility physicians are able to help her achieve a successful pregnancy but that she should completely surrender her body to her physician to achieve this goal. Indeed, many women report that they feel a lack of control during fertility treatment. Women undergoing fertility treatment feel they have little choice but to succumb to the invasive investigations and procedures the doctors prescribe. A very private aspect of their lives, namely reproduction, becomes medicalized. As a result of this process, feelings of depersonalization may emerge. Even after successful treatment, many women retrospectively describe fertility treatment as being physically and emotionally painful, while some women even reported feeling "hurt" or "damaged" [2].

Undergoing fertility treatment also has an impact on the woman's social and professional life. Social activities are often put on hold during a treatment cycle, as many women are not able or willing to share their experiences with others. Furthermore, the frequent hospital visits may result in absence from work. The demands of treatment also put pressure on the marital relationship. Partners often cope differently with treatment related strain and this may lead to disagreement about whether to continue treatment or not. Being diagnosed with infertility may evoke strong feelings of deficiency in a woman, who feels that motherhood is the norm. She may feel social pressure to reproduce from her family, friends, or even society. Thus, a person's social background shapes their experience of infertility.

The psychological consequences of IVF treatment

Results of quantitative research show that women who are about to start IVF may be more anxious than control populations, although in some studies no differences are found. During treatment, women often experience symptoms of anxiety, especially at oocyte pick-up and just before pregnancy testing. Even though men show the same pattern of emotional reactions during IVF treatment as women, their emotions are usually less intense. Most women adjust well to unsuccessful IVF treatment. However, up to 25% of women report clinically relevant levels of depression after failed IVF [3]. Negative emotions usually disappear after IVF pregnancy, which could suggest that depression related to IVF treatment

How to Improve Your ART Success Rates, ed. Gab Kovacs. Published by Cambridge University Press.

results from the inability to become pregnant rather than treatment itself. However, IVF treatment itself has been shown to evoke psychological symptoms in women [4].

Distress and IVF outcome

In lay etiology, psychological problems are often believed to have a negative effect on fertility. The origin of this belief can be dated back to the 1950s. During this period, a number of psychodynamic writings were published, in which infertility was considered to be the result of unconscious conflicts in the infertile woman, including the fear of motherhood and sexuality. The full psychogenic model of infertility has been the main perspective on the relation between infertility and psychological functioning in biomedicine until the 1980s [5]. Although nowadays most researchers reject the full psychogenic model of infertility, a modified version of this model is still popular in studies on IVF. The cyclical model of stress proposes that infertility leads to distress and distress has a negative influence on pregnancy chance [5]. According to this concept, distress has a direct effect on IVF pregnancy outcome through stress-related hormones or immunological mechanisms, by modulating T cell activity. Also, distress is believed to have an indirect negative effect on IVF outcome through adverse health-related behavior, such as unhealthy eating habits, smoking, and alcohol consumption.

Although IVF treatment is known to increase distress, the evidence for an association between distress and IVF outcome is inconclusive. In a recent meta-analysis by Boivin *et al.*, a significant effect of distress on the chance of achieving a positive pregnancy test was found, but no clear effect on ongoing pregnancy or live birth rates was evident [6] (Figure 44.1). Surprisingly, we found that women who reported few feelings of anger, depression, uncertainty and/or anxiety, e.g., negative affect, before treatment were less likely to achieve term live birth after a first IVF or intracytoplasmic sperm injection (ICSI) cycle than women who expressed a moderate level of negative affect [7]. Still, as the majority of participating women did not meet the criteria for either clinical depression or anxiety, these results do not rule out

	Pregnant			Non-pregnant				Std. mean difference
Study or subgroup	Mean	SD	Total	Mean	SD	Total	Weight	IV, fixed, 95% CI
3.6.3 Positive scan/live birth								
Anderheim et al. 2005	21	4.7	58	21.8	4.8	81	4.5%	−0.17 [−0.50, 0.17]
de Klerk et al. 2008	5.1	3.9	73	5	3.4	216	7.3%	0.03 [−0.24, 0.29]
Demyttenaere et al. 1998	52.8	8.8	23	52.4	10.1	75	2.3%	0.04 [−0.43, 0.51]
Ebbesen et al. 2009	7.2	6.1	215	7.2	6.5	566	20.7%	0.00 [−0.16, 0.16]
Klonoff-Cohen et al. 2001	14.2	5.1	46	15.5	6.01	90	4.0%	−0.23 [−0.58, 0.13]
Lee et al. 2006	13.7	10.2	364	13.2	11	440	26.5%	0.05 [−0.09, 0.19]
Lintsen et al. 2009	17.6	4.7	196	17.7	5	494	18.7%	0.02 [−0.19, 0.15]
Merari et al. 2002	43	15.5	23	39.2	10.6	90	2.4%	0.32 [−0.14, 0.78]
Sanders & Bruce, 1999	35.9	9.2	15	37.8	10.7	75	1.7%	−0.18 [−0.73, 0.38]
Verhaak et al. 2001	35.6	8.3	59	38	10.9	148	5.6%	−0.23 [−0.54, 0.07]
Subtotal (95% CI)			**1072**			**2275**	**93.7%**	**−0.01 [−0.09, 0.06]**
Heterogeneity: $Chi^2 = 7.49$, df = 9 ($P = 0.59$); $I^2 = 0\%$								
Test for overall effect: $Z = 0.37$ ($P = 0.71$)								
3.6.4 Positive pregnancy test								
Akyuz et al. 2006	45	4.6	39	47.6	7.8	41	2.6%	−0.40 [−0.84, 0.04]
Boivin & Takefman, 1995	34.1	8.2	17	37.9	12.4	23	1.3%	−0.34 [−0.98, 0.29]
Demyttenaere et al. 1992	42	8.54	10	47.4	9.31	30	1.0%	−0.58 [−1.31, 0.15]
Lancastle & Boivin, 2005	36	12.3	13	41	11.2	63	1.4%	−0.43 [−1.04, 0.17]
Subtotal (95%CI)			**79**			**157**	**6.3%**	**−0.42 [−0.71, −0.14]**
Heterogeneity: $Chi^2 = 0.25$, df = 3 ($P = 0.97$); $I^2 = 0\%$								
Test for overall effect: $Z = 2.91$ ($P = 0.004$)								
Total (95%CI)			**1151**			**2432**	**100.0%**	**−0.04 [−0.11, 0.03]**
Heterogeneity: $Chi^2 = 15.15$, Df = 13 ($P = 0.30$); $I^2 = 14\%$								
Test for overall effect: $Z = 1.09$ ($P = 0.28$)								
Test for subgroup differences: $Chi^2 = 7.41$, df = 1 ($P = 0.006$), $I^2 = 86.5\%$								

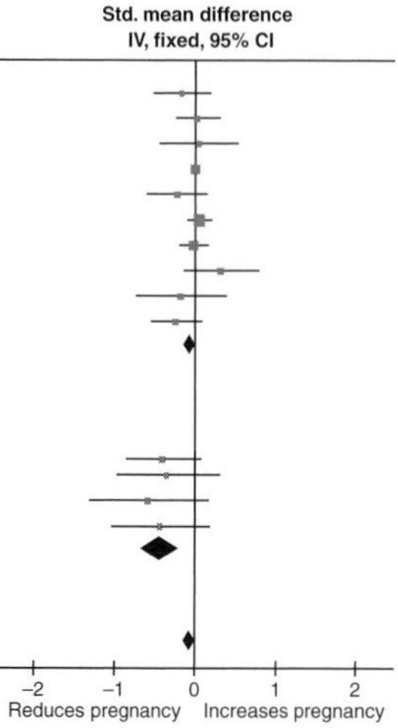

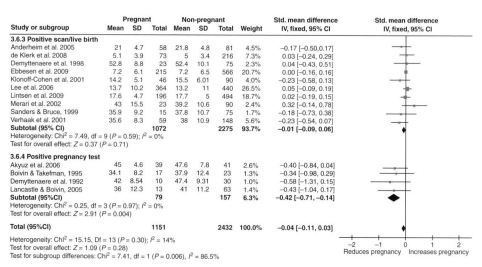

Figure 44.1 A meta-analysis of studies investigating the impact of psychological stress on IVF outcomes. Those studies in which the end-point was limited to the achievement of a positive pregnancy test indicate a negative effect. However, no significant effect of stress on the chance of achieving an ongoing pregnancy or live birth was demonstrated (reproduced with permission, Boivin J *et al.*, *BMJ* 2011).

that high patient distress leads to worse IVF outcomes than moderate distress. Our study is not the first to find a positive association between distress and IVF outcomes. Apparently, the relation between patient distress and IVF success rates might be curvilinear, rather than linear. One might argue that some distress is required for changing unhealthy lifestyle habits, such as smoking. The expression of extreme low levels of distress may also reflect a tendency to repress awareness of negative emotions caused by IVF treatment.

In conclusion, the relation between distress and IVF success rates seems more complex than commonly believed. The popular belief that distress adversely affects IVF outcome may cause feelings of shame and guilt in IVF patients who do not conceive. Physicians should explore such beliefs in their patients and reassure them that distress before and during IVF treatment has no significant influence on live birth rates.

Psychosocial counseling in IVF

Nowadays, psychological problems are considered to be an effect of infertility rather than a cause. Since the psychological consequences model of infertility became popular in the 1980s, professionals in the infertility field have recommended the provision of psychosocial counseling to couples with fertility problems. Infertility counseling helps people explore, understand and cope with issues related to infertility and its treatment. According to the Code of Practice of the UK Human Fertilisation and Embryology Authority, several tasks of counseling can be distinguished in the context of fertility treatment. A psychosocial counselor may help couples to collect and comprehend all information that is needed to make treatment-related decisions, as well as the emotional and social implications of these decisions, e.g., implications and decision-making counseling. When IVF treatment is causing emotional distress in patients, counselors should offer emotional support to help them cope more effectively with treatment strain, e.g., support counseling. Therapeutic counseling should be offered, when specific issues concerning infertility or treatment need more working through. Although many couples embarking on IVF may welcome some form of psychosocial counseling, studies addressing the effectiveness of psychosocial interventions for this population are scarce.

We evaluated a psychosocial counseling intervention for couples undergoing their first cycle of IVF treatment. Counseling was offered to both partners before the start of the first treatment cycle, during the waiting period, which previous studies have suggested is the most stressful phase of treatment, and then again after completion of the first cycle. Couples were randomized to receive either counseling in line with the principles of the experiential psychosocial therapy, in which the central focus is the way individuals relate to others, or no counseling. Consistent with some previous studies, our counseling intervention had little effect on the amount of distress women experienced during their first cycle of IVF treatment [8]. Furthermore, counseling did not influence distress experienced by male partners either. At pregnancy testing however, women who had received additional psychosocial counseling tended to express less negative affect than women who had received routine care only, suggesting that our psychosocial counseling intervention succeeded in reducing unrealistic expectations women might have about IVF success rates. Interestingly, many of the couples invited to participate in the study did not express any need for counseling in order to cope with the procedural distress of IVF treatment. Furthermore, most participating women did not experience clinically significant psychological distress during their first IVF cycle. Therefore, our results do not favour routine psychosocial counseling for all first-time IVF couples. Counseling might be more beneficial for couples who already experience high levels of distress at the start of their first IVF cycle. Future research should therefore be aimed at identifying couples that are particularly vulnerable to distress during treatment.

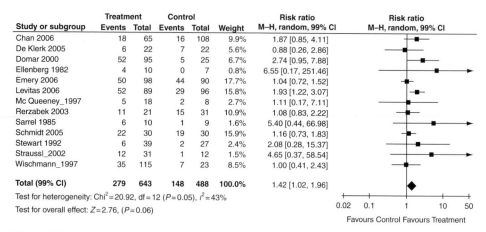

Study or subgroup	Treatment Events	Treatment Total	Control Events	Control Total	Weight	Risk ratio M–H, random, 99% CI
Chan 2006	18	65	16	108	9.9%	1.87 [0.85, 4.11]
De Klerk 2005	6	22	7	22	5.6%	0.88 [0.26, 2.86]
Domar 2000	52	95	5	25	6.7%	2.74 [0.95, 7.88]
Ellenberg 1982	4	10	0	7	0.8%	6.55 [0.17, 251.46]
Emery 2006	50	98	44	90	17.7%	1.04 [0.72, 1.52]
Levitas 2006	52	89	29	96	15.8%	1.93 [1.22, 3.07]
Mc Queeney_1997	5	18	2	8	2.7%	1.11 [0.17, 7.11]
Rerzabek 2003	11	21	15	31	10.9%	1.08 [0.83, 2.22]
Sarrel 1985	6	10	1	9	1.6%	5.40 [0.44, 66.98]
Schmidt 2005	22	30	19	30	15.9%	1.16 [0.73, 1.83]
Stewart 1992	6	39	2	27	2.4%	2.08 [0.28, 15.37]
Straussl_2002	12	31	1	12	1.5%	4.65 [0.37, 58.54]
Wischmann_1997	35	115	7	23	8.5%	1.00 [0.41, 2.43]
Total (99% CI)	**279**	**643**	**148**	**488**	**100.0%**	1.42 [1.02, 1.96]

Test for heterogeneity: Chi^2 = 20.92, df = 12 (P = 0.05), I^2 = 43%

Test for overall effect: Z = 2.76, (P = 0.06)

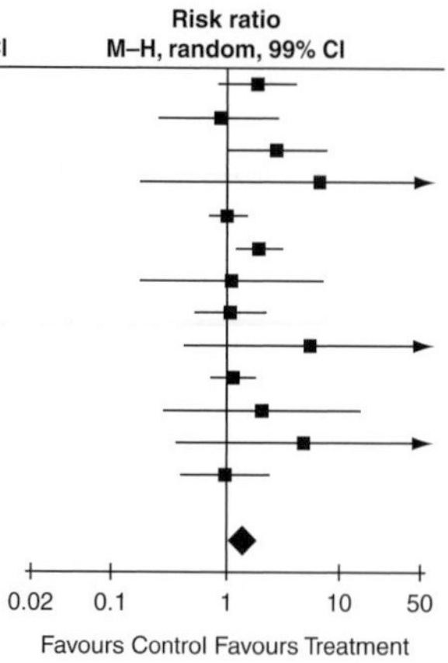

Figure 44.2 A meta-analysis of the impact on IVF outcomes of counseling interventions aimed at reducing stress. An overall beneficial effect is evident (reproduced with permission of Oxford University Press, from Hämmerli K *et al.*, *Hum Reprod Update* 2009).

Educational interventions which focus on information provision and skills training lead to more positive changes in people with fertility problems than counseling interventions, which focus on emotional expression and support [9]. In contrast to counseling interventions, educational interventions are often carried out in a group format with a higher number of structured sessions. Each of these unique characteristics could explain why educational interventions are more beneficial to people's well-being than psychosocial counseling. However, Hämmerli *et al.* concluded in their meta-analysis that psychological interventions do not affect mental health outcomes in people suffering from infertility, although they may increase pregnancy rates, possibly by impacting disrupted sexual activity [9] (Figure 44.2). Hence, alternative ways to decrease distress related to IVF treatment should be considered, such as brief interventions aimed at optimizing day-to-day interactions between physicians and patients.

References

1. Kalbian AH. Narrative ARTifice and women's agency. *Bioethics* 2005;**19**:93–111.
2. Redshaw M, Hockley C, Davidson LL. A qualitative study of the experience of treatment for infertility among women who successfully became pregnant. *Hum Reprod* 2007;**22**:295–304.
3. Verhaak CM, Smeenk JM, *et al.* Women's emotional adjustment to IVF: a systematic review of 25 years of research. *Hum Reprod Update* 2007;**13**:27–36.
4. de Klerk C, Heijnen EM, Macklon NS, *et al.* The psychological impact of mild ovarian stimulation combined with single embryo transfer compared with conventional IVF. *Hum Reprod* 2006;**2**:721–7.
5. van Balen F. The psychologization of infertility. In: Inhorn MC, Balen van F, eds. *Infertility around the Globe: New thinking on childlessness, gender and reproductive technologies.* Berkeley: University of California Press, 2002:79–98.
6. Boivin J, Griffiths E, Venetis CA. Emotional distress in infertile women and failure of assisted reproductive technologies: meta-analysis of prospective psychosocial studies *BMJ* 2011;**342**:d223.
7. de Klerk C, Hunfeld JA, Heijnen EM, *et al.* Low negative affect prior to treatment is

associated with a decreased chance of live birth from a first IVF cycle. *Hum Reprod* 2008;**23**:112–6.

8. de Klerk C, Hunfeld JA, Duivenvoorden HJ, *et al.* Effectiveness of a psychosocial counselling intervention for first-time IVF couples: a randomized controlled trial. *Hum Reprod* 2005;**20**:1333–8.

9. Boivin J. A review of psychosocial interventions in infertility. *Soc Sci Med* 2003;**57**:2325–41.

10. Hammerli K, Znoj H, Barth J. The efficacy of psychological interventions for infertile patients: a meta-analysis examining mental health and pregnancy rate. *Hum Reprod Update* 2009;**15**:279–95.

Chapter 45

Future fertility for young women with cancer: Protection, preservation, or both?

Kate Stern

Introduction

With improvements in cancer treatments over the last few decades comes the expectation that the majority of young women diagnosed with cancer will be cured. Thus, as well as provision of a "disease-free state", medical specialists must also strive for the preservation of an optimum "quality of life" following chemotherapy treatment including preservation of fertility. This has led both to the development of protocols for cancer treatment which minimize the reproductive risks without reducing the efficacy of the chemotherapy and to the provision of options to protect and preserve fertility.

How big is the problem? Cancer risk for young women

While cancer becomes more common with increasing age, the risk of cancer in young women is not insignificant. Data from the National Cancer Institute shows that in 2007 in the USA, the incidence of cancer was 16/100 000 in females less than 20 years and 184/100 000 in those 20–39 years (http://www.seer.cancer.gov/faststats/selections.php?#Output) (see Figure 45.1).

The commonest cancers affecting young women include breast cancer, hematological malignancy including Hodgkin's lymphoma and non-Hodgkin's lymphoma, and brain tumors. Figure 45.2 highlights the conditions determining referral to the Fertility Preservation Service at the Royal Women's Hospital and Melbourne IVF in Melbourne (2003–2009).

Risk of damage from cancer treatment

Many anticancer drugs exert their actions predominantly on dividing cells. The toxic effects of chemotherapy treatments may include inhibition of cell division and adverse effects on DNA function within the dividing granulosa and theca cells of the ovary, as well as the oocytes contained within the follicle.

Furthermore, it has been confirmed that exposure to various alkylating agents during chemotherapy treatment (in particular cyclophosphamide and procarbazine) and the resultant effects on the ovaries, are age-dependent [1, 2]. As the number of oocytes declines with advancing age, the ovaries of older individuals become more vulnerable to gonadal toxins relative to the ovaries of younger women and girls. An individual's chance of developing ovarian failure is related to increasing age, diagnosis, and the specific treatment modalities used. Radiotherapy and chemotherapy and the use of alkylating agents in particular, all

How to Improve Your ART Success Rates, ed. Gab Kovacs. Published by Cambridge University Press. © Cambridge University Press 2011.

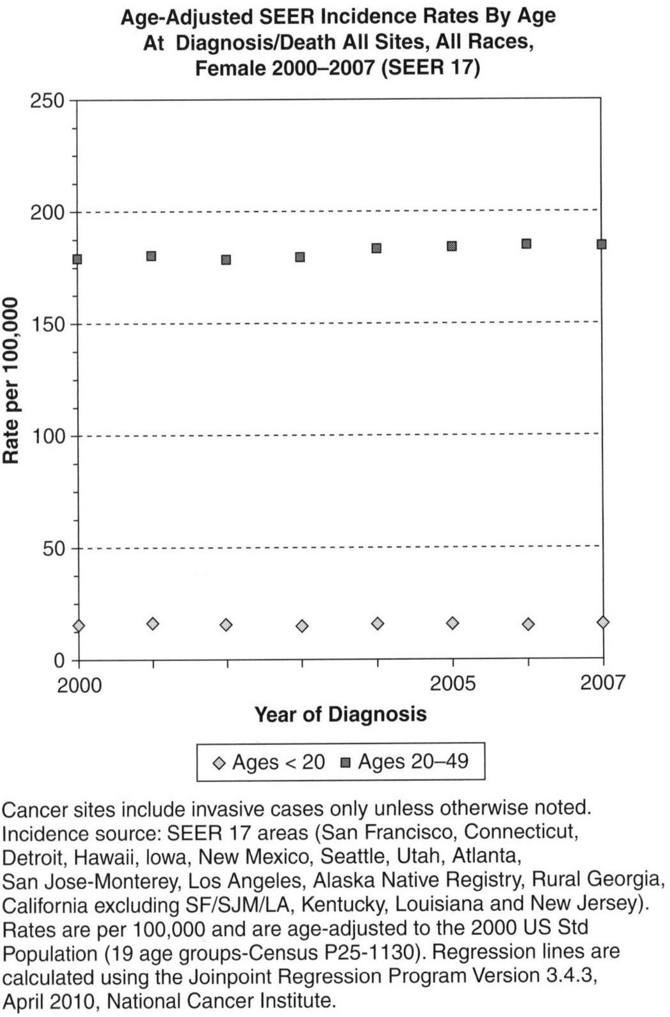
Age-Adjusted SEER Incidence Rates By Age
At Diagnosis/Death All Sites, All Races,
Female 2000–2007 (SEER 17)
250
200
150
100
50
0
Rate per 100,000
2000
2005
2007
Year of Diagnosis
Ages < 20
Ages 20–49
Cancer sites include invasive cases only unless otherwise noted.
Incidence source: SEER 17 areas (San Francisco, Connecticut, Detroit, Hawaii, Iowa, New Mexico, Seattle, Utah, Atlanta, San Jose-Monterey, Los Angeles, Alaska Native Registry, Rural Georgia, California excluding SF/SJM/LA, Kentucky, Louisiana and New Jersey).
Rates are per 100,000 and are age-adjusted to the 2000 US Std Population (19 age groups-Census P25-1130). Regression lines are calculated using the Joinpoint Regression Program Version 3.4.3, April 2010, National Cancer Institute.

Figure 45.1 Age-adjusted SEER incidence rates by age at diagnosis/death.

increase risk. Radiotherapy to the pelvis can also cause serious damage to the uterus, particularly the endometrium and the myometrium. Cranial radiation may also affect pituitary hormone production and release.

Table 45.1 illustrates the range of risks associated with chemotherapy and radiotherapy treatment of the commonest cancers [3]. However, given the scarcity of data regarding rates of infertility following most cancer treatments, oncologists may have difficulty in providing specific and accurate data to patients about their particular risks for infertility.

The clinical and endocrinological response to chemotherapy agents, particularly alkylating agents, can be extremely variable. Commonly during and/or after chemotherapy there is a temporary cessation of menstrual and ovulatory function [1], with hot flushes and amenorrhoea. This may persist into more "permanent" ovarian failure and premature menopause, or may resolve over 6 to 18 months, and thus be diagnosed as "temporary" only in retrospect! Sometimes however, ovarian function may appear to persist normally, as evaluated by clinical

Table 45.1 Representative rates of ovarian failure after treatment of common childhood and young adult cancers [3]

Disease	Likelihood of premature ovarian failure
Breast cancer: standard chemotherapy	
Age < 30	< 10%
Age 30–40	20–40%
Sarcoma	< 10–40%
Hodgkin's lymphoma	< 10% unless intensive therapy
non-Hodgkin's lymphoma	10–40%
Leukemia (early stage)	< 10%
High-dose therapy and stem-cell transplantation	> 80–90%

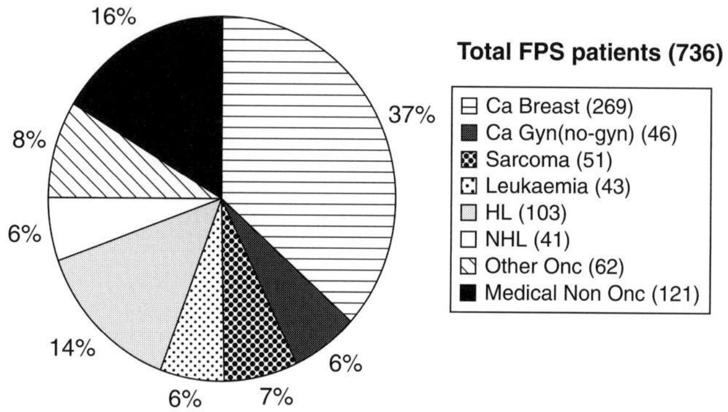

Figure 45.2 Cancer in young women (Melbourne IVF referral data 2003–2009 presented at ESHRE 2010).

or hormonal measures. In many of the young patients who continue to menstruate regularly after chemotherapy, or who resume menses after a time of amenorrhoea, morphological and ultrasound assessment demonstrates reduced follicle numbers, and endocrine assessment shows alterations in follicle-stimulating hormone (FSH), anti-mullerian hormone (AMH), inhibin B, and luteinizing hormone (LH)[2] indicating likelihood of premature ovarian failure. Thus reporting of resumption of ovarian function after cancer treatments may incorrectly reassure physicians and their patients, with potentially serious long-term fertility consequences.

Options for fertility preservation and protection

Given the toxic effects of chemotherapy agents on the ovary, with the resultant risk of temporary and more permanent ovarian failure, the availability of options to preserve and protect fertility is of great importance to these young women and their families. Current options to preserve fertility in this patient population of women who undergo chemotherapy treatment are limited, but include preservation of embryos, oocytes, or ovarian tissue prior to cancer treatment, and ovarian protection with the use of GnRH analogues throughout the duration of treatment [4].

Embryo freezing

Cryopreservation of embryos in an IVF cycle prior to the onset of cytotoxic treatment offers the best chance of a subsequent pregnancy should a woman subsequently become infertile after chemotherapy. The survival rate of embryos after freezing and thawing is in the range of 75–90%, and implantation rates (clinical pregnancy rate for each individual embryo transferred) are between 30–37% currently (National Perinatal Statistics Unit, Australia 2008), approximating spontaneous fertility. If multiple embryos are available, the cumulative pregnancy rate can be more than 60%.

Unfortunately, there are sometimes barriers to the use of this technique in the oncology setting. Often, commencement of chemotherapy is required forthwith after diagnosis, so there is not enough time for the 10–16 days required to initiate and complete an IVF cycle. Additionally, younger women or adolescents may not have a stable partner and for young women it may not be appropriate to consider donor sperm. In some jurisdictions, if a relationship subsequently dissolves, the woman may not be able to utilize the embryos if her ex-partner refuses to give permission. In addition, many women with a malignancy do not respond well to standard ovarian stimulation regimens, perhaps because of intense physical and psychological stress associated with the cancer diagnosis, such that the numbers and/or quality of oocytes obtained may not be optimal. Finally, there are theoretical concerns that the controlled ovarian hyperstimulation (COH) with high levels of estrogens required to produce suitable oocytes may have an adverse effect on hormonally sensitive tumors. For women with estrogen-receptor positive breast cancer who, in consultation with their oncologist, decide to pursue ovarian stimulation, there may be some protective effect from concomitant use of tamoxifen or letrozole, although long-term follow-up data is not yet available.

Oocyte freezing

An alternative to embryo freezing is to freeze mature oocytes after ovarian stimulation. Whilst still experiencing the problems of COH, this maintains autonomy, as there is no requirement for a partner or sperm donor. For many years the fragility of the oocyte, compared with the embryo, hampered success rates with viability after thawing (see Figure 45.3), but with recent improvements in freeze-thaw protocols including vitrification, this is a much more viable option with reports of over 60% of mature oocytes surviving the thaw, and subsequent fertilization rates now approximating those for fresh oocytes during IVF [6] (see Table 45.2).

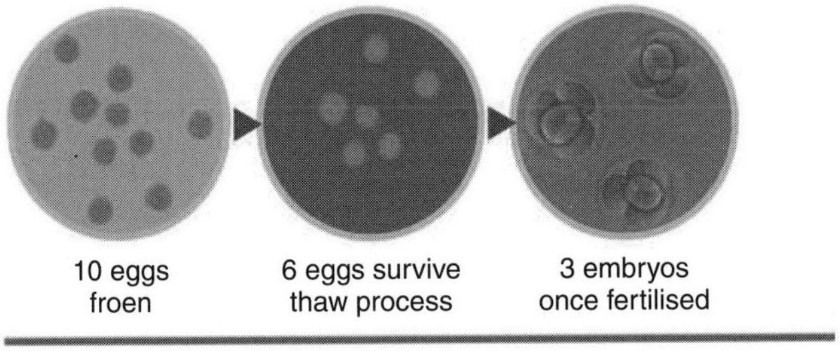

Figure 45.3 Survival of oocytes after freezing. (Reproduced with permission Melbourne IVF).

Table 45.2 Mature oocyte utilization rate

	Mature oocyte freezing results					
	Slow			Vitrification		
	0.1 Msuc	0.2 Msuc	0.3 Msuc	EG	EG+DMSO	EG+PROH
Survival rate%	51	71	73	85	93	80
Fert rate%	54	80	73	77	87	70
Embryos/100 thawed	23	53	48	62	75	30
Imp rate%	10	17	6	14	14	13
Imp/100 thawed	2	9	3	9	11	4

Fert rate = fertilization rate, imp rate +implantation rate, imp/100 thawed = implantation rate per 100 embryos thawed, suc = sucrose, DMSO = dimethylsulphoxide, PROH = 1,2 propanediol, EG = ethyleneglycol.

By the end of 2009, over 930 births had been reported from oocyte freezing, with no major increase in complication rates such as miscarriage or congenital abnormalities [7]. Like embryo freezing however, the requirement for hormonal stimulation and time may preclude the use of oocyte freezing for some young women about to embark on chemotherapy.

Ovarian tissue freezing and grafting

In some centers, patients may be offered the opportunity to harvest and freeze ovarian tissue prior to the commencement of cancer treatment. The tissue is obtained laparoscopically, with the surgeon usually taking up to one-third of one ovary, or a whole ovary if high dose chemotherapy or pelvic radiotherapy is planned for cancer treatment.

This option has the advantage of speed (versus the time required to stimulate and harvest oocytes). However, it exposes the patient to the risk of laparoscopy, which carries approximately a 0.5–2% chance of conversion to open laparotomy and a 1 in 12 000 chance of death.

To date there have only been 14 live births reported worldwide following the reimplantation of thawed ovarian tissue (ESHRE 2010). Follicular development from grafted ovarian tissue does not always follow typical cyclical patterns, making spontaneous fertility, and IVF more difficult than in the conventional setting. The major impediments to success include an extremely high attrition rate of the tissue and the follicles, and difficulties with development of good quality oocytes and embryos. Factors contributing to limited graft function and survival include age of patient at time of tissue excision, prior chemotherapy, the graft site, and the volume of grafted tissue, ischemic damage to follicles and stroma, and low inhibin A and AMH [8].

Although the harvested tissue is rigorously and repeatedly tested by histological and other immunohistochemical and molecular techniques, there is some concern that intraovarian small vessels or even the ovarian tissue itself may occasionally harbour malignant cells, particularly in acute leukemia.

It is hoped that further improvements in freeze-thaw technology may allow frozen ovarian tissue to be a more dependable form of fertility preservation in the near future.

Table 45.3 Oocyte and ovarian tissue freezing: a) numbers of oocytes and tissue slices obtained in cancer patients; b) comparison of practicalities of different processes

a)

	Tissue freeze slices	Oocyte freeze	Embryo freeze
Average no.	140	14.6	6.8
Range	28–538	3–45	3–15

b)

	Oocyte freezing	Ovarian tissue freezing
Invasiveness	Minimal	Moderate
Time required	2+ weeks	1 day
Expectation of success	Moderate if enough oocytes frozen	low currently

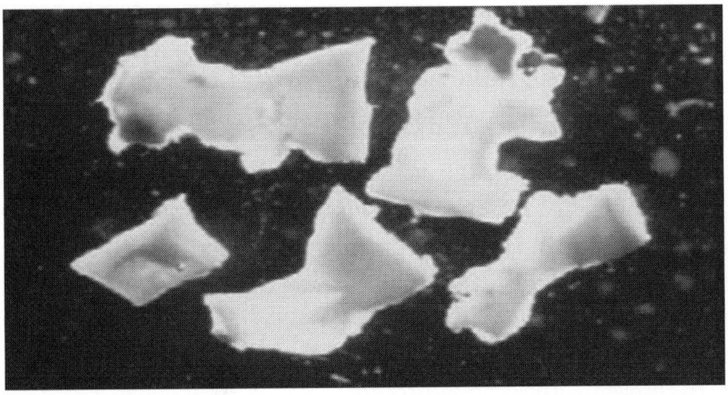

Figure 45.4 Thin slices of ovarian tissue prepared for freezing. (Courtesy of Dr Deb Gook, Melbourne IVF).

This field is rapidly evolving, so patients should be counseled that while currently this technique is highly experimental, there is the potential to preserve a large number of follicles within the tissue, and the results to date are very encouraging.

Protection of the ovaries during chemotherapy

Gonadotropin-releasing hormone (GnRH) analogues may be agonists or antagonists (working by down-regulation or competitive inhibition respectively). In women they induce a temporary and reversible medical state of hypoestrogenism by decreasing pituitary FSH and LH. They are commonly used in the treatment of endometriosis, in some infertility treatments to prevent the LH surge, and as adjuncts to chemotherapy in hormonally sensitive breast and prostate cancers. In children they have also been utilized in the treatment of central precocious puberty.

Recently, GnRH analogues have been shown to protect the ovary from damage during chemotherapy in some animal models. The mechanism of this protective effect is poorly understood, particularly as the early phases of follicle development are thought to be gonadotrophin-independent. Possibly the protective effect could be mediated either by reduction of blood flow to the ovary or through modulation of AMH activity.

Most human studies of GnRH analogues to date involving cancer patients have been uncontrolled and/or retrospective. Thus there is little prospective data specifically addressing the issues for those women of reproductive age who are at highest risk of infertility from chemotherapy. However, despite the above limitations, there is now increasing evidence from clinical studies to suggest a therapeutic benefit from GnRH agonists for ovarian protection.

Two recent reviews, by Beck-Fruchter *et al.* [8] and Blumenfeld *et al.* [9] evaluated the clinical evidence regarding the use of GnRH agonists as ovarian protectors during chemotherapy. These reviews both concluded that the published studies did provide evidence that GnRH analogues provided ovarian protection benefit (which was statistically significant in one paper); however, the limitations of the data analyzed precluded making a definitive conclusion as to the usefulness of the agonists.

Recently, Badawy *et al.* [10] reported their findings of a randomized controlled trial which demonstrated a statistically significant benefit of ovarian protection in patients with breast cancer who received GnRH agonist with chemotherapy versus chemotherapy alone.

This randomized trial, and the reviews cited above, provide support for the role of GnRH analogues for ovarian protection. They also lay the groundwork for further prospective studies. Other medications including immunomodulators are also being trialed as ovarian protectors in animal models.

Assessment of ovarian function and ovarian reserve

Assessment of ovarian function and ovarian reserve is not a simple task. Traditionally menstrual cycle regularity and the presence or absence of menses has been used as a guide to the functionality of the ovaries, but clearly this is not sufficiently accurate, due to the enormous variability in menstrual cyclicity and the fact that ovarian compromise can occur in the presence of regular menses.

As the most extensively investigated endocrine marker, serum FSH has been the most useful parameter for assessment of ovarian reserve. Other modalities for assessment of ovarian reserve such as inhibin B, AMH, and biophysical assessments including antral follicle count (AFC) and ovarian volume, have emerged as useful and potentially superior methods of ovarian reserve assessment. In particular, AMH, which is unaffected by cyclicity and is a marker of smaller follicles, is becoming acknowledged as an extremely reliable indicator of ovarian reserve (Chapter 1). It appears that a combination of endocrine and biophysical parameters provides the best insight currently available into current and future ovarian function

How to choose between the different preservation options

It is impossible to be dogmatic about which fertility-preserving option offers the best chance for a robust reproductive future (see Figure 45.5). The particular circumstances, time restraints associated with commencement of impending cancer treatment, prior reproductive history, and future aspirations will all interact to lead women to make the best choice for their individual situation. Some women may choose more than one option.

The diagnosis of a potentially life-threatening malignancy requiring chemotherapy is an extraordinarily traumatic and shattering experience for young women and their families. Discussion of further evaluation, therapeutic choices, and the short- and longer-term implications of these, as well as discussion of prognosis, is extremely challenging for

Balance of risk

- risk to patient from doing procedure:
  - delay in commencement of cancer treatment
  - medical risks of procedure
  - potential risk of hormones
  - suboptimal response to fertility-preserving treatment
  - risk of false hope/insurance for future fertility
- risk to patient from not doing procedure:
  - reduced fertility/sterility
  - potential childlessness
  - lack of confidence in survival

Figure 45.5 Factors to consider in decision-making for fertility preservation.

oncologists and their teams. Figure 45.5 lists some of the issues that need to be considered when making decisions about fertility preservation. Often counseling requires several consultations, despite the pressure of time for commencement of treatment. Incorporation of discussion about threats to future fertility, and options to preserve and protect fertility, can potentially add an extra layer of complexity and often confusion to an already fraught interaction. However, patients and their families invariably welcome the information imparted regarding future fertility. This information, and perhaps most importantly, the referral for fertility discussion, can give young women and their families optimism about future survival and quality of life. It can also provide an opportunity for them to feel more in control of their situation and to make choices, which suit their individual life situation. Counseling is of paramount importance, as many young people will choose not to avail themselves of any interventionist options, but will appreciate being informed of both the implications of their cancer and its treatment on future fertility and the choices available.

Conclusions

It is now acknowledged that discussion of future fertility options should be considered an essential part of the treatment plan for young women having gonadotoxic therapy. Increasing research and clinical collaboration and cooperation between reproductive medicine specialists and oncological teams will allow us to provide our patients with information which can help them to have more control over their reproductive future.

For those who wish to be more active regarding preserving fertility, we can now offer the various options with increasing confidence and optimism.

References

1. Meirow D. Ovarian injury and modern options to preserve fertility in female cancer patients treated with high dose radio-chemotherapy for hemato-oncological neoplasias and other cancers. *Leuk Lymphoma* 1999;**33**:65–76.
2. Anderson RA, Themmen AP, Al-Qahtani A, Groome NP, Cameron DA. The effects of

chemotherapy and long-term gonadotrophin suppression on the ovarian reserve in premenopausal women with breast cancer. *Hum Reprod* 2006;**21**:2583–92.

3. Stern CJ, Toledo MG, Gook DA, Seymour JF. Fertility preservation in female oncology patients. *Aust N Z J Obstet Gynaecol* 2006; **46**:15–23.
4. Levine J, Canada A and Stern CJ. Fertility preservation in adolescents and young adults with cancer. *J Clin Oncol* 2010;**28**: 4831–41.
5. Gook DA, Edgar DH. Human oocyte cryopreservation. *Hum Reprod Update* 2007;**13**:591–605.
6. Noyes N. Over 900 oocyte cryopreservation babies born with no apparent increase in congenital anomalies. *RBM Online* 2009;**18**:769–76.
7. Demeestere P, Simon S, Emiliani A, *et al.* Orthotopic and heterotopic ovarian tissue transplantation. *Hum Reprod Update* 2009;**15**:649–65.
8. Beck-Fruchter R, Weiss A, Shalev E. GnRH agonist therapy as ovarian protectants in female patients undergoing chemotherapy: a review of the clinical data. *Hum Reprod Update* 2008;**14**: 553–61.
9. Blumenfeld Z, von Wolff M. GnRH-analogues and oral contraceptives for fertility preservation in women during chemotherapy. *Hum Reprod Update* 2008;**14**: 543–52.
10. Badawy A, Elnashar A, El-Ashry M, Shahat M. Gonadotropin-releasing hormone agonists for prevention of chemotherapy-induced ovarian damage: a randomized prospective study *Fertil Steril* 2009, **91**: 694–7.

Chapter 46

How to report IVF success rates

Elizabeth A. Sullivan and Yueping A. Wang

Introduction

In the most recent world report on monitoring ART/IVF was available in 54 countries worldwide [1]. There was wide variation in ART practice by country and region and in the measures used to quantify ART treatment success [1]. There was no data on what an individual woman, couple, community, or country would define as successful ART treatment.

There is no single measure or universal, standard definition of success for ART. This is evident from the differences in practice guidelines, regulatory processes, and government and private sector policies on access and funding/reimbursement of patient costs of fertility treatment between countries and professional organizations. This chapter defines success from a medical and population paradigm and does not take into account cultural or ethnic specific measures of success.

Key concepts

Success can be defined as a favourable or desired outcome. When used in a medical paradigm it is a composite measure of several *indicators of benefit* including efficacy, patient safety, quality, and cost. The key components for a measure of ART treatment success are: efficacy – the capacity of the treatment to produce the desired effect, a liveborn baby; patient safety – defined as "the reduction of risk of unnecessary harm associated with health care to an acceptable minimum" [3]; and quality – defined as "the degree to which health services for individuals and populations increase the likelihood of desired health outcomes and are consistent with current professional knowledge" [3]. An additional parameter that should be added to this composite measure of success is the *absence of disability*, where disability is defined as "any type of impairment of body structure or function, activity limitation and/or restriction of participation in society", in this case associated with ART treatment [3].

Success rate

The success rate is a fraction which is a *number* that can represent part of a *whole*. This rate consists of two components, the numerator and denominator. The numerator represents a number of equal parts and the denominator informs how many of those parts make up a whole. For ART treatment, the numerator is usually the number of a specified outcome, e.g., clinical pregnancy, and denominator is the number of treatments, e.g., initiated cycles. The success rate of ART treatment is usually presented as a percentage, e.g., number of clinical pregnancies per 100 initiated cycles.

How to Improve Your ART Success Rates, ed. Gab Kovacs. Published by Cambridge

There are a number of reasons for reporting IVF success rates. These include: providing an evidence base for couples/individuals seeking to make informed decisions about IVF treatment; benchmarking of clinical practice; regulatory purposes; policy evaluation; commercial activities such as marketing services; and monitoring the safety and quality of IVF treatment and maternal and perinatal outcomes at a clinic, national or international level.

International definition of success of ART

There are a range of definitions for procedures and outcomes of ART treatment used internationally. The lack of internationally accepted standard definitions has made it difficult to compare ART treatment and outcomes at a clinic and population level. In 2009, the International Committee Monitoring Assisted Reproductive Technologies (ICMART) and the World Health Organization *Revised Glossary on ART Terminology* was released [6]. The glossary standardized ART terminology with definitions of pregnancy and perinatal outcomes including: clinical pregnancy, spontaneous abortion/miscarriage, delivery, live birth, preterm birth, low birthweight, and perinatal mortality (to seven completed days post birth) [6]. These standard terms are used in the computation of success rates of ART. Standardized terminology is more informative to patients, health professionals, government and non government organizations, and allows comparative analysis between clinics, countries, and regions. However, the glossary does not include specific measures of success which would take into consideration the well-being of babies and their mothers, the absence of disability, and survival of the neonate beyond seven days.

Currently used measures of success of ART treatment

The three most commonly used denominators to measure the success of ART treatment are initiated cycles, aspirations, and embryos transferred. The three main numerators are clinical pregnancy, delivery, and live delivery. These are used in national and regional reports and the peer literature. "Take home" baby, term liveborn singleton, BESST (singleton, term gestation, live birth rate per cycle initiated) and healthy baby (term singleton neonatal survivor [≥28 days] with normal birthweight and no identified congenital anomaly) are mainly computed by registries or research studies as they include composite measures of treatment and perinatal outcome data which may not be available at the treating clinic [2, 4].

Clinical pregnancy is the most widely used measure of the success of ART treatment. However, clinical pregnancy is not the endpoint of ART treatment but an interim measure. About 15–20% of clinical pregnancies following ART treatments end in spontaneous abortions or miscarriages. Live delivery and live births are other frequently used measures of success for ART and are aligned with vital statistics reporting of birth registrations. The latter does not take neonatal outcomes into consideration. Similarly, the parameters of the take home baby measure do not include neonatal mortality or disability.

Term liveborn singleton and healthy baby are measures of singleton birth outcomes, thus differentiating singletons from multiples. Term liveborn singleton takes gestation and birth status into consideration while healthy baby summarizes better perinatal outcomes. However, both measures have the potential to under- and over-estimate success due to quality of data and ascertainment of perinatal outcomes. These measures are not well accepted in settings where twins are considered a better outcome than singletons.

Selection bias is a potential issue when determining the denominator for ART success measures. For example, the exclusion of cancelled cycles from the denominator by presenting

Table 46.1 Comparative outcomes of autologous fresh cycles by women's age group

	Age group (years)				
Stage/outcome of treatment	< 30	30–34	35–39	40–44	≥ 45
Initiated cycles	1,000	1,000	1,000	1,000	1,000
Aspirations	931	934	916	891	861
Embryo transfers	796	823	799	731	592
Clinical pregnancies	342	314	246	109	18
Clinical pregnancies per initiated cycle (%)	34.2	31.4	24.6	10.9	1.8
Clinical pregnancies per aspiration (%)	36.7	33.7	26.8	12.2	2.1
Clinical pregnancies per embryo transfer (%)	42.9	38.2	30.8	14.9	3.0

Source: Rates based on data available on ART in Australia and New Zealand 2008 available at www.aihw.gov.au/publications/per/49/11525.pdf

pregnancies per 100 aspirations will positively impact pregnancy success rates. Table 46.1 demonstrates how clinical pregnancy rates of autologous fresh cycles differ dependent upon the denominator. The selection of transfer cycles as the denominator over-estimates the success rate of ART compared to a denominator of initiated cycles. For example, among patients aged 45 years or older, the clinical pregnancy rate per embryo transfer was 1.7 times the rate per initiated cycle. This compares to 1.2 times the rate per initiated cycle for cycles among patients aged 30–34 years. Conversely, the choice of initiated cycle as the denominator is limited to differentiate the success rates between some ART procedures such as IVF or intracytoplasmic sperm injection (ICSI).

Reporting success rates of cryopreserved embryos

Cryopreservation of embryos is now routine practice. The dilemma is how to present success rates of ART treatment following transfer of thawed embryos. Ideally, the subsequent success following thawed embryo transfer should be credited back to the initiated aspiration and a cumulative success rate calculated. Cumulative success rate per aspiration is measured by the number of successes resulting from one aspiration for a patient, e.g., number of clinical pregnancies per 100 aspirations. Cumulative success rate per patient is measured by the number of successes resulting from a specified number of treatments of a patient or during a specified period, e.g., number of clinical pregnancies per three treatment cycles (one fresh cycles plus two thaw cycles), or number of clinical pregnancies per patient over one year.

The success rate is the chance of success of each individual treatment cycle. The cumulative success rate summarizes the overall chance of success for several cycles or over a specified time period. Where data are available, cumulative success rates are more relevant in the settings where single embryo transfer and thaw cycles are the dominant practice.

Other factors

A number of demographic factors should be taken into consideration when measuring the success of ART treatment. In general, access to the ART treatment at a younger age is related to higher success rates of pregnancy and live births. Patients with a diagnosis of tubal infertility or male factor infertility usually have better outcomes. A higher success rate is also experienced with patients undertaking their first treatment cycle or who have a history of a live birth.

It is difficult to have a single measure of success of ART treatment when there is a continuum of outcomes extending from assisted conception to live birth, to a surviving infant without disability. Firstly, the concept of success for fertility specialists, obstetricians, neonatologists, and patients may not be a shared concept. It may differ by clinical setting, country, culture, or ethnicity and by whether it is an individual couple or population perspective. Secondly, for most clinics accurate follow-up of babies born to patients whose pregnancy care is delivered in settings other than the fertility center is logistically difficult and resource intensive resulting in under ascertainment and bias regarding perinatal outcomes. Thirdly, even if accurate information is available on birth outcomes not all congenital anomalies or developmental disabilities are diagnosed or recognized in the perinatal period. One solution is to develop an indicator of *absence of disability* using robust, reliable standard measures of perinatal outcomes derived from data collected through clinics, and national and regional collections.

Measures of success of ART treatment

The baseline measures of success for ART remain the clinical pregnancy rate (the number of clinical pregnancies per 100 initiated cycles, aspiration cycles or embryo transfer cycles) and the delivery rate (number of deliveries per 100 initiated cycles, aspiration cycles or embryo transfer cycles) as defined in the ICMART glossary [6].

Live birth is the central component of any primary measure of success of ART treatment. Live birth delivery rate is also defined in the ICMART glossary as "the number of deliveries that resulted in at least one live born baby per 100 initiated cycles, aspiration cycles or embryo transfer cycles" [6]. It is the summary measure of ART success. Multiple embryo transfer, multiple pregnancies, and multiple births all contribute to the excess risks and complications of ART treatment through higher rates of adverse pregnancy and perinatal outcomes. Intrauterine growth restriction, preterm birth, and/or low birth weight are all markers of perinatal morbidity. Additional to birth status, clinically relevant information on plurality, gestational age, and birthweight should be incorporated into primary measures of ART success. These data items should be available in the majority of data collections and provide a composite proxy measure of ART success. Measures of success of ART treatment that restrict the numerator to exclude preterm or low birthweight babies provide a proxy measure of preferred outcome at a population level. These success rates are based on live born singleton babies of term gestation (37–42 completed weeks of gestation) and normal birthweight (≥2500 g).

Three numerators for primary measures of success of ART treatment are:

1. Number of: live born singletons, twins and higher order multiples.
2. Number of: term, live born singletons and live born twins at > 34 weeks.
3. Number of term, live born singletons of normal birthweight.

The objective of reporting success rates determines denominator (initiated, aspirated, or embryo transfer cycles). In settings where single embryo transfer is routine practice or government policy, the primary measure of ART success should be stratified by the number of embryos transferred to differentiate singletons from twins and higher order multiples, e.g., for points 2 and 3. In places where double embryos transfers are routine or in cultures where twins are considered an optimal outcome this should still be considered as a way of monitoring safety. For patients of advanced age or those with a history of recurrent pregnancy loss the first primary success measure may be more relevant.

In settings where longitudinal treatment data are available on women, cumulative success rates should be calculated. The preferred primary outcome is the total delivery rate with at least one live birth, this is the total number of deliveries with at least one live born baby resulting from one (initiated or aspirated) fully utilized ART cycle including all fresh and frozen/thaw ART cycles [6].

The primary measures described above use information available at the birth event. The ideal ART success measure includes information collected outside the birth event and is defined as a live birth, neonatal survivor (> 28 days) of normal birthweight with an *absence of disability*. Disability as described earlier is a broader, more encompassing concept than congenital anomalies, as many minor congenital anomalies cause no disability. Congenital anomalies need to be considered when developing a secondary measure of success of ART as they are important causes of perinatal mortality and morbidity and are over represented in multiple births and selectively among ART babies. However, the inclusion of congenital anomalies is not feasible in most data collections due to poor ascertainment, diagnostic complexity, and the lack of congenital anomaly registries in many settings. Data on disability is even more limited and is currently only available from research data sets. However, in registries that have information on congenital anomalies, a secondary measure of ART success should be the number of term live born singleton survivors (> 28 days) of normal birthweight with no major congenital anomalies. This measure could also be modified to report on twin births. Again, the choice of denominator should reflect the objective of reporting the success rates and the availability of longitudinal data on treatment of women.

Conclusion

The measure used to assess the success of any given ART treatment is dependent upon whose perspective the outcome is being determined and the quality of the data available to populate the measure. The interpretation of success of ART treatment by a patient may be totally different from that of government. In all settings, the described baseline and primary measures should be reported and where possible secondary success measures that include congenital anomalies and survival to 28 days.

References

1. International Committee for Monitoring Assisted Reproductive Technology, Nygren KG, Sullivan E, Zegers-Hochschild F, Mansour R, *et al.* World collaborative report on Assisted Reproductive Technology 2003. *Fertil Steril* 2011 In press.
2. Min JK, Breheny SA, MacLachlan V, Healy DL. The singleton, term gestation, live birth rate per cycle initiated: the BESST endpoint for assisted reproduction. *Hum Reprod* 2004;**19**:3–7.
3. Runciman W, Hibbert P, Thomson R, *et al.* Towards an International Classification for Patient Safety: key concepts and terms. *Int J Qual Health Care* 2009;**21**: 18–26.
4. Wang YA, Chapman M, Costello M, Sullivan EA. Better perinatal outcomes following transfer of fresh blastocysts and blastocysts cultured from thawed cleavage embryos: a population-based study. *Hum Reprod* 2010;**25**:1536–42.

5. Wang YA, Chambers GM, Sullivan EA. Assisted reproductive technology in Australia and New Zealand 2008. *Assisted reproduction technology series no*. 14. 2010, Canberra: Australian Institute of Health and Welfare.

6. Zegers-Hochschild F, Adamson GD, de Mouzon J, *et al.* International Committee for Monitoring Assisted Reproductive Technology (ICMART) and the World Health Organization (WHO) revised glossary of ART terminology. *Hum Reprod* 2009;**24**:2683–7.

Chapter 47

Why RCTs and how to design them

Johannes L. H. Evers

Parkinson's disease is a disorder of the ageing brain. At least 27 observational studies (22 case-control, 4 cohort, 1 cross-sectional) have shown that persons who smoke develop Parkinson's less frequently. Nefzger and co-workers [5] were among the first to draw attention to the presumed protective effect of smoking on the development of Parkinson's disease. Benedetti and co-workers [1] not only found that ever-smokers had a 50% reduced risk of Parkinson, but also that there is a significant dose-effect relationship: the more pack-years of cigarette smoking the less Parkinson's disease. From these findings people have concluded that perhaps nicotine in tobacco smoke may have neuroprotective effects. However, also a completely different conclusion may be drawn: reduced dopamine levels (as in Parkinson's disease) may diminish the rewarding effects of nicotine on the brain and hence reduce the reward and thereby diminish the inclination to smoke in patients with preclinical Parkinson's disease. Not developing addiction to smoking might be an early prodromal effect of the disease. A classical example of a cause-and-effect reversal. Observational studies are not capable of detecting this.

Observation shows, experiment teaches

Observational studies can never prove a causal relation between two factors, they may at best establish an association and provide information for designing a future experimental intervention study. Or, to paraphrase Claude Bernard [2], observation shows, experiment teaches: "Only within very narrow boundaries can man observe the phenomena which surround him; most of them naturally escape his senses, and mere observation is not enough". The value of observation however may increase if a large signal-to-noise ratio exists [3], or, in medicine, if the cure rate with treatment (the signal) is many-fold higher than the spontaneous recovery rate. Examples are: blood transfusion for hemorrhagic shock, condoms to prevent AIDS, and smallpox vaccination. When the effect of an intervention is spectacular, the chance of unknown confounders being important is so small that it can be disregarded. A daily medical practice example is the so-called "parent's-kiss-technique" in case of obstruction of a child's nostril by a foreign object, e.g., a marble. The technique consists of occluding the unblocked nostril, followed by having the parent blow into the child's mouth. The object easily dislodges and mother and child are delighted, a convincing $n = 1$ observational study. When repeated in a prospective observational cohort study [6], the results were confirmed, the technique was successful in 20 out of the 31 children (64.5%) in the study group. Only one child required general anaesthesia for removal of the nasal foreign body (3%). This compares favourably

How to Improve Your ART Success Rates, ed. Gab Kovacs. Published by Cambridge University Press.

with a rate of 32.5% requiring removal under general anaesthesia in the preceding 6-month period, reflecting a convincingly high signal-to-noise ratio. The larger the signal-to-noise ratios the greater the chance that an observational study design will suffice. Hefty signal-to-noise ratios make randomized controlled studies (RCTs) redundant, an RCT of the parent's kiss procedure has not yet been performed, and probably never will. Unfortunately in assisted reproduction large signal-to-noise ratios are exceedingly rare, although IVF itself was introduced by a now famous $n = 1$ observational study by Steptoe and Edwards [9].

Hierarchy of study designs

Table 47.1 gives the hierarchy of study designs, with the experimental studies on top, the narrative observational studies at the bottom, and the analytical observational studies in between.

Narrative studies *generate* a hypothesis, analytical studies *test* a hypothesis, and experimental studies *prove* a hypothesis, or prove it wrong. Although narrative observational studies (case reports, case series) are easy to write and often fun to read, they offer little or no rigor, except when the signal far exceeds the noise. The noise, spontaneous pregnancy, in a woman with absent Fallopian tubes is extremely small, so the signal (a pregnancy following IVF) does not have to be very strong to offer convincing evidence. Randomized controlled studies (RCTs) comparing tubal surgery and IVF in case of tubal pathology have never been performed, which made the authors of a 2008 Cochrane review conclude: "Any effect of tubal surgery relative to expectant management and IVF in terms of live birth rates for women with tubal infertility remains unknown. Large trials with adequate power are warranted to establish the effectiveness of surgery in these women," and " Live birth rates in relation to the severity of tubal damage, and different techniques used for tubal repair including microsurgery and laparoscopic methods should also be reported," according to Pandian and colleagues [10]. This cry of despair illustrates the many advantages of well-designed prospective experimental studies, they can establish causation, they may measure relative effectiveness, allow for economic comparisons, and reveal which lifestyle and other factors might influence the outcome of the treatment under investigation. It also illustrates that RCTs are not always feasible, or at least that they are less likely to be performed. If the signal-to-noise ratio of a new treatment is considered to be at least reasonable and the old treatment is very cumbersome, expensive, hazardous or time-consuming (for example the IVF-surgery discussion, or the term breech trial), clinicians may adopt the new treatment on a massive

Table 47.1 Hierarchy of study designs

1. Experimental studies
a. Randomized Controlled Trial, RCT
2. Observational studies
a. Analytical
i. Cohort study
ii. Cross-sectional study
iii. Case-control study
b. Narrative
i. Case series
ii. Case report

scale in a very short period of time, the well-informed infertility patients will demand the procedure, and an RCT will never be performed. *Not* doing an RCT in the introduction phase of a new treatment – when equipoise still exists – may be considered *un*ethical. Once patients are aware of the new treatment and convinced of its beneficial effects they may decline to be entered into an RCT, especially if they run the risk of no-treatment in the control arm of the trial. For example, the effect of surgical obstruction of the spermatic vein in subfertile male patients with a varicocele will probably never be tested in a (highly needed) RCT, since couples with difficulty conceiving will demand to be treated with intracytoplasmic sperm injection (ICSI), a fast, cheap, easy and successful way to achieving a pregnancy, especially when compared to surgery, recovery (men are pusillanimous), followed by 6 or 12 months of expectant management, and maybe still ICSI after all.

Case-control study design

Before addressing RCTs, in short a few words about observational study designs. A case-control study has a retrograde direction of enquiry, it starts with the outcome and looks back at the exposure. Case-control studies are fast and only require a small sample size, e.g., five children with retinoblastomas resulting from 15 500 IVF pregnancies compared to eight children with retinoblastomas from 180 000 spontaneous pregnancies, reflected in a relative risk of 7.2 (95% CI 2.4–17.0; [4]). Apart from needing few subjects, they are most appropriate for detecting trends and effects of rare diseases, for diseases or conditions that develop slowly and/or have a long lag time. To study the risk of e.g., ovarian cancer in IVF patients is only feasible in an observational study, and a case-control design will be the easiest and fastest way of obtaining an impression of the association between IVF and ovarian malignancies. The weakness of case-control studies is their inherent biases and confounding: index case bias, recall bias, inaccurate or incomplete records, sampling bias in the controls. Moreover they only study one single outcome and cannot establish causality.

Cross-sectional study design

Cross-sectional studies are also fast and cheap; however, since they consist of an observation at a set point in time (they have no direction of enquiry), long-term follow-up is not a requirement and they can provide insight into the prevalence of a disease (e.g., of tubal pathology in infertility patients undergoing laparoscopy). They are unsuitable for rare diseases, however, and they can only establish an association, not causality. They are most appropriate for obtaining clinical information before embarking on more elaborate types of study.

Cohort study design

The strength of cohort studies is that their direction of enquiry is prospective, so they can help determining the prevalence and the course of a disease or disorder, they may suggest a cause-and-effect relationship, and, since they are prospective, they allow for complete and accurate collection of data. Moreover, they can include some degree of blinding of the patient, the doctor and even the outcome assessor. Their weaknesses consist of proneness to losses to follow-up, especially in long-term studies. They are less suitable for rare or slowly developing diseases or diseases with a long lag time, and they may face problems to include sufficient controls if the therapy under investigation is very popular or in case of a high exposure in the population to a certain factor. Confounding (a factor that correlates, either positively or negatively, with both the dependent variable and the independent variable) and bias are major problems in observational studies. The fact that fires and fire engines are often observed at the same time at the same location does not necessarily mean that fire engines cause fires. The conclusion that many people really like filling questionnaires may result from an erroneous interpretation of the answers to a question like "Do you like filling questionnaires?" Forms of bias that we may encounter in research in assisted reproduction are chanelling bias (a treatment is prescribed depending on the severity of the disease or its prognosis, e.g., medical treatment in mild endometriosis and surgery in severe, leading to the conclusion that medical therapy results in more spontaneous pregnancies than surgery), surveillance bias – doctors tend to look more carefully for a given outcome (e.g., endometriosis) in one group (e.g., infertility patients) than in the other (patients undergoing laparoscopic sterilization), recall bias – patients with an adverse outcome (e.g., ovarian cancer) are more likely to remember the exposure (fertility drugs), index case bias (the index cases, with outcome plus exposure, are included in a small group), verification bias – the test outcome (performing a laparoscopy) is related to performing the reference test (hysterosalpingography), and publication bias (a positive outcome is more likely to get published). Retrospective cohort studies, sometimes referred to as 'trohoc' studies, add incomplete data collection to these forms of bias.

Randomized clinical trial study design

Figure 47.1 offers a schematic representation of issues involved in RCT design. In fact in an RCT two randomization procedures take place, the first (r1) is the random drawing of a representative sample from the general population, and the second (r2) random allocation of these individuals to either of (most often) two treatment arms. Next, the outcome of treatment is studied and compared between arms.

Allocating patients randomly to one of two treatments eliminates bias and confounding in treatment assignment, allows for blinding the patient, the doctor and the outcome assessor to treatment allotment (allocation concealment), and it allows for applying the probability theory to estimate the likelihood that a difference in outcome between the two groups is more than merely due to chance [8]. The key concepts here are *randomization* and *allocation concealment*. Proper randomization serves to generate an unpredictable succession of allocations to either of the two treatment options, allocation concealment serves to guarantee that the assignment of a patient to a treatment arm remains concealed from especially the

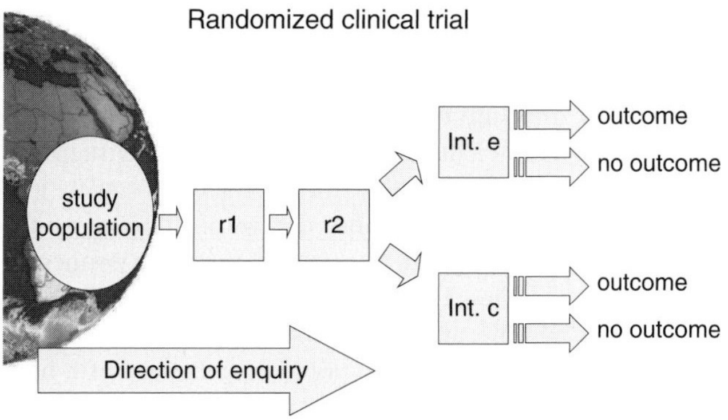

Figure 47.1 Schematic representation of issues involved in randomized clinical trial design.

treating physician until inclusion in the treatment group is definitive. Alternating allocation, allocation based on birth date or patient chart number or day of the week is sometimes referred to as pseudo- or quasirandomization, although, in fact, it is not randomization at all. Every randomization procedure that differs from fair coin tossing creates the risk of contamination by confounding and selection bias. Generation of a proper randomization sequence takes little time and effort but affords big rewards in scientific accuracy and credibility. Investigators should devote appropriate resources to the generation of properly randomized trials and reporting their methods clearly [7]. The US National Institutes of Health has developed a website, at http://clinicaltrials.gov, in collaboration with the US Food and Drug Administration to allow doctors, investigators and patients to access the following information in abstracts of clinical study protocols: a summary of the purpose of the study, its recruiting status, the criteria for patient participation, the location of the trial centers, and specific contact information, study design, phase of the trial, disease or condition, and drug or therapy under study. Editors of many scientific journals have made it mandatory for publication that a trial has been registered beforehand with this or similar registries. Another website, www.equator-network.org, is created by the EQUATOR network, an international initiative of the CONSORT group. It seeks to improve reliability and value of medical research literature by promoting transparent and accurate reporting of research. It offers resources to authors, editors, and peer reviewers to produce high quality research publications and it promotes good reporting of scientific studies. Among many other things the CONSORT group offers a statement, a checklist and a format for a flow diagram (Figure 47.2) of the progress through the four phases of a parallel randomized trial of two groups (enrolment, intervention allocation, follow-up, and data analysis).

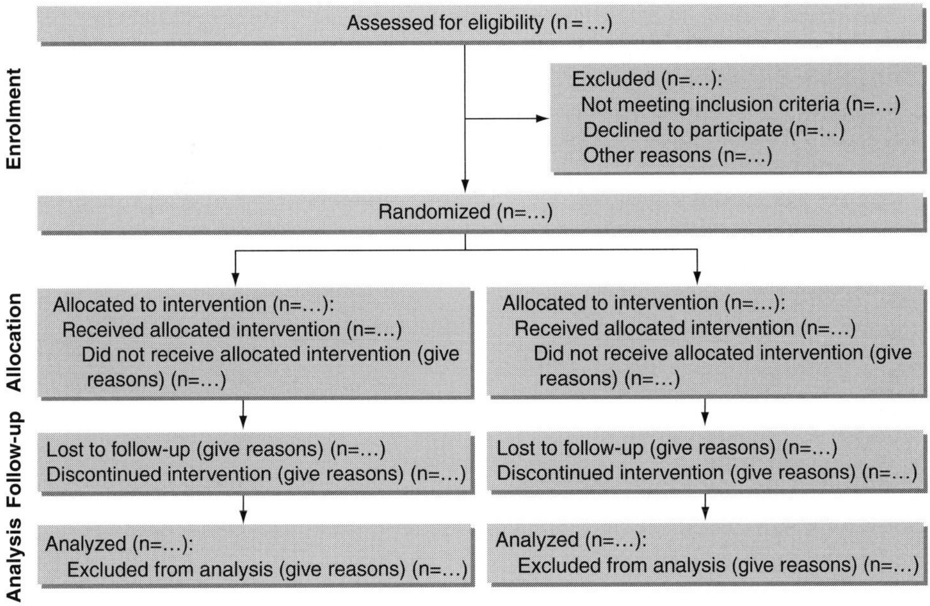

Figure 47.2 Flow diagram of the progress through the phases of a parallel randomized trial of two groups: enrolment, intervention allocation, follow-up, and data analysis (adapted from: Schulz KF, Altman DG, Moher D; CONSORT Group. CONSORT 2010 statement: updated guidelines for reporting parallel group randomised trials. *BMJ*. 2010;340:c332. doi: 10.1136/bmj.c332).

Many scientific journals require inclusion of such a flow diagram in a (clinical) research report nowadays. The checklist allows for checking that all important issues of an RCT are addressed in the eventual publication. It assists authors to write a study report according to a logical and transparent structure and helps scientific journal editors ascertaining that the reporting of the study includes all essential details.

"We believe"

In conclusion, appropriately designed RCTs are pivotal for the clinical evaluation of new treatments, but also of new diagnostic tests. If however not performed at the very introduction of such a treatment (when equipoise still exists), the chance to do so may be foregone, doctors (and patients) may be prejudiced, and it may take years (and thousands of patients) before a presumed positive treatment effect will be disproven and abandoned again. In assisted reproduction acupuncture, varicocelectomy, medical treatment of endometriosis, or – in IVF – co-medication with corticosteroids, aspirin, heparin, or DHEA are but a few recent examples. Some *believe* that they work and that you cannot deny your patients their benefit, but it will take a properly designed RCT to convince the rest of us.

References

1. Benedetti MD, Bower JH, Maraganore DM, *et al.* Smoking, alcohol, and coffee consumption preceding Parkinson's disease: a case-control study. *Neurology* 2000;**55**:1350–8.
2. Bernard C. *An Introduction to the Study of Experimental Medicine*, 1865. First English translation 1927, McMillan & Co Ltd, London.
3. Glasziou P, Chalmers I, Rawlins M, McCulloch P. When are randomised trials unnecessary? Picking signal from noise. *BMJ* 2007;**334**:349–51.
4. Moll AC, Imhof SM, Cruysberg JR, *et al.* Incidence of retinoblastoma in children born after in-vitro fertilisation. *Lancet* 2003;**361**:309–10.
5. Nefzger MD, Quadfasel FA, Karl VC. A retrospective study of smoking in Parkinson's disease. *Am J Epidemiol* 1968;**88**:149–58.
6. Purohit N, Ray S, Wilson T, Chawla OP. The 'parent's kiss': an effective way to remove paediatric nasal foreign bodies. *Ann R Coll Surg Engl* 2008;**90**:420–2.
7. Schulz KF, Altman DG, Moher D; CONSORT Group. CONSORT 2010 statement: updated guidelines for reporting parallel group randomised trials. *BMJ* 2010;**340**:c332.
8. Schulz KF, Grimes DA. Generation of allocation sequences in randomised trials: chance, not choice *Lancet* 2002;**359**:515–9.
9. Steptoe PC, Edwards RG. Birth after the reimplantation of a human embryo. *Lancet* 1978;**2**:366.
10. Pandian Z, Akande VA, Harrild K, Bhattacharya S. Surgery for tubal infertility. *Cochrane Database Syst Rev* 2008;**16**(3): CD006415.

Chapter 48

How to read a Cochrane Review

Cynthia Farquhar

Setting the scene

You are a fertility specialist consulting with Susan and Tim who are planning on having their first IVF cycle. They need to decide whether or not to have single or double embryo transfer. Susan is 32 years old and Tim is 34 years old and Susan has tubal infertility secondary to adhesions following peritonitis as a child. They have had one ectopic pregnancy and one tube has been removed. They have no other pregnancies. They have been trying to conceive for the past three years. You wish to explain to them the advantages and disadvantages of double and single embryo transfer. The Cochrane Library (www.cochrane.org) has a review comparing the two options which you use to discuss the options with the couple [3].

> Title of Cochrane Review: Number of embryos for transfer following in-vitro fertilization or intra-cytoplasmic sperm injection
>
> Authors: Pandian Z, Bhattacharya S, Ozturk O, Serour G, Templeton A.
>
> Cochrane Database of Systematic Reviews 2009, Issue 2.

For every review there are three major considerations

Are the results valid?
What are the results?
Are the results applicable to this couple?

Are the results valid?

There is no point looking at the results if they are clearly not valid. The answers to this section are all in the methods section of the review.

a. *Did the review address a clearly focused issue? Did the review describe which infertile couples they included, what they meant by single embryo transfer and how they measure the pregnancy outcomes? You can find the answer by first reading the objective of the review. This is contained in both the abstract and the main body of the review. Further information is contained in the study selection criteria.*

How to Improve Your ART Success Rates, ed. Gab Kovacs. Published by Cambridge University Press.

In this review the objective is "To evaluate the effectiveness and safety of different policies for the number of embryos transferred". The participants were "couples undergoing assisted reproductive technologies" and the interventions compared were "different policies for the number of embryos transferred" and the primary outcomes were "live birth rate, multiple pregnancy rate".

A description of single embryo transfer (SET) including subsequent frozen embryo transfers (FZET) in an assisted reproductive technology (ART) cycle was provided and live birth and multiple pregnancy were defined.

b. *Did the authors select the right sort of studies for the review? Does the review describe the study design they included. Ideally this should be randomized controlled trials as this is an intervention study and non randomized studies have many inherent biases and in particular selection bias.*

In the Cochrane review the authors limited the studies to only randomized controlled trials (RCTs) that compared the effectiveness and safety of different policies for the number of embryos transferred. Non randomized studies were not included as they are considered likely to have underlying reasons for selecting some patients for SET or double embryo transfer (DET) such as age or previous IVF failures. This is known as selection bias and usually results in patients in each group with different baseline characteristics that influence the outcomes. For example, some clinics encourage older women and couples who have had previous failed cycles to transfer more than one embryo as they consider that they are more likely to conceive. This will mean that the patients in the two arms of the study will be different and may influence the overall results.

c. *Do you think the important, relevant studies were included? This question relates to the search strategy. Did the authors of the review describe which databases they used and which search terms they used? There should be no restrictions on whether or not the paper was published or not as unpublished results are often negative (this is known as publication bias). There should be no language restrictions as there may be studies in languages other than English.*

In the Cochrane review the keywords were provided in the text with dates and the search strategy is available in the appendices. There was no language restriction. Unpublished studies are included. All major databases were searched and these include The Cochrane Central Register of Controlled Trials, Medline, Embase, PsychINFO, and Cinahl.

d. *Did the authors do enough to assess the quality of the included studies? Did they consider how the randomization sequence was generated, did they conceal the allocation of the patients to the study groups and did they blind the researchers and the patients from the allocation. Did they account for all the couples who were randomized? Did the study authors report all the important outcomes – in this case live birth and multiple pregnancy?*

All studies were assessed for risk of bias and presented in a table for each study and summarized in the risk of bias figures (Figure 48.1 and Figure 48.2). Important domains for the risk of bias that were considered were randomization, concealment of allocation, blinding and missing data because of withdrawals or losses to follow up [2]. Figure 48.1 contains a summary of the risk of bias and Figure 48.2 provides the information for each domain for each included study.

In this review fewer than half of the studies reported that the allocation to each of the study groups was concealed from the researchers. Blinding was also reported only by 25% of the studies. All studies reported live birth and multiple pregnancy (which were the primary outcomes of the review) and therefore considered free of selective reporting. In

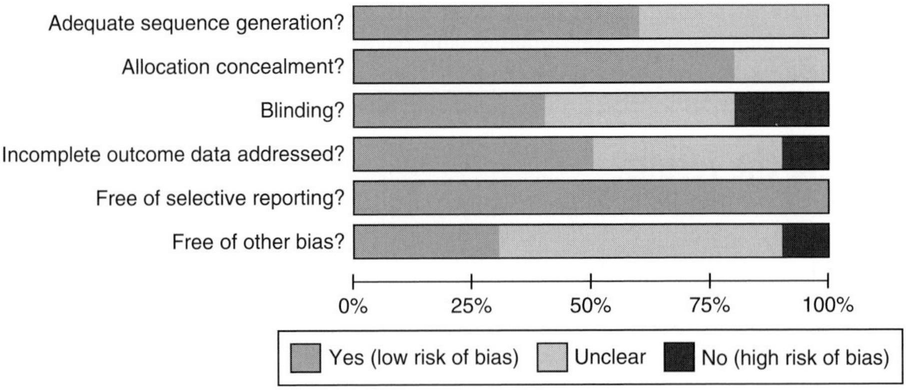

Figure 48.1 Summary of risk of bias table for the included studies.

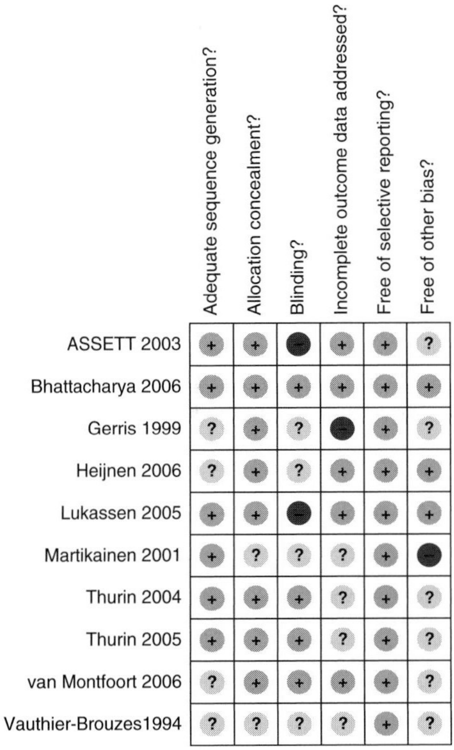

Figure 48.2 Risk of bias for each of the included studies.

many cases the authors have failed to report relevant information and therefore are "unclear" for a particular domain. All of these domains are important in determining if the studies in the review are likely to be "biased" and in some way influencing the study results.

Overall for the eight included studies the risk of bias was moderate as there is incomplete reporting on several domains. This risk of bias should be taken into consideration when considering the results of the review.

What were the results?

a. *Were the results similar from study to study? If not what are the reasons for variations between the studies discussed?*

For the first comparison in the Cochrane review (SET versus DET) the results for live birth and multiple pregnancy have been summarized into a Forest plot in Figures 48.3–48.5. A visual inspection of the figures suggests that the results are similar in that the data is overlapping and there are no major outliers. A statistical measure of how similar the results are is provided by the heterogeneity which is in the left-hand side of the figure near the bottom. In all the figures the chi-squared test for heterogeneity is not significant and the I^2 statistic for inconsistency is 0–1% which is very low. Therefore, it can be concluded that the results are similar. If there had been heterogeneity present then the authors of the review would need to discuss the possible reasons such as clinical differences between the studies.

b. *What is the overall result of the review? Is there a clinical bottom line? What is it? What is the numerical result?*

The overall result of the Cochrane review is presented in the black diamond at the bottom on the right hand side of each figure. The black diamond is the synthesis of all the results from the individual studies and if it is on the right-hand side of the vertical line (which represents the odds ratio of 1, i.e., no effect) and does not include the vertical line then there is evidence of an effect. In this review the black diamond suggests a two fold increase in live births (OR 2.00, 95% CI 1.59–2.51) with a single cycle of DET compared to a single cycle of SET (Figure 48.3) but when the comparison is between a single cycle of DET with SET plus frozen embryo transfer (Figure 48.4) there is no evidence of a difference in cumulative live birth (OR 1.21, 95% CI 0.89–1.64). However, for the outcome of multiple pregnancies there is a marked reduction in SET cycles (OR 0.06, 95% CI 0.02–0.15) (Figure 48.5).

	DET		SET			Odds ratio
Study or subgroup	Events	Total	Events	Total	Weight	M-H, fixed, 95% CI
ASSETT 2003	5	14	3	13	1.9%	1.85 [0.34, 10.05]
Bhattacharya 2006	6	12	6	11	3.0%	0.83 [0.16, 4.30]
Gerris 1999	19	27	9	26	2.6%	4.49 [1.41, 14.25]
Lukassen 2005	19	53	14	54	8.5%	1.60 [0.70, 3.65]
Martikainen 2001	28	70	22	75	12.2%	1.61 [0.81, 3.20]
Thurin 2004	142	331	91	330	50.0%	1.97 [1.43, 2.73]
Thurin 2005	7	22	4	20	2.7%	1.87 [0.45, 7.69]
van Montfoort 2006	59	154	32	154	19.0%	2.37 [1.43, 3.93]
Total (95% CI)		**683**		**683**	**100.0%**	**2.00 [1.59, 2.51]**
Total events	285		181			

Heterogeneity: $Chi^2 = 4.09$, df = 7 ($P = 0.77$); $I^2 = 0\%$
Test for overall effect: $Z = 5.91$ ($P < 0.00001$)

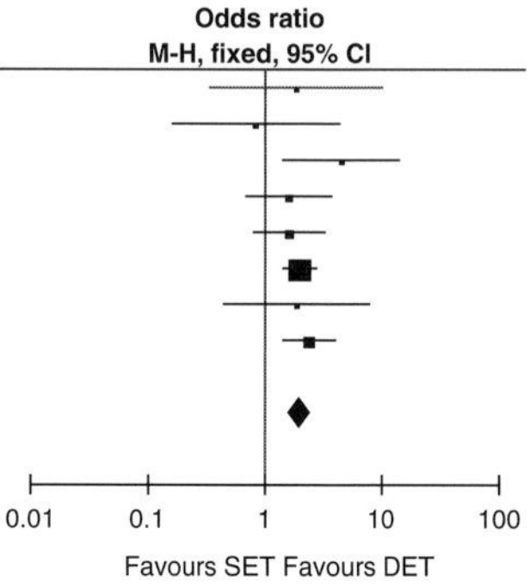

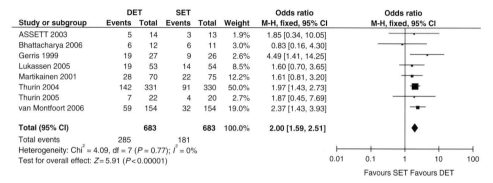

Figure 48.3 Forest plot comparing double embryo transfer (DET) versus single embryo transfer (SET) for the outcome of live birth.

Study or subgroup	DET Events	DET Total	SET+1FZET Events	SET+1FZET Total	Weight	Odds ratio M-H, fixed, 95% CI
2.1.1 DET versus SET pluz 1 FZET						
Thurin 2004	140	323	123	332	89.7%	1.30 [0.95, 1.78]
Thurin 2005	9	30	9	18	10.3%	0.43 [0.13, 1.44]
Subtotal (95% CI)		**353**		**350**	**100.0%**	**1.21 [0.89, 1.64]**
Total events	149		132			
Heterogeneity: $Chi^2 = 3.03$, df = 1 ($P = 0.08$); $I^2 = 67\%$						
Test for overall effect: $Z=1.24$ ($P=0.22$)						
2.1.2 DET versus 2 fresh SET						
Lukassen 2005	22	54	19	54	100.0%	1.27 [0.58, 2.76]
Subtotal (95% CI)		**54**		**54**	**100.0%**	**1.27 [0.58, 2.76]**
Total events	22		19			
Heterogeneity: Not applicable						
Test for overall effect: $Z=0.59$ ($P=0.55$)						
2.1.3 DET plus FZET versus SET plus FZET						
ASSETT 2003	4	14	4	13	100.0%	0.90 [0.17, 4.70]
Subtotal (95% CI)		**14**		**13**	**100.0%**	**0.90 [0.17, 4.70]**
Total events	4		4			
Heterogeneity: Not applicable						
Test for overall effect: $Z=0.12$ ($P=0.90$)						

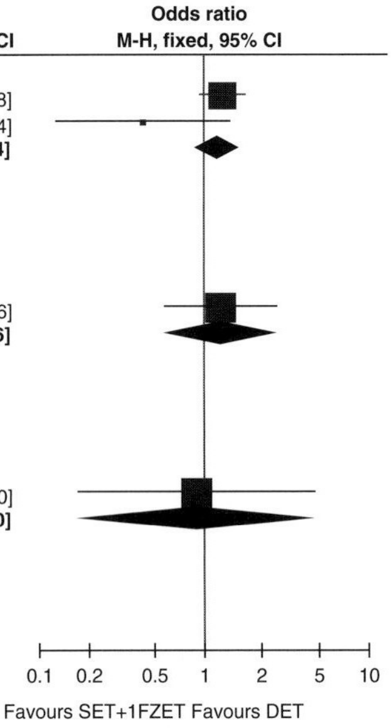

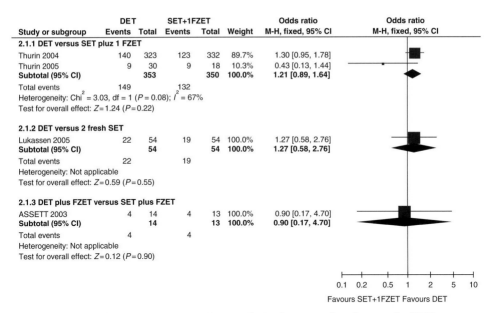

Figure 48.4 Forest plot comparing double embryo transfer (DET) versus single embryo transfer (SET) (two or more cycles) for the outcome of cumulative live birth.

Study or subgroup	SET Events	SET Total	DET Events	DET Total	Weight	Odds ratio M-H, fixed, 95% CI
ASSETT 2003	0	3	0	5		Not estimable
Bhattacharya 2006	0	6	0	6		Not estimable
Gerris 1999	1	9	6	19	5.3%	0.27 [0.03, 2.68]
Lukassen 2005	0	14	7	19	9.6%	0.06 [0.00, 1.11]
Martikainen 2001	1	22	11	28	14.2%	0.07 [0.01, 0.63]
Thurin 2004	1	91	46	142	54.8%	0.02 [0.00, 0.17]
Thurin 2005	0	4	1	7	1.6%	0.48 [0.02, 14.70]
van Montfoort 2006	0	32	13	59	14.5%	0.05 [0.00, 0.92]
Total (95% CI)		**181**		**285**	**100.0%**	**0.06 [0.02, 0.15]**
Total events	3		84			
Heterogeneity: $Chi^2=4.05$, df=5 ($P=0.54$); $I^2=0\%$						
Test for overall effect: $Z=5.70$ ($P<0.00001$)						

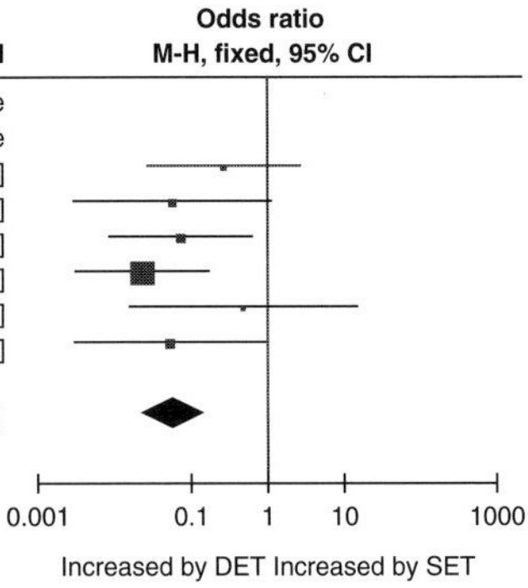

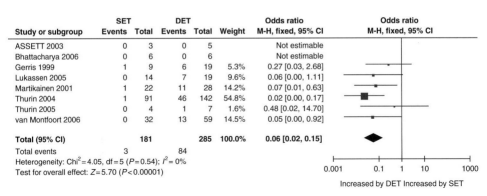

Figure 48.5 Forest plot comparing double embryo transfer (DET) versus single embryo transfer (SET) for the outcome of multiple pregnancy.

The bottom line is that if a clinic has a policy of SET with subsequent FZET then the multiple pregnancy rate will be reduced by 94%.

c. *How precise are the results? Is there a confidence interval?*

The confidence intervals for all outcomes are narrow suggesting reasonable precision. For the outcome of cumulative live birth the confidence intervals include 1 and there is no evidence of a negative effect of SET with FZET on this outcome.

Can I use the results to help Susan and Tim decide about single or double embryo transfer?

a. *Can I apply the results to this couple? Are they any different from the patients who were included in the studies in this review?*

Table 48.1 Study details including prognostic factors

Study author and year	Participants	Intervention	Duration of infertility (mean ± SD)	Previous ART cycle	Frozen cycles
Gerris 1999	Women aged < 34 years old	SET versus DET	3.5 years	First cycle	Not included
Heijnen 2007	Women aged 38–45 years	DET versus TET	DET: 3.7 (± 2.5) years TET: 3.2 (± 2.4) years	First or previous successful cycle	Not included
Lukassen 2005	Women aged <35 years	DET versus SET (2 cycles)	SET: 3.1 (±1.5) years DET: 3.5 (±1.9) years	First or previous successful cycle	Not included
Martikainen 2001	Women aged 22–40 years	SET versus DET	Not stated	Women who had /not had more than one previous failed treatment.	Frozen cycles included
Moustafa 2008	Women aged less than 30 years	SET plus FZET versus DET plus FZET	SET: 3.5 (±3.1) years DET: 2.9 (± 2.6) years	First cycle (one exception)	26 cycles had subsequent 2nd FZET (SET: 10, DET: 16)
Thurin 2004	<36 years	SET plus FZET versus DET	0–12 years	First or second cycle	Frozen cycles included
van Montfoort 2006	no criteria	SET versus DET	SET: 3.3 (±1.8) years DET: 3.3 (± 2.1) years	First cycle	Not included
Vauthier-Brouzes 1994	<36 years	DET versus FET	Not stated	First or previous successful cycle	Frozen cycles included

SET = single embryo transfer; DET = double embryo transfer; TET = triple embryo transfer; FET = four embryo transfer; FZET = frozen embryo transfer.

Susan and Tim would appear to be very similar to the couples in this review. Table 48.1 provides a summary of the prognostic factors of the studies. There is no reason that the clinical results from this Cochrane review will not apply to this couple who are young and are having their first cycle of IVF.

b. *Should I apply the results to this couple? How great would the benefit of therapy be for this particular couple? Is the intervention consistent with their values and preferences? Were all the clinically important outcomes considered? Are the benefits worth the harms and costs?*

There is good evidence that if this couple have SET then they will reduce the likelihood of multiple pregnancies to 1%. This benefit is worth it as there is no accompanying reduction in live birth rate if they have SET with subsequent FZET. Multiple pregnancy is associated with adverse events for both the baby and mother, including miscarriage, preterm birth, perinatal death, admissions to neonatal intensive care, increased maternal pre-eclampsia, and caesarean birth. Although some couples express a desire to have a multiple pregnancy once the risks are fully explained to them they are likely to agree.

c. *What is the absolute likelihood of Susan and Tim having a baby following SET compared to DET? And what is the absolute likelihood of them having a multiple pregnancy with single and double ET?*

If Susan and Tim have one cycle of SET then the likelihood of having a live birth is 27% compared to 41% with DET. However, if they have two cycles of SET (with either a subsequent FZET or another fresh cycle of SET) then the absolute likelihood of having a live birth is 38% compared with 43% with DET. The multiple pregnancy rate with DET is 29% of pregnancies compared with 1.6% of pregnancies with SET which is similar to the multiple pregnancy rate in the general population.

d. *How much extra will it cost them? And how much more will it cost the funder (public or private) if they choose one or two embryos?*

There is a small additional cost with a SET policy providing that remaining embryos are frozen and subsequently transferred. Most clinics will freeze embryos at a relatively low cost and it has been suggested that all clinics should provide cryopreservation of embryos [4]. The cost of freezing is offset by the cost savings if multiple pregnancy is reduced. Cost savings were considerable in a cost-effectiveness analysis reported by one of the RCTs in this review – "each additional successful pregnancy in the DET group will cost €19096 extra" because of the increased multiple pregnancy rate [1].

Acknowledgements

This chapter was developed from the Cochrane Journal Club approach to reading a Cochrane Review. The author is grateful to the authors of the Cochrane Review for updating the review for this chapter.

References

1. Fiddlers AAA, van Montfoort APA, Dirksen CD, *et al.* Single versus double embryo transfer: cost-effectiveness analysis alongside a randomized controlled trial. *Human Reproduction* 2006;**21**:2090–7.
2. Higgins JPT, Green S. *Cochrane Handbook for Systematic Reviews of Interventions* Version 5.0.2 [updated September 2009]. The Cochrane Collaboration, 2008. Available from www.cochrane-handbook.org.
3. Pandian Z, Bhattacharya S, Ozturk O, Serour G, Templeton A. Number of embryos for transfer following in-vitro fertilisation or intra-cytoplasmic sperm injection. *Cochrane Database Syst Rev* 2009; CD003416. DOI: 10.1002/14651858.CD003416.pub3.
4. Thurin-Kjellberg A, Olivius C, Bergh C. Cumulative live-birth rates in a trial of single embryo or double embryo transfer. *New Engl J Med* 2009;**361**:18–19.

Index

Page numbers in *italics* denote a table those in **bold** a figure.